D0597446

The Complete Guide To KETO

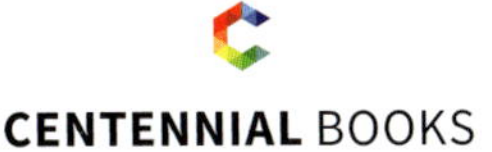

CENTENNIAL BOOKS

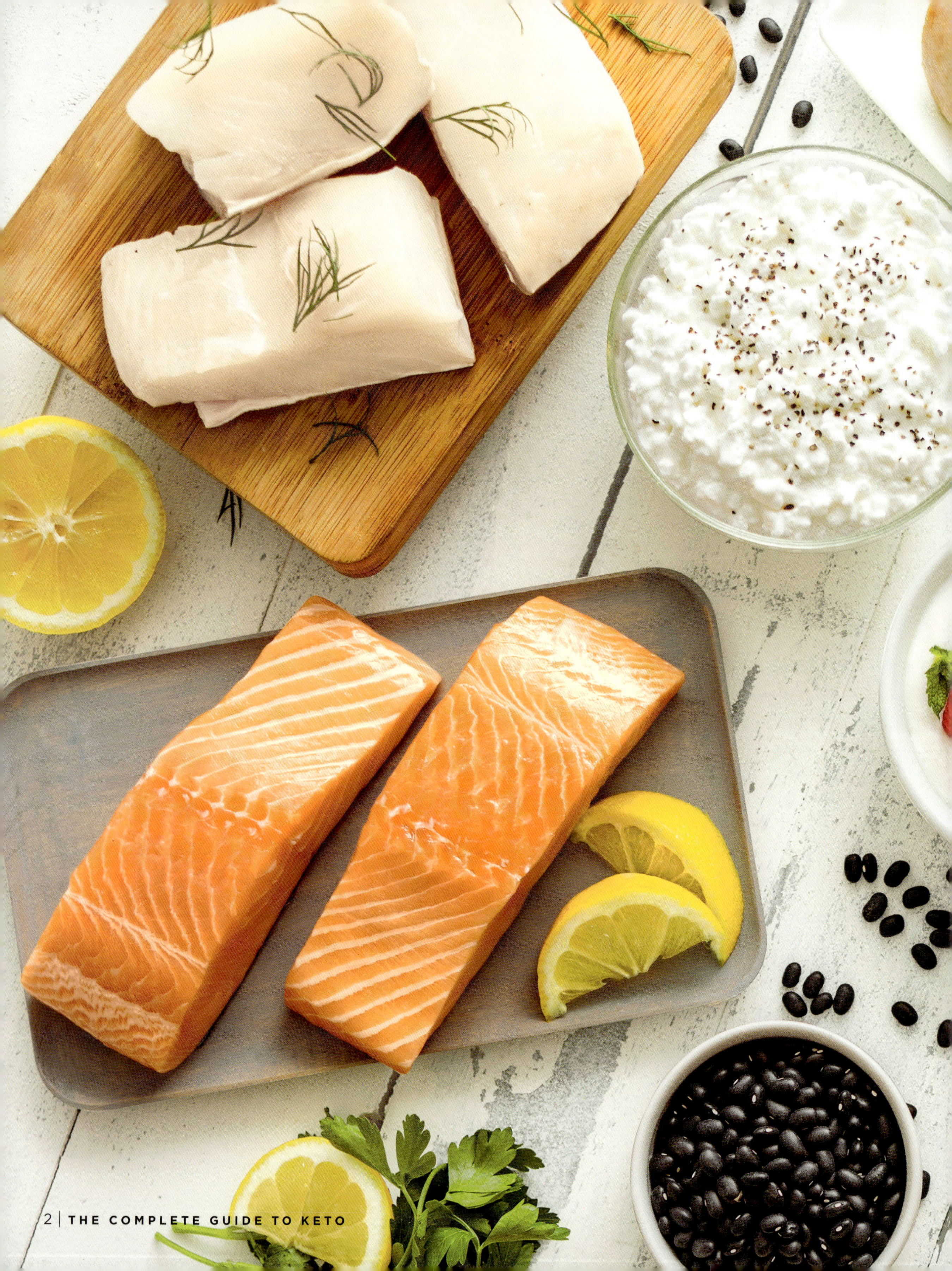

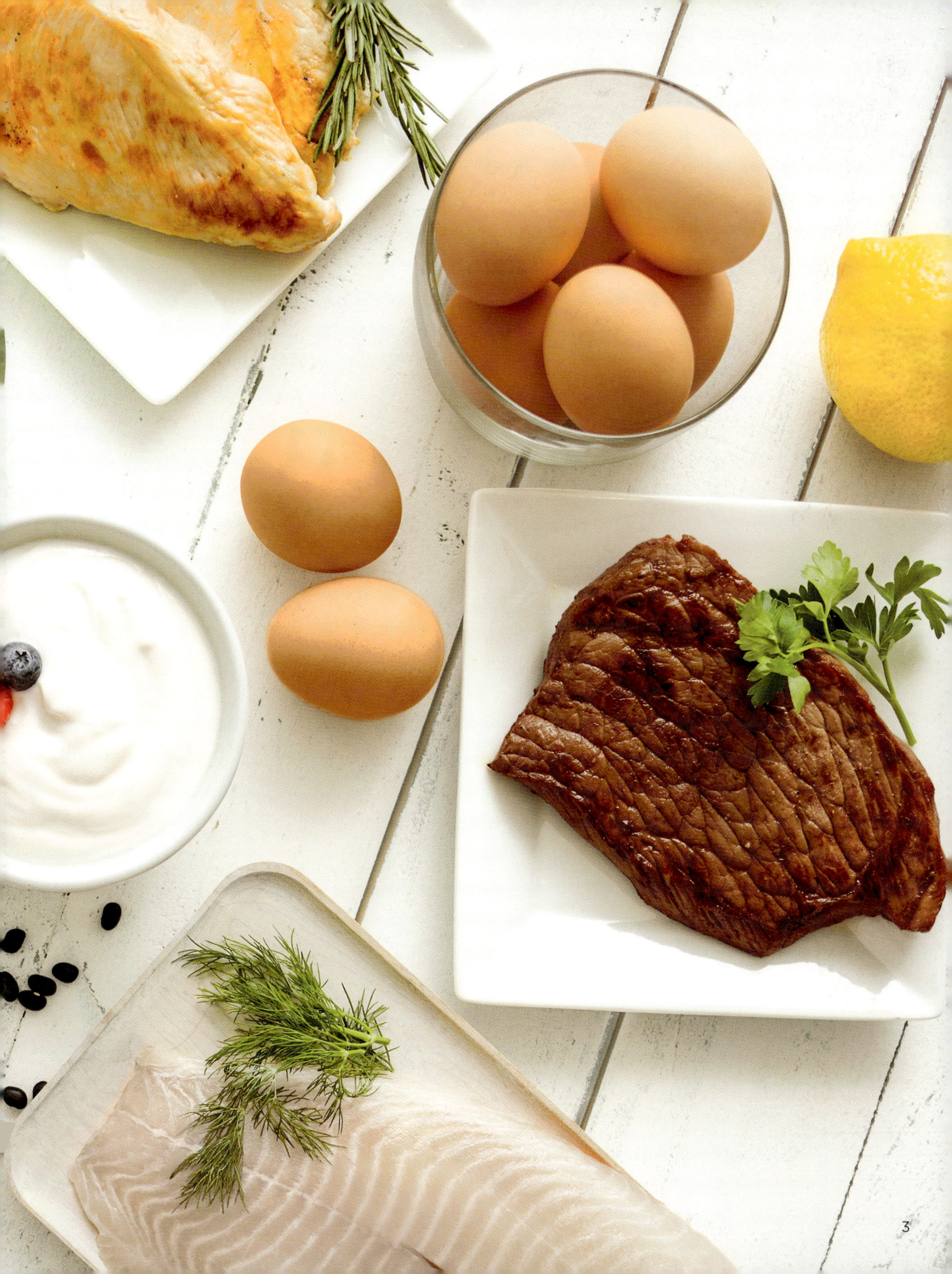

Contents

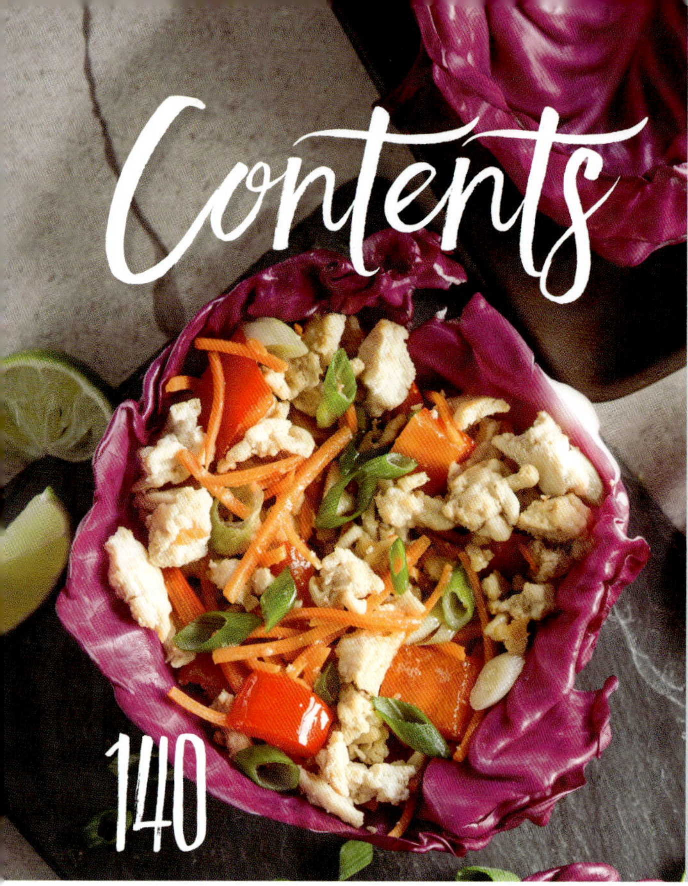

140

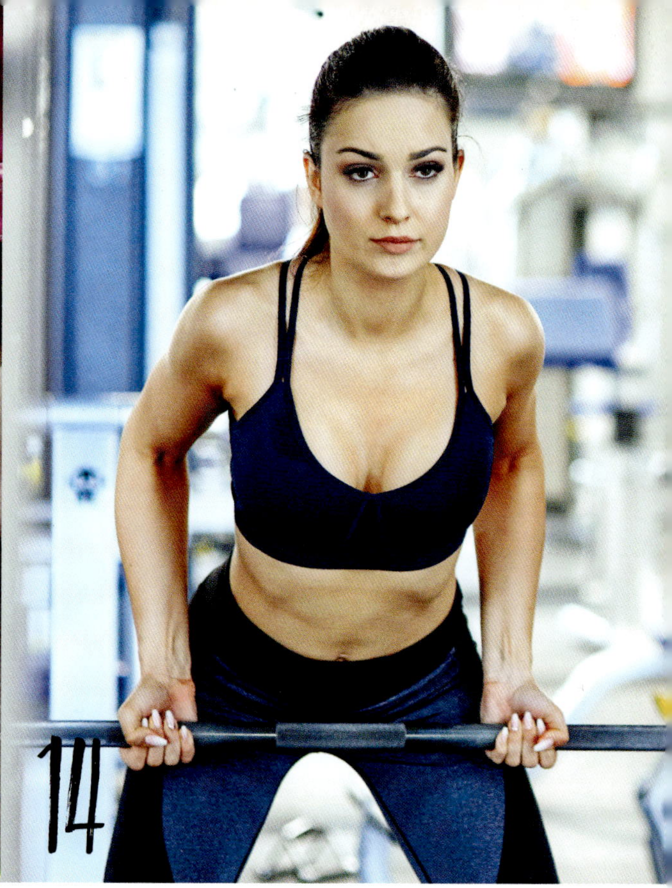

14

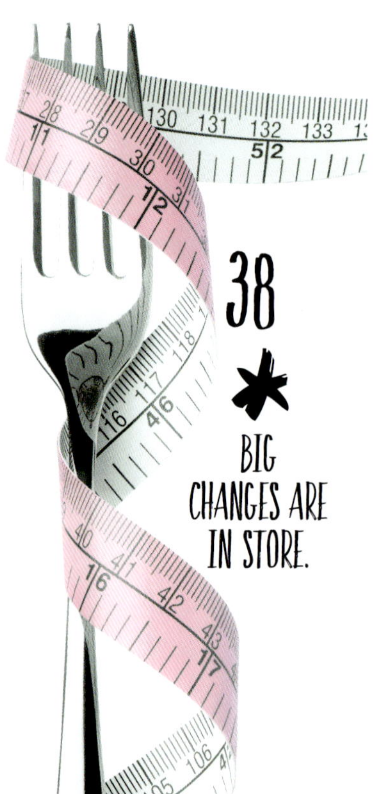

PART 1: KETO 101

PART 2: READY, SET, KETO

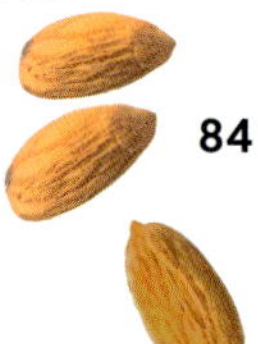

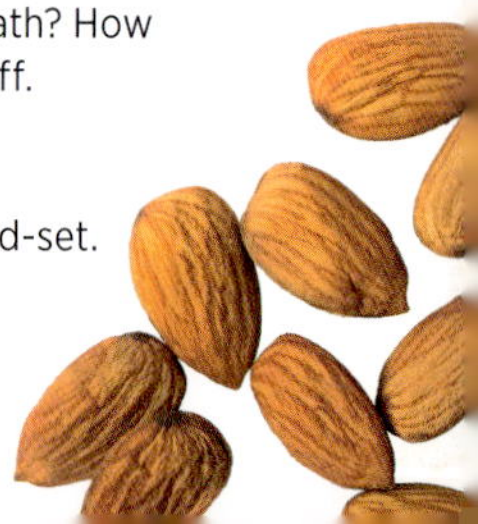

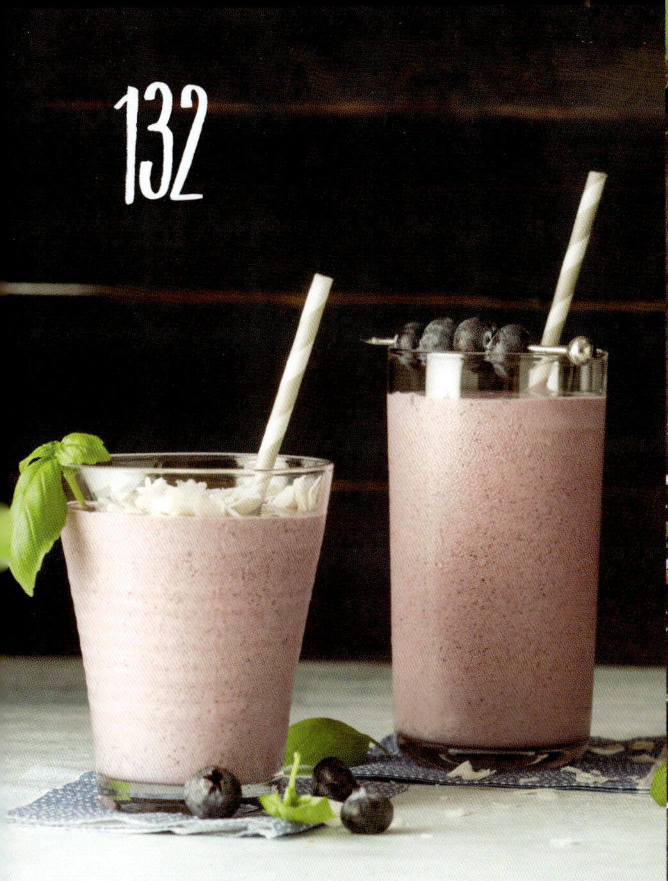

132

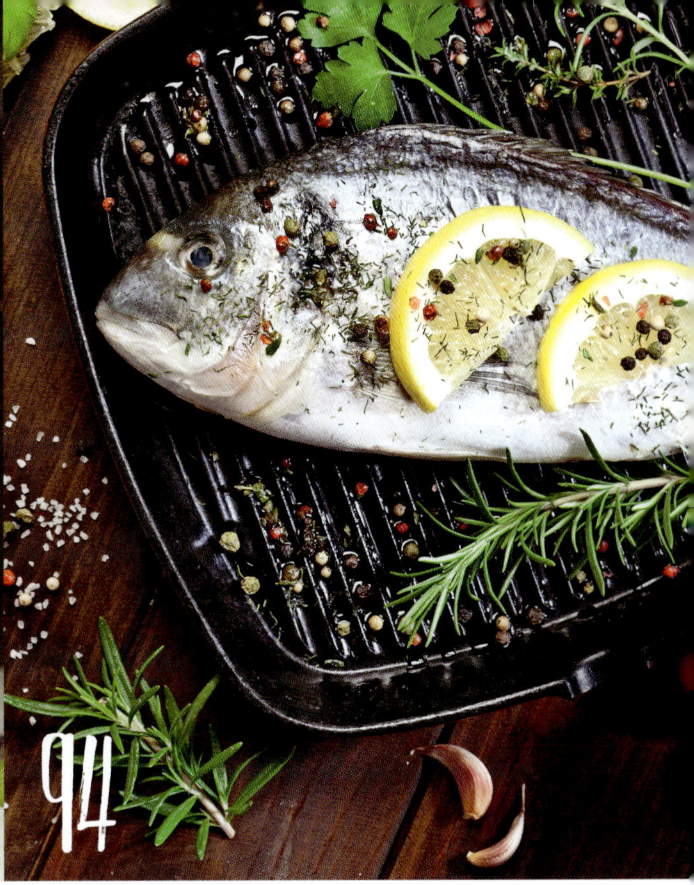

94

PART 3: COOK KETO

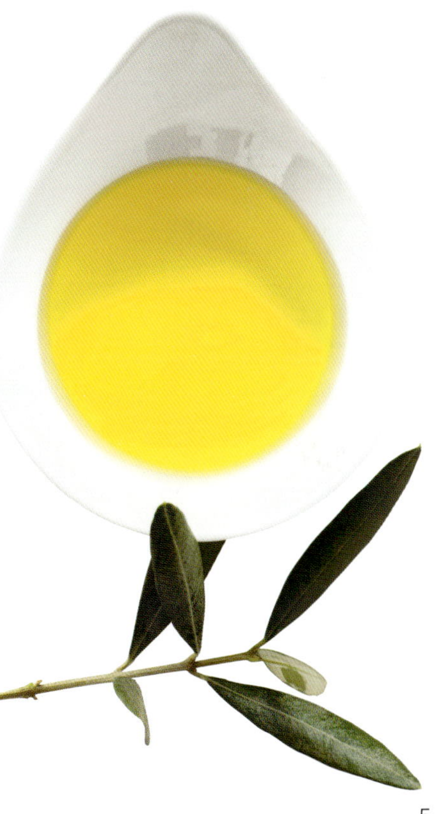

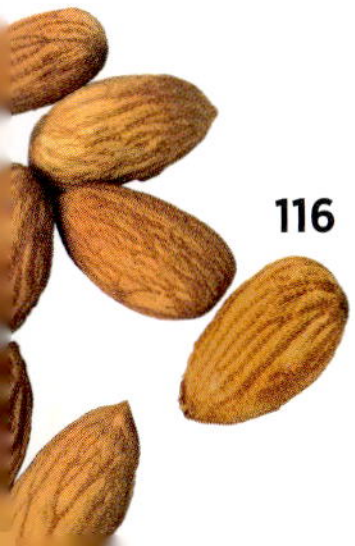

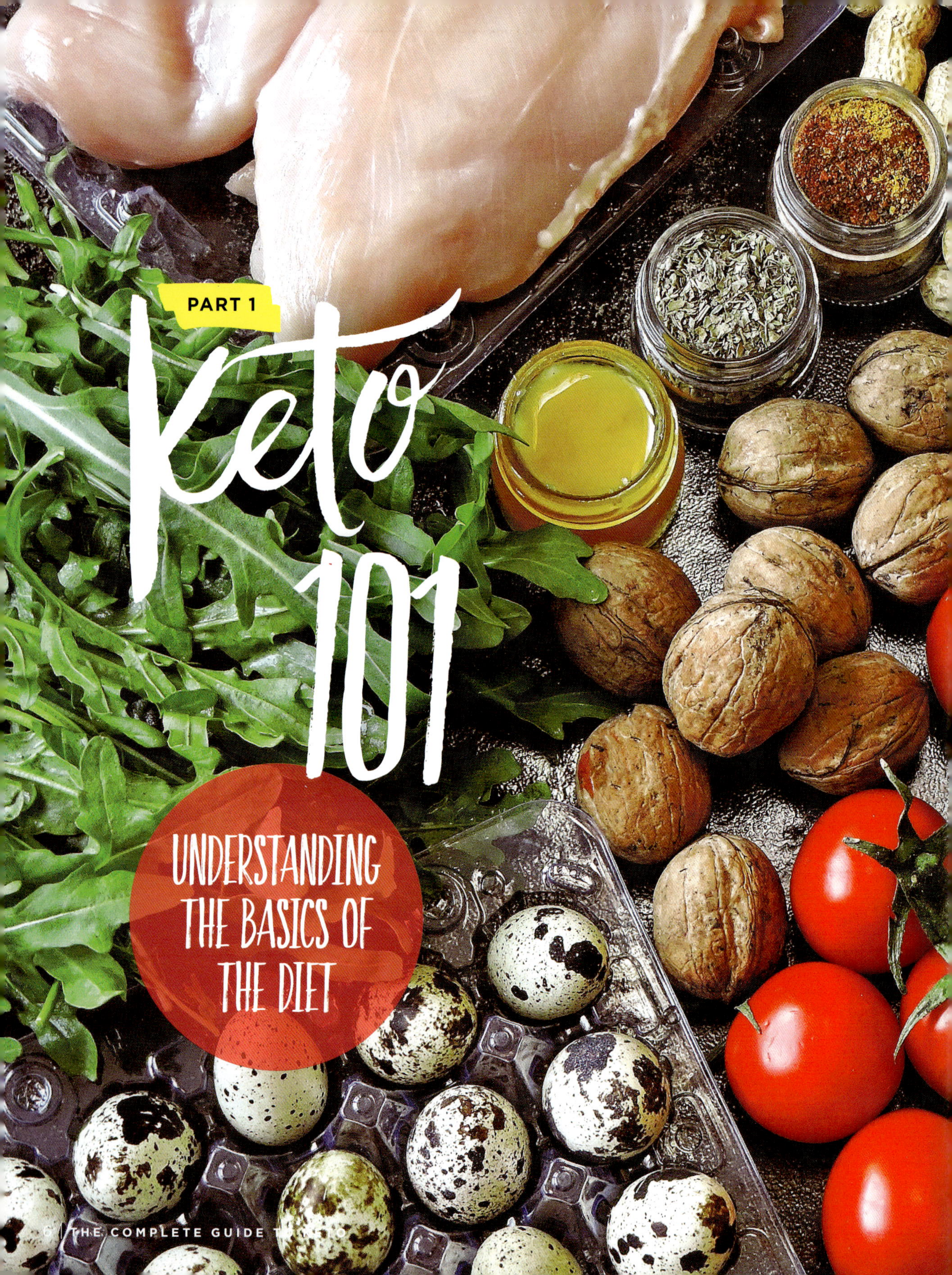

PART 1

Keto 101

UNDERSTANDING THE BASICS OF THE DIET

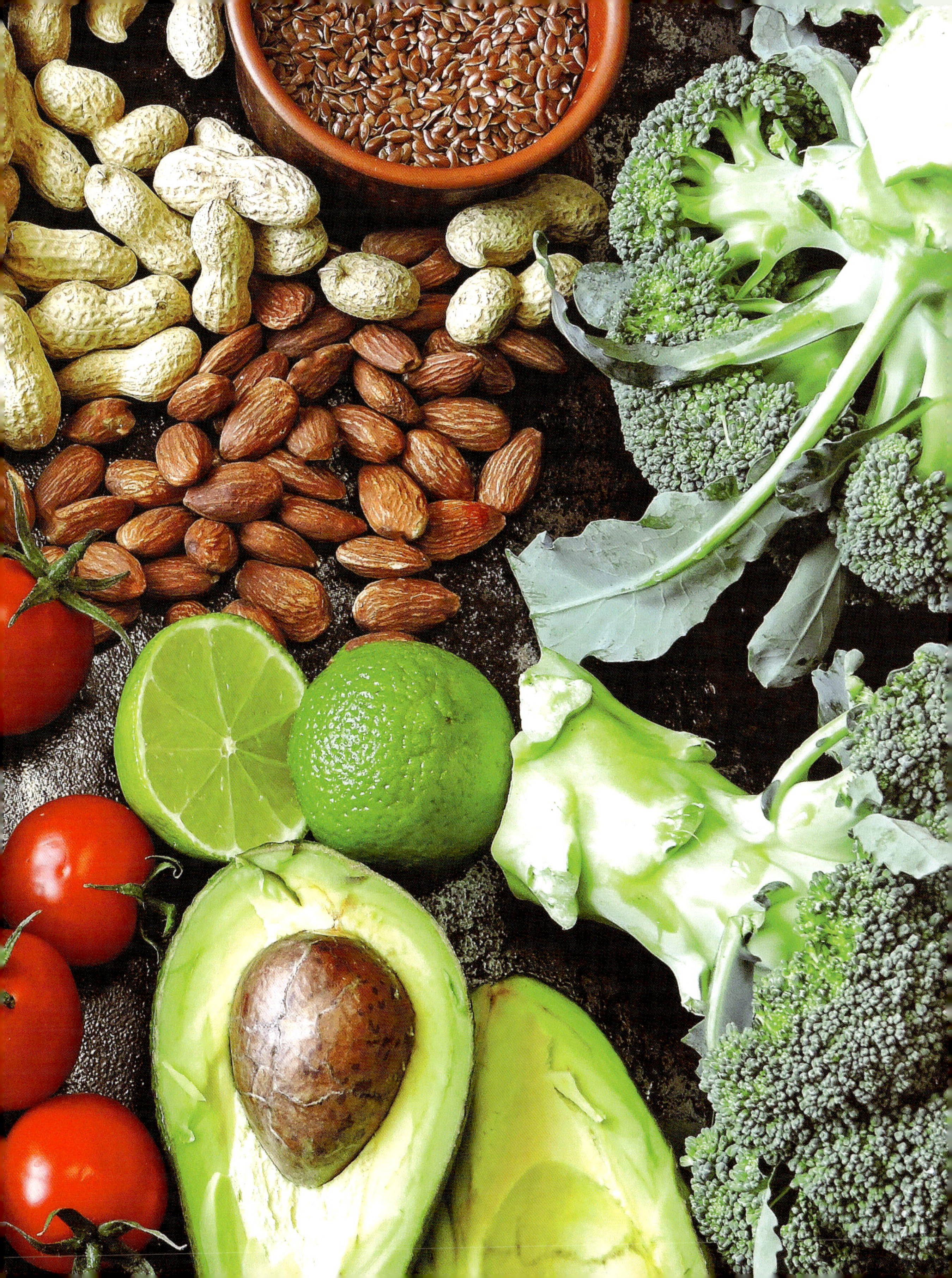

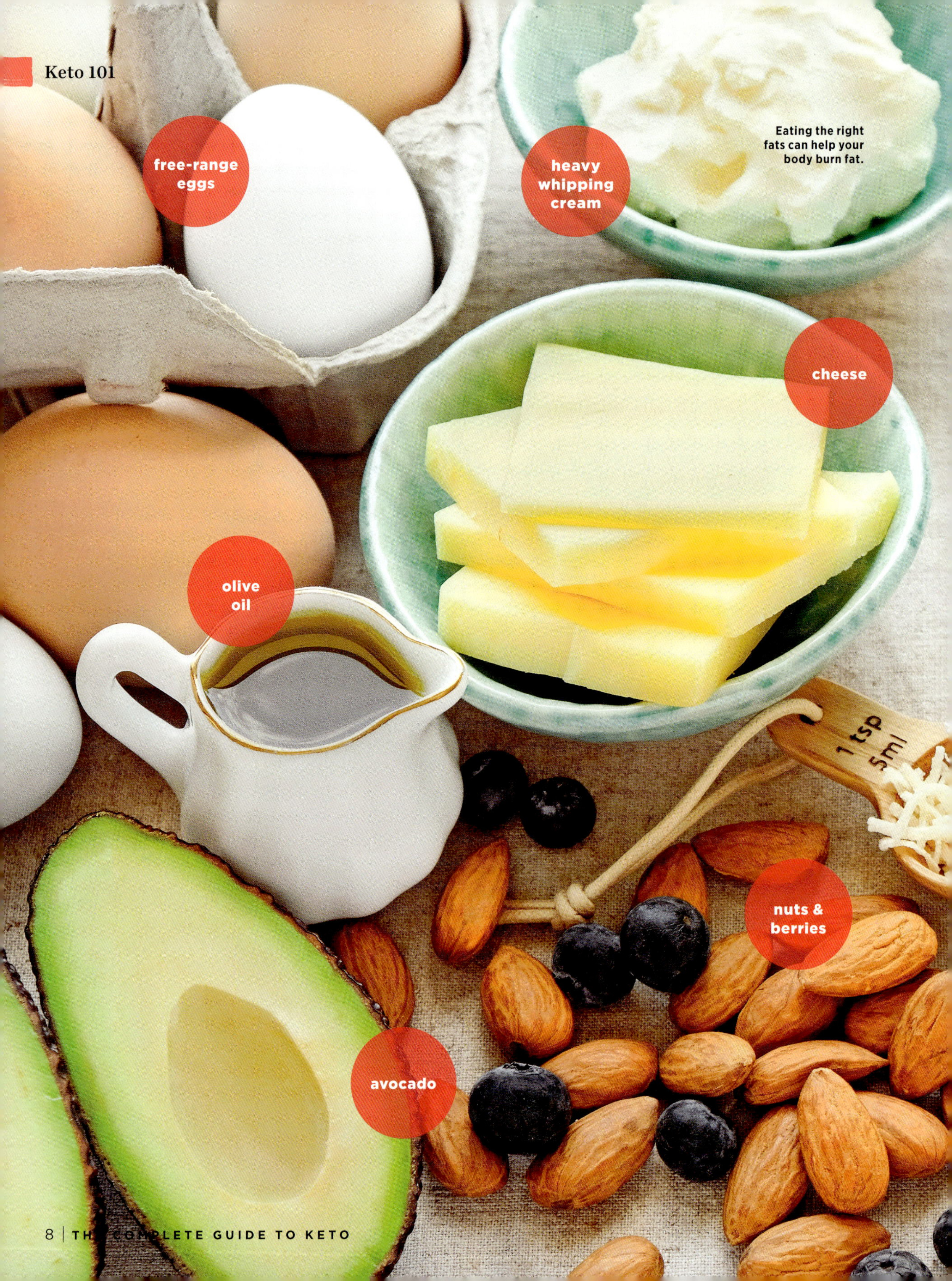
free-range eggs
heavy whipping cream
Eating the right fats can help your body burn fat.
cheese
olive oil
1 tsp
5ml
nuts & berries
avocado

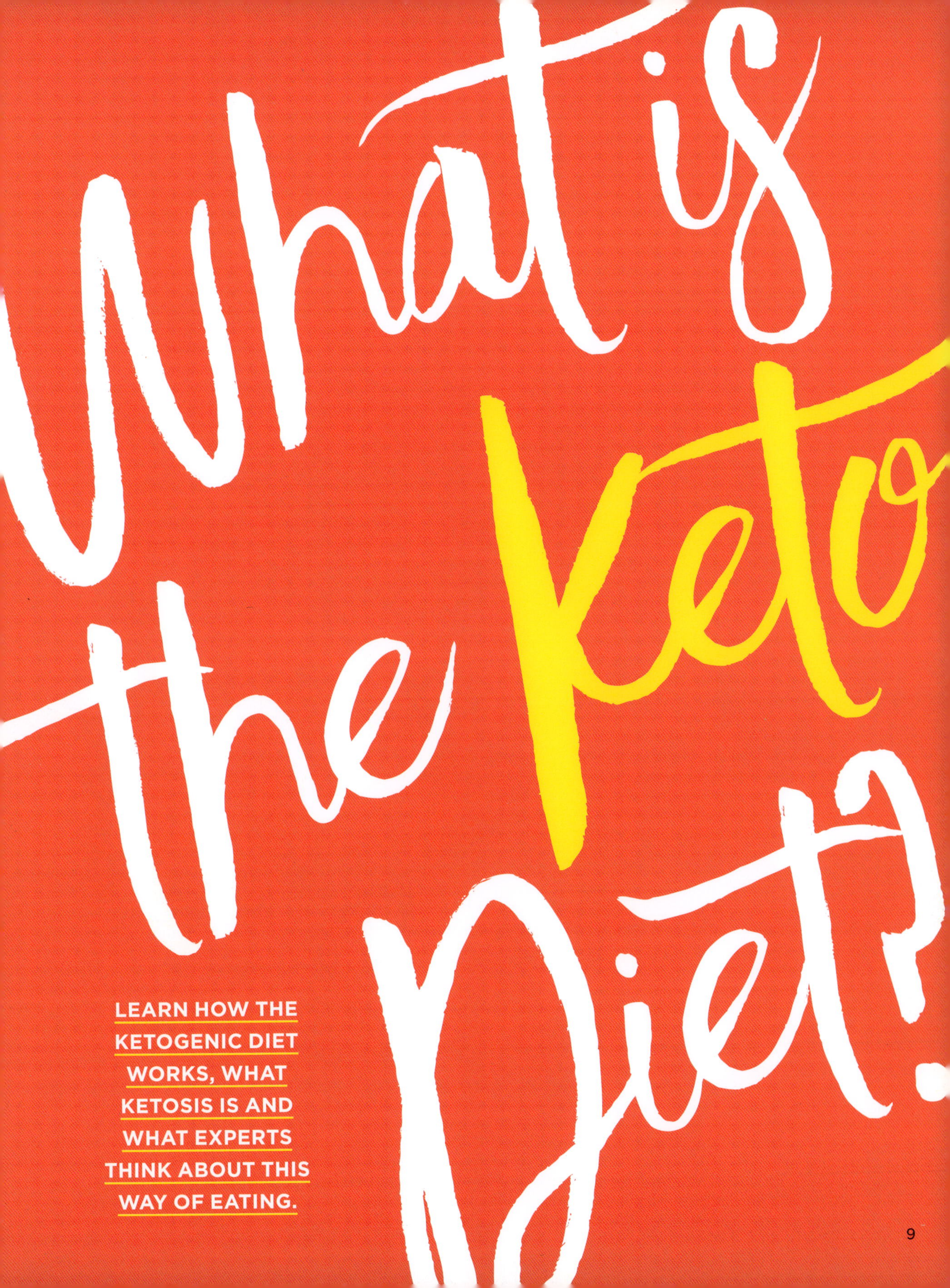

What is the Keto Diet?

LEARN HOW THE KETOGENIC DIET WORKS, WHAT KETOSIS IS AND WHAT EXPERTS THINK ABOUT THIS WAY OF EATING.

THE TENETS OF THE KETO DIET ARE simple, even if the science is not: The ultra-low-carb diet alters the way your body burns fuel for energy. Rather than churning through carbs, your body taps into stored body fat or fat from food to spur a process known as ketosis.

The general population's been turning to it as a means for fast weight loss in recent years. Keto has also become popular with endurance athletes, who believe using fat for energy will keep them from running low on blood sugar midrace (aka bonking).

Intrigued? Consider this your primer on the keto diet. Here's everything you need to know, from food rules to possible setbacks.

What Is the Keto Diet?

The keto diet works by nearly eliminating carbs.

"This removes your body's first choice of energy, which is glucose," says Jim White, RD, owner of Jim White Fitness and Nutrition Studios. "The body will first use its stores of glycogen for energy before it switches to using fat. Then the liver will convert fatty acids to ketone bodies, which the body can use for energy as an emergency backup."

This is a process known as ketosis. You're not relying on sugar (or carbs) for energy but, rather, fat. Your body uses those ketone bodies for energy you need to get through the day.

Ultimately, you're cutting your carb intake to fewer than 50 grams per day, but this number varies from person to person (some people go as low as 20 grams per day). Roughly 5 percent of your daily calories will come from carbs, 20 percent from protein, and 75 percent from fat. The idea is to find the threshold that keeps you in ketosis.

How Do You Know If You're Making Ketones?

They'll usually show up within the first two weeks, says Colin E. Champ, MD, who specializes in integrative medicine. That's typically how long it takes to burn through your glycogen stores and begin ketosis. Use urine test strips to help detect ketones.

"Once you start using the ketones effectively, they'll no longer spill over into your urine—you'll burn them for energy. Some people use a finger prick to detect ketones in their blood, but most people rely on what they're eating at that point," says Champ.

"A very light state of ketosis measures .5–1.0 mmol/L, a light state is 0.6–1.5 mmol/L, a medium state hovers around 1.6–3.0 mmol/L, and a strong state is greater than 3.1 mmol/L," says Jordan Mazur, RD, the coordinator of performance nutrition for the San Francisco 49ers. "Aim for a range that indicates you're in a state of ketosis, but don't aim for an 'optimal ketone threshold' every time."

When Did the Diet Become Popular?

"There's mention of the keto diet in ancient texts," says Champ. Well, kind of. "Hippocrates mentioned that when epileptics fasted, they stopped having seizures," he explains. "Then, in the late 1800s or early 1900s, people realized it wasn't necessarily the fasting that did it—any diet very high in fat, low in carbs and moderate in protein could benefit those with epilepsy, because it promotes ketones."

Researchers aren't exactly sure why, but ketone bodies seem to have an "anticonvulsant" effect on patients, according to research published in the *Journal of*

IN ORDER TO TRULY KNOW WHEN YOU'RE MAKING KETONES, START WITH URINE TEST STRIPS DAILY TO DETECT THEIR PRESENCE AND CONCENTRATION.

Keto-Friendly Foods

FATS

Eat saturated fat (**grass-fed butter**), monounsaturated fat (**avocados**, **olive oil**) and polyunsaturated omega-3s (**salmon**). Certain low-carb nuts and seeds are also fair game, like **almonds**, **macadamias** and **walnuts**, plus **sunflower seeds**, **pumpkin seeds** and **flaxseeds.** Skip refined oils or fats (**canola oil**) or trans fats (**margarine**). While full-fat cream and milk are high in saturated fat, they're also high in lactose sugar, so watch your consumption. Hard **cheese** is fine, though.

PROTEIN

Keep protein intake moderate (otherwise, it can kick you out of ketosis), emphasizing **grass-fed beef** and **free-range poultry** and **eggs**—which are higher in omega-3 fatty acids—**pork** (go easy on the bacon), **wild-caught fish** and **tofu**. You can also supplement your diet with keto-friendly **protein powders** for low-carb shakes.

FRUITS & VEGETABLES

Whole grains and refined carbs are out, but you can consume **nonstarchy veggies**, like **leafy greens** (**kale**, **Swiss chard**, **spinach**), **asparagus**, **broccoli** and **mushrooms**. Fruit options are limited to **berries**, **lemons**, **olives**, **coconuts** and **tomatoes**, as they're relatively low-carb.

BEVERAGES

You're permitted to drink **unsweetened tea** and **coffee**—and, depending on how strict your diet is, you can occasionally drink a **low-carb alcoholic beverage**. "One glass of **red wine** is fine," Champ says. "Two will decrease ketones."

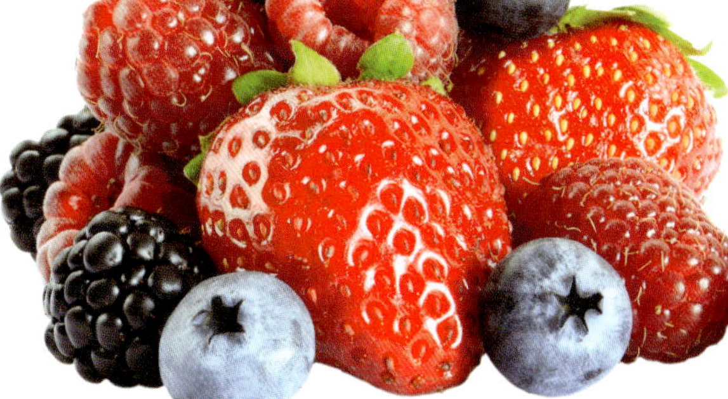

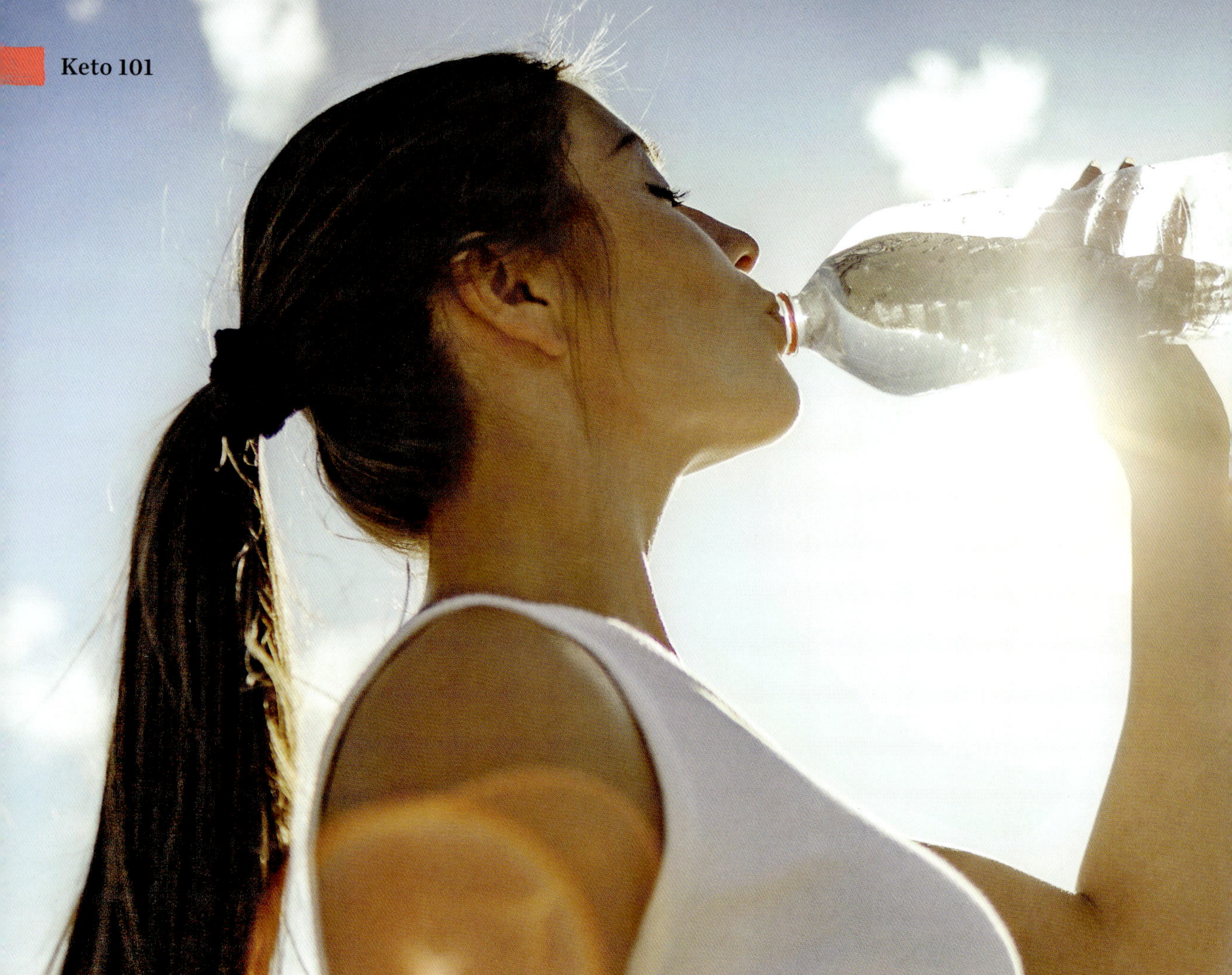

Neurochemistry. Johns Hopkins even has a Pediatric Ketogenic Diet Center, to help treat kids and adults with the condition.

Ketones could have a role in cancer prevention too, which is a topic of Champ's research. "It's a little premature to say. We don't know if it can help treat cancer or not. But we know it's pretty good for decreasing sugar levels and helping people with diabetes," he adds. By reducing carbs, you limit spikes in blood sugar and the need for insulin.

Celebrity endorsements quickly skyrocketed the keto diet's popularity as well, with prominent names like LeBron James, Kim Kardashian and Halle Berry touting the benefits of the meal plan. And the speedy weight-loss results are why many Americans are trying it.

Food Rules: What You Can and Can't Eat

"The keto diet doesn't allow most fruits, grains, beans, sugars, alcohol or low-fat dairy products," White says. "This essentially leaves you with animal and plant fats, meat, eggs, high-fat dairy, a few vegetables, berries, nuts and seafood."

If you're trying to lose weight or improve your body composition, use a nutrition tracker, an app or the USDA database to calculate carbs per serving. This will help you stay in the correct range for ketosis.

What Does Science Say?

The keto diet is thought to promote weight loss, because extreme carb restriction depletes glycogen stores in the body, causing people to

The correct carb range for ketosis is different for every individual.

What Your Brain Feels Like on Keto

"Most of the body can use glucose, amino acids or fatty acids for fuel—but 99.9 percent of the time, your brain can use only glucose," Jim White, RD, says. "It's the preferred and primary energy source, because it's the easiest to convert to energy; the body wants to maximize efficiency. But in cases where the body is starved of glucose, it can use ketones from fat." When you first make the shift, you can anticipate the "keto flu"—side effects of carb restriction that mirror the actual flu. "They can include nausea, vomiting, diarrhea, fatigue, headache, cravings, muscle cramps and soreness, dizziness and trouble concentrating," White says. These symptoms usually last for just a few days, but sometimes they can linger longer, especially if you were consuming a lot of carbs before going on keto. You might feel "run-down and lethargic," Colin Champ, MD, adds. "Because high-carb diets are tied to high amounts of insulin in the blood, the kidneys hold on to a lot of sodium. When you stop eating those foods, you pee out a lot of your sodium—which can lead to dehydration and brain fog." Add salt to your food, consume bone broths, and supplement your diet with magnesium and potassium, Champ suggests.

lose a lot of water weight. Once dieters see the scale move in the right direction, they can become more motivated. People are also eating more fats and protein, which are naturally more satiating than carbs, so they feel less hungry and eat fewer calories.

There are few long-term studies revealing the efficacy of the keto diet for long-term weight loss. However, studies do suggest it's effective in helping people shed the pounds quickly. Compared to a moderate-carb diet, the keto diet helped obese men lose more weight and fat in the first six months, according to research from the *American Journal of Clinical Nutrition.*

What the Experts Say

Even though it's been proven to deliver fast results, there are some things to keep in mind when you go keto. For one, because you are eliminating whole grains and many fruits and vegetables, your fiber levels may be low, which can effect your gastrointestinal health, says White. (Eating plenty of high-fiber green vegetables, like asparagus, broccoli and spinach, or taking a keto-friendly fiber supplement, can help.)

And most experts say you don't need to stay on a keto diet for years on end. "Even the strongest ketogenic diet believers don't think 100 percent of the population should be on a ketogenic diet 100 percent of the time," says Champ. "There are certainly benefits for carbs in the diet." Many proponents of keto eventually increase their carbs once they reach their weight-loss goals.

However, the keto diet can help reinforce a healthier lifestyle, because people see the results on the scale and in how their clothes fit. Sweet cravings begin to go away, and people learn to supplement their diets with wholesome foods rather than processed carbs, which drive the majority of Americans' diets.

By using keto to jump-start weight loss and eliminate unhealthy foods in your diet, you may be on your way to long-term, lasting success.

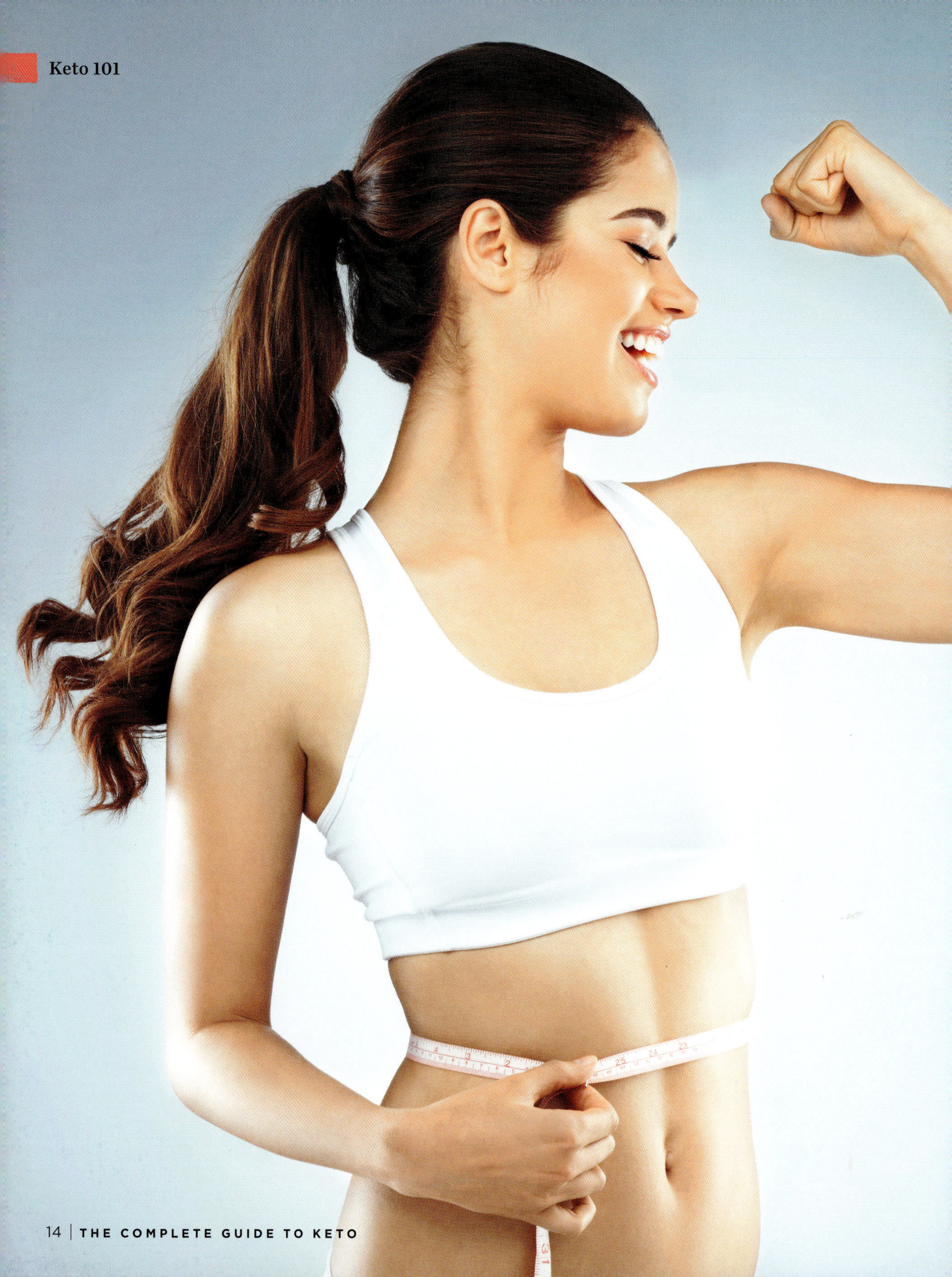

Keto Science, Simplified

UNDERSTANDING WHAT FUELS KETO'S FAT-BURNING FURNACE WILL HELP YOU MASTER THE PLAN. HERE'S A BASIC KETOSIS PRIMER.

WITH HUNDREDS OF STORIES OF weight-loss transformations swirling on social media, we really don't need a study to tell us that the keto diet is effective. Still, it's good to know that research consistently gives keto followers a distinct advantage when it comes to shedding pounds. A recent study in the *Journal of Endocrinology and Metabolism* found that people who followed a keto diet lost a stunning 2.2 times more weight than those on low-fat, low-calorie diets. And compared to other low-carb diets or the popular Mediterranean diet, keto resulted in decidedly faster slimdowns, according to a Harvard Health report.

What's more, you don't just lose more weight on keto, you also feel less hungry—which is great for sustaining the plan. "Keto keeps you satiated much longer, and you rarely feel hungry," says Maria Emmerich, a nutritionist, certified keto coach and bestselling author. "Over time, you'll experience additional benefits, like mental clarity, improved moods, better memory, more energy and much more."

The Basics

We know the goal in the keto diet is to get your body to use fat instead of carbs for energy. But when your body "burns fat," what's really going on? How exactly does the keto diet work?

For most people on a Western diet, the body gets energy by burning sugar, which comes from carbs. Your muscles and brain like running on sugar (glucose), and they are naturally efficient at burning it. But something interesting happens when your carb intake drops low enough, say, 20 to 50 grams a day. Because your body is starved for glucose, it starts reaching into its fat cells and switches over to burning fat for energy. The state your body enters when it starts converting stored fat into fuel for your cells is called ketosis.

Some parts of your body, especially your brain, can't use unrefined fatty acids for energy. So your system has to refine them into a usable fuel. Think of the gasoline you put in your car: It's refined from crude oil that comes from the Earth. Our refining process takes place in the liver, where "fat is turned into ketones, another fuel source for the body and, primarily, for the brain," explains Emmerich.

In other words, the liver, like an oil refinery, breaks down the fatty acids into digestible nuggets, or ketones. The process is called ketogenesis, the root for the name "keto" diet.

Kicking Into Ketosis

The good news about ketosis is that it's a natural state for your body to be in. The human anatomy automatically goes there when your food doesn't contain enough carbs to fuel your metabolic processes. In a biological shift, the body burns fat and makes ketones in the process.

But putting your body into a state of nutritional ketosis isn't always easy at first. "The transition can be uncomfortable, because ketone levels are still rising and the body is somewhat experiencing carb and sugar withdrawal," says Josh Axe, DNM, a leading nutrition expert and the author of *Keto Diet: Your 30-Day Plan to Lose Weight, Balance Hormones, Boost Brain Health, and Reverse Disease*. "Side effects, which have been nicknamed the keto flu, can include fatigue, constipation, cravings, headaches and more, depending on the person." Discomfort is temporary and typically lasts just one to two weeks. "Once the body is fat-adapted and more accustomed to using fat rather than carbs for energy," says Axe, "people usually experience not only weight loss but improved digestion, appetite suppression and enhanced cognitive performance."

The Payoff

When your body converts into the ketogenic state through diet, it goes through three phases of adaptation. "If you restrict carbs enough, to 20 grams or below, your body will show elevated blood ketones in two to three days—but your body isn't efficient at using fat as its primary

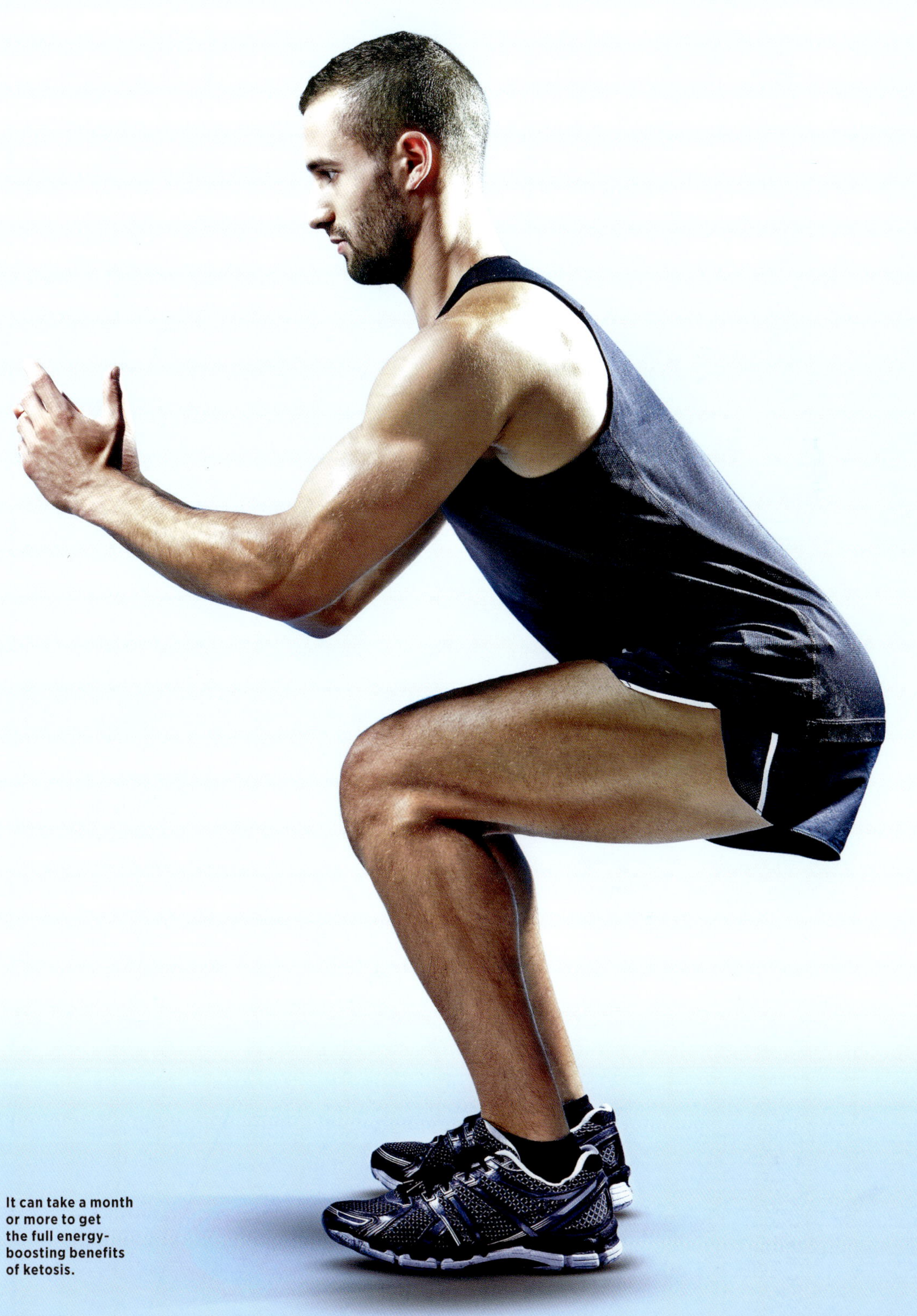

It can take a month or more to get the full energy-boosting benefits of ketosis.

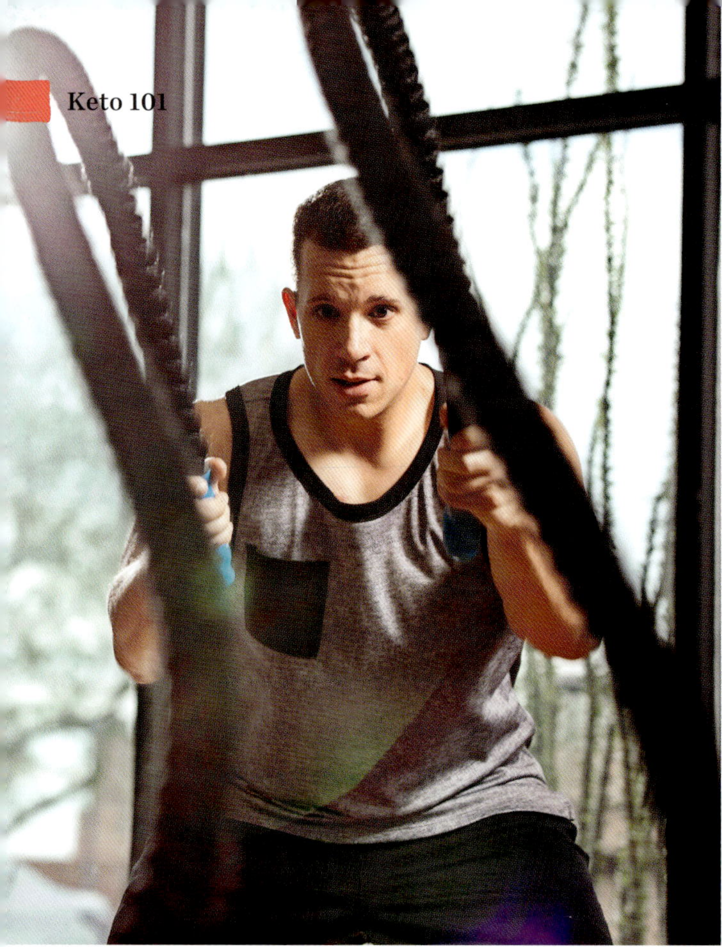

A Word About Water Weight

Keto diets produce fast results at first because we shed water weight as we deplete glycogen (glucose the body holds in storage; about two days' worth). The science makes sense: "Carbohydrates make you retain water, but when you cut them way back, your body releases much of the water," explains Emmerich. "Unfortunately, along with this water go electrolytes [sodium, potassium and magnesium]. It's important to replenish these minerals when you go keto by adding extra salt to food, and maybe a magnesium supplement." While you're not yet burning fat, losing water weight helps jump-start the process and provides extra motivation to keep going.

fuel yet," says Emmerich. "It takes most people four to six weeks to get that big boost in energy, mental clarity and hunger control, which is the second phase. The third phase is the continued improvement in health you see after several months of keto—most of our clients stay keto for the healthy improvements, like getting off medications, not for the weight loss. That is just a bonus to how good they feel."

It's true, you can use keto just for the short term, say, until you reach your weight-loss goal. But once you're in the habit, most experts suggest that you'll feel so good—and the results in your waistline and vitals will be so improved—you won't want to stop. "I see this as a lifestyle, as do most of my clients, when they experience how good they can feel. They never want to go back to feeling tired, hungry and foggy," says Emmerich. "I started this for my own health issues. I had IBS, acid reflux and 50-plus extra pounds. Now I no longer have health issues and have lost all the extra weight."

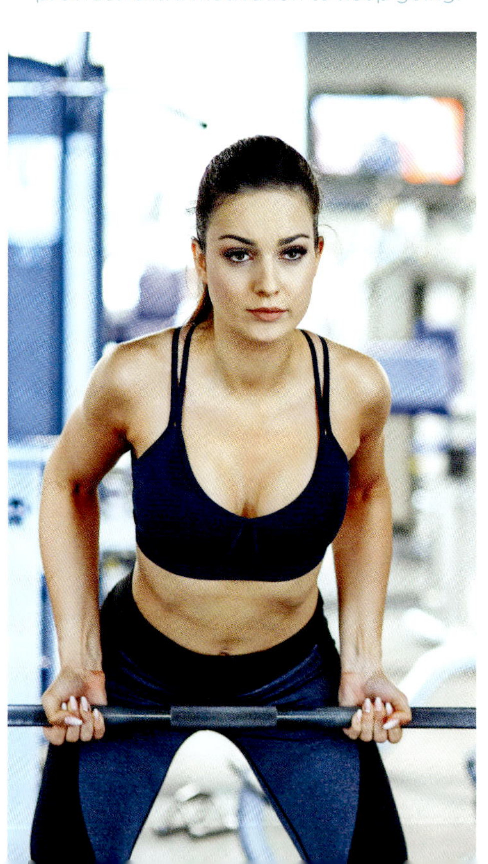

The Macronutrient Ratios of Keto

Macronutrients, or "macros," as keto aficionados call them, are energy-providing nutrients—carbohydrates, fats and proteins—that your body needs in order to function properly. The keto diet recommends different ratios from what many traditional medical experts suggest. While a standard healthy diet wants to ensure you get a certain balance of nutrients, the goal of keto is different—it's designed to force your body into ketosis, the state in which it's using fat, not glucose, to fuel you. This causes you to burn more fat, thereby losing excess weight, boosting energy and increasing focus, all of which can contribute to an overall healthier lifestyle.

CARBS
5 to 10%

PROTEIN
20 to 30%

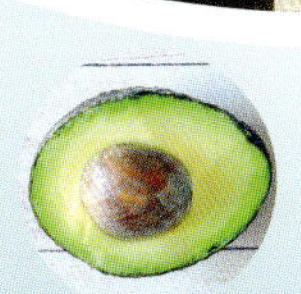

FATS
70 to 80%

Full Fat Story

THE GOOD, THE BAD, AND THE (OCCASIONALLY) UGLY OF KETO'S NO. 1 NUTRIENT.

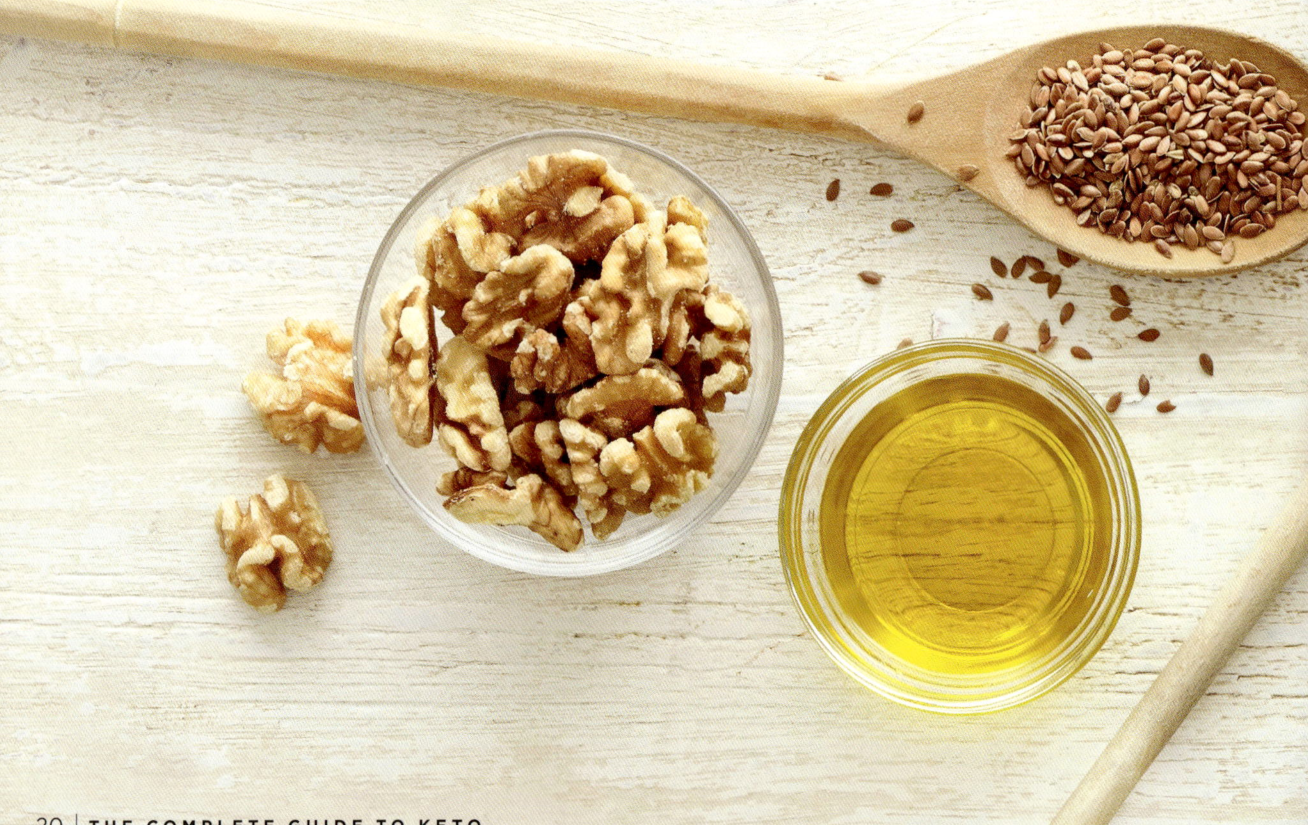

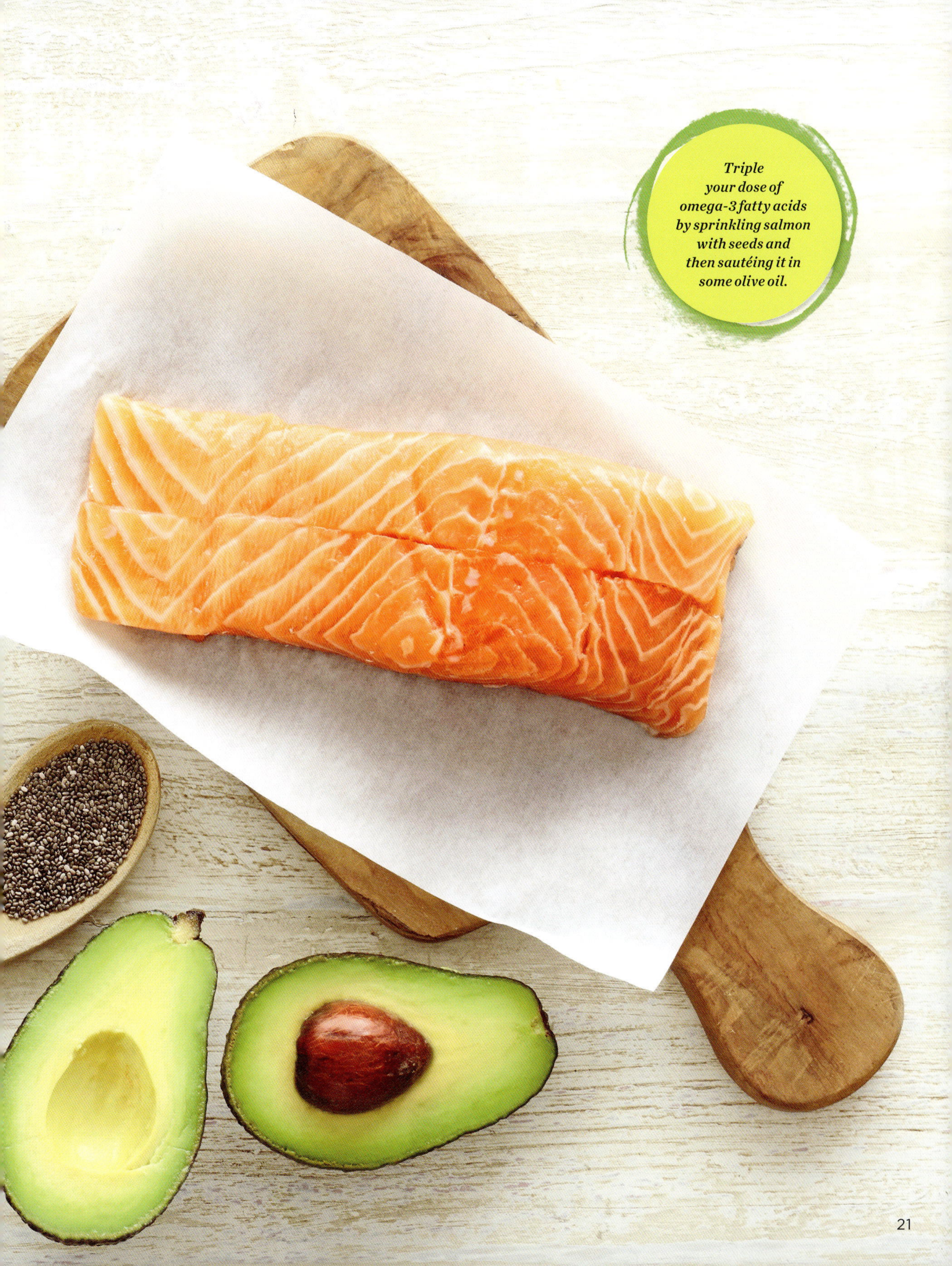
Triple your dose of omega-3 fatty acids by sprinkling salmon with seeds and then sautéing it in some olive oil.

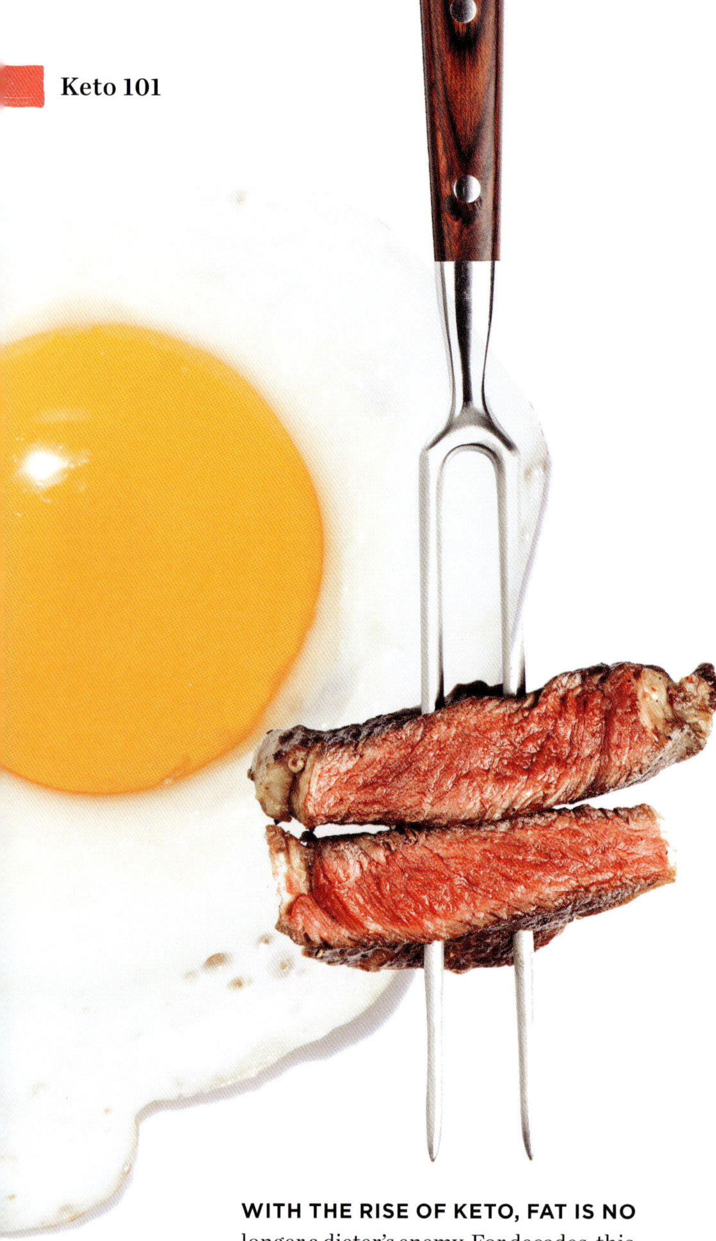

WITH THE RISE OF KETO, FAT IS NO longer a dieter's enemy. For decades, this essential macronutrient has been dissed and downgraded, accused of causing ailments like obesity and heart disease. Food labels everywhere have touted "Non-Fat!" and "Reduced Fat!" as selling points. Now, keto has returned fat to the menu, but many people remain confused about which kinds are the best to eat—and whether some are still considered unhealthy. Luckily, new research in just the past few years has revealed a lot more about how fat works in the body and which types to choose. Following is a breakdown of the various categories and the bottom line on each.

Saturated Fats

These types of fats, which are solid at room temperature and mostly derived from animal sources (think meat, cheese, butter, lard), were long blamed for raising blood cholesterol and contributing to heart disease. But the tide has been turning, says David Ludwig, MD, PhD, a professor of nutrition at the Harvard T. H. Chan School of Public Health. "Saturated fat used to be public-health enemy No. 1," he explains, "but it's neither that nor exactly a health food. Overall, it's rather neutral, depending on what other foods are eaten with it or substituted for it."

Research is backing that up. A report in *Annals of Internal Medicine* analyzed 76 studies and concluded there was no evidence for avoiding saturated fats in favor of unsaturated. Another meta-analysis, in *The American Journal of Clinical Nutrition*, has found no support for the idea that saturated fat increases the risk of heart disease or stroke. Despite those and similar findings, the American Heart Association still recommends severely limiting saturated fats to 6 percent of total calories per day. So what gives?

Well, it's complicated, says Ludwig. "For instance, saturated fats do somewhat raise LDL, the so-called 'bad' cholesterol. But at the same time, they raise the 'good' HDL cholesterol, which is protective, and they also lower triglycerides." And the higher your HDL, the better. Balance is the key, says Kendra Whitmire, a nutritionist and dietitian in Laguna Beach, California, who practices functional and therapeutic nutrition. "You don't want to eat only saturated fats," she says. "You'll want to balance those with omega-3 fatty acids and other forms. But if you're getting your saturated fat from whole-food sources—butter, meat, eggs—in addition to taking in some fish oils and vegetable and nut oils, it's not going to be a problem."

Unsaturated Fats

These fats come in two forms, monounsaturated and polyunsaturated, and many healthy foods naturally contain some of each. These are the fats you'll hear characterized as "healthy," because in general, they've been shown to raise HDL cholesterol and lower LDL.

Monounsaturated fats are abundant in olives, avocados and many nuts, such as walnuts—and also in their resulting oils when pressed into liquid form. These are generally "good-for-you" fats, especially the heart-healthy, HDL-boosting olive oil, though there are some exceptions (see "On the 'Out' List," page 24).

On the polyunsaturated side, one type, in particular, has been found to be especially beneficial: the now world-famous omega-3 fatty acids, which have come to be seen almost as a kind of wonder fat. In addition to their cardiovascular benefits, omega-3s have been found to reduce inflammation in the body, help fight depression and anxiety, lower blood pressure, reduce cancer risk, improve sleep quality and skin health, possibly reduce risk of dementia and more. Omega-3s are abundant in fatty fish, like salmon, mackerel and herring, and also in some plant sources, such as flaxseed and chia seeds.

But, just to muddy the waters a bit, another form of polyunsaturated fats, omega-6, is a little less golden. This type, which includes many vegetable oils like soybean, corn and safflower, is also essential to health—in moderation. Because these oils are widely used in restaurant and packaged-food preparation and have also benefited from a reputation as heart-healthy and superior to saturated fats, we now consume many more of them than we did a century ago. Here, the devil may be in the dose—or, more precisely, in the ratio.

Humans evolved on a diet with a ratio of omega-6 to omega-3 fatty acids of about 1 to 1, according to many evolutionary and Paleolithic-nutrition studies. But in the typical Western diet today, the ratio is 15 or 16 to 1—a staggering difference that is thought to promote many common ailments, including cardiovascular disease, cancer and autoimmune disorders. Research has shown that lowering the ratio down to 3 or 4 to 1 can help prevent those conditions.

Trans Fats

The fourth category is man-made fats—and here, the answer is simple: Just say no. Trans fats came about when food manufacturers in the early 20th century found a way to make liquid fats shelf-stable (and thus useful for packaged goods, like crackers and breads) by transforming them into solid fats through hydrogenation. This processing, though, made them dangerous, and trans fats were ultimately found to increase LDL cholesterol, reduce HDL, create inflammation and cause insulin resistance—all of which greatly raise the risk of heart disease. Trans fats are now banned by the FDA in the U.S., but always look for them on the label; if you see trans fats listed, put the item back on the shelf.

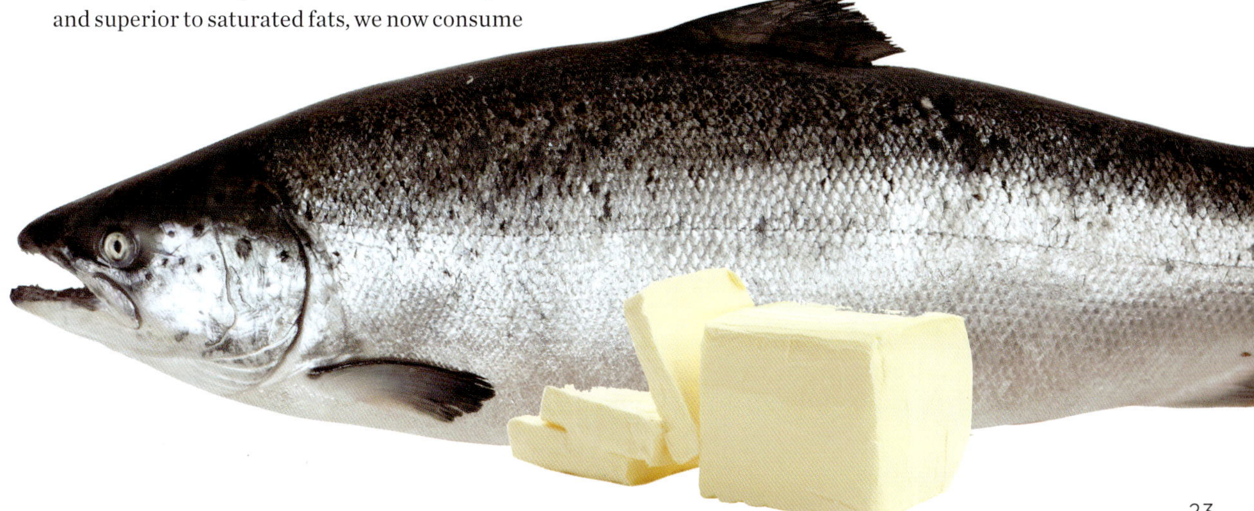

COOKING WITH FAT

All the Oils You Need

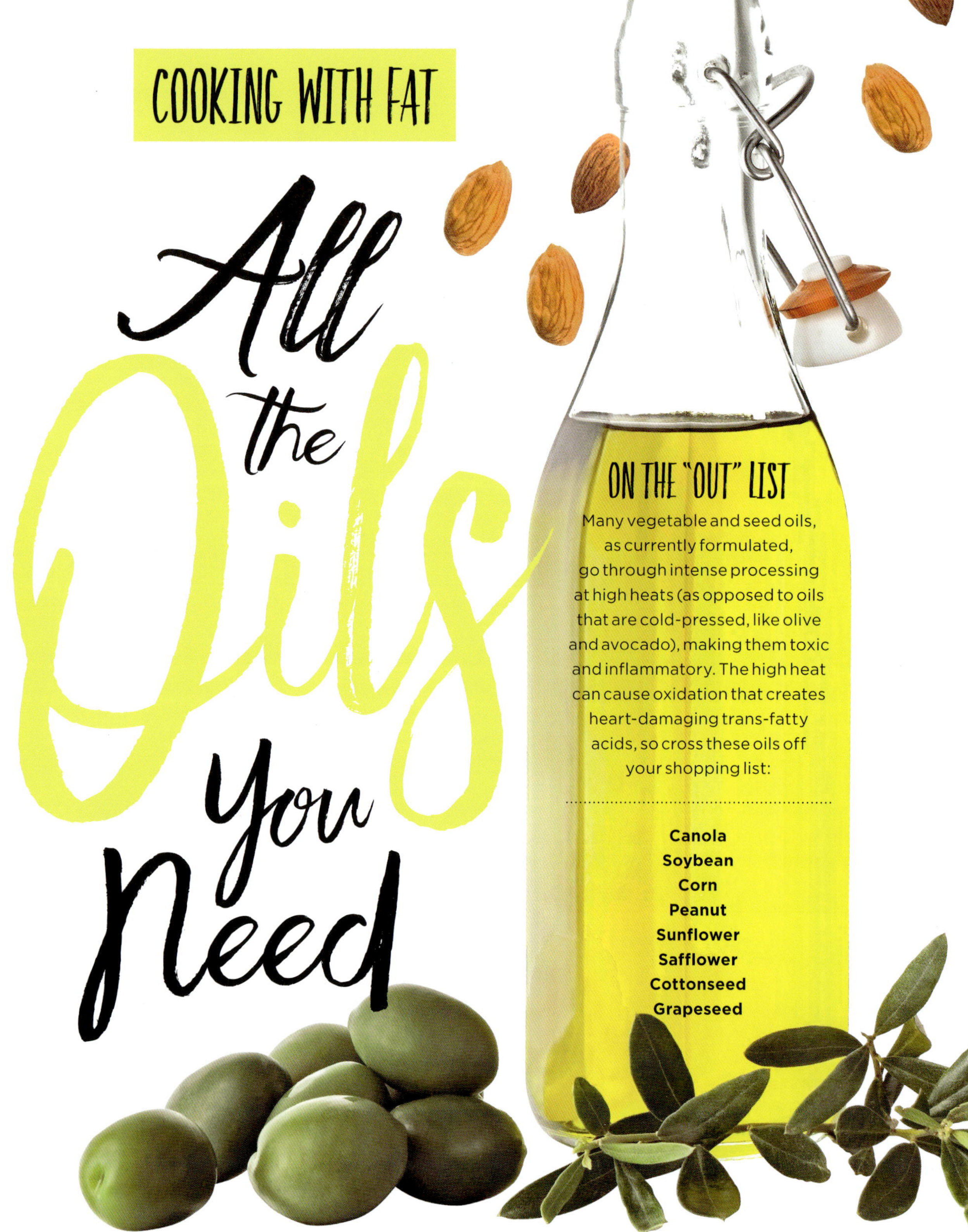

ON THE "OUT" LIST

Many vegetable and seed oils, as currently formulated, go through intense processing at high heats (as opposed to oils that are cold-pressed, like olive and avocado), making them toxic and inflammatory. The high heat can cause oxidation that creates heart-damaging trans-fatty acids, so cross these oils off your shopping list:

Canola
Soybean
Corn
Peanut
Sunflower
Safflower
Cottonseed
Grapeseed

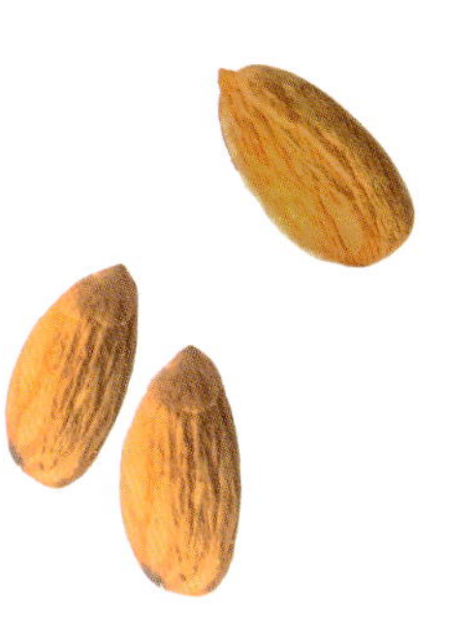

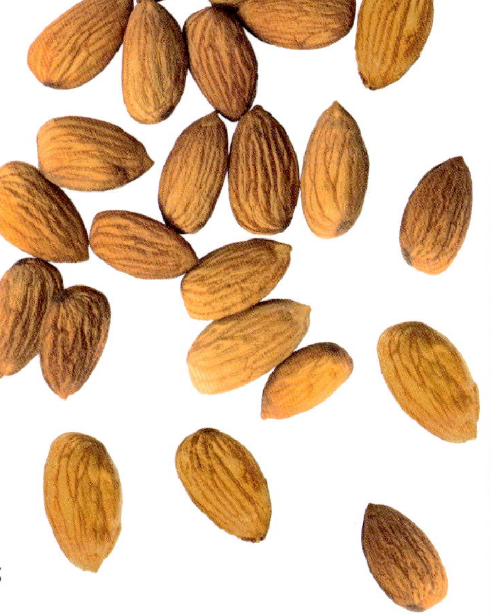

Extra-Virgin Olive Oil

The benefits of this mainly monounsaturated fat are many: It is antioxidant, anti-inflammatory and anti-bacterial; protects against heart disease; and raises HDL cholesterol. It has a medium smoke point (the heat at which an oil starts to degrade), so it's fine for sautéing but not for cooking at very high temperatures. It excels in sauces and salad dressings.

Coconut Oil

While coconut oil is saturated, it's a type that operates differently in your body than animal-based saturated fats. It also may have special benefits: It boosts fat burning and contains medium-chain triglycerides (MCTs), which go straight to the liver to be used as a quick source of energy or turned into ketones.

Butter

Now that margarine has been banished to the neverland of trans fats, butter has made a slow, steady comeback. Butter can create magic in cooking and is completely keto-friendly. But it has a low smoke point, so if you want to cook at higher heats, use ghee (clarified butter) instead. (You can buy ghee or make your own.)

Avocado Oil

Whole avocados are keto gold, and the oil pressed from the fruit is equally healthful. It's also incredibly versatile, with just about the highest smoke point of any oil—520°F—meaning that you can cook at very high heat without having it break down or burn.

Sesame Oil

Sesame seeds have been pressed to extract their oils for thousands of years. They bring a distinctive flavor, particularly savory in Asian-inspired dishes, along with hefty omega-3 values and compounds called phytosterols that reduce cholesterol uptake in the body.

Walnut Oil

Walnuts are stars of a keto diet, and so is the oil they provide—which is rich in omega-3 fatty acids as well as vitamins like manganese, niacin, potassium and zinc. It doesn't cook well at high heats; its rich, nutty flavor is better served as a standout ingredient in sauces, salad dressings or toppings for grilled meats.

FATS IN FOODS

EAT THESE FREELY

Fish

Poultry
(look for free-range and organic)

Meats
(look for grass-fed and unprocessed beef, lamb, pork, venison)

Eggs

High-Fat Dairy
(cream, sour cream, full-fat cheese, cottage cheese, mayonnaise, cream cheese)

Avocados

Olives

Nuts
(pecans, almonds, walnuts, hazelnuts, cashews, macadamias)

Seeds
(sunflower, chia, flaxseed, pumpkin)

EAT THESE CAREFULLY

Processed and Cured Meats
(bacon, salami, ham)

AVOID THESE

Margarine
(full of trans fat)

Fast Food Meats
(often cooked in unhealthy oils)

THE TRUTH

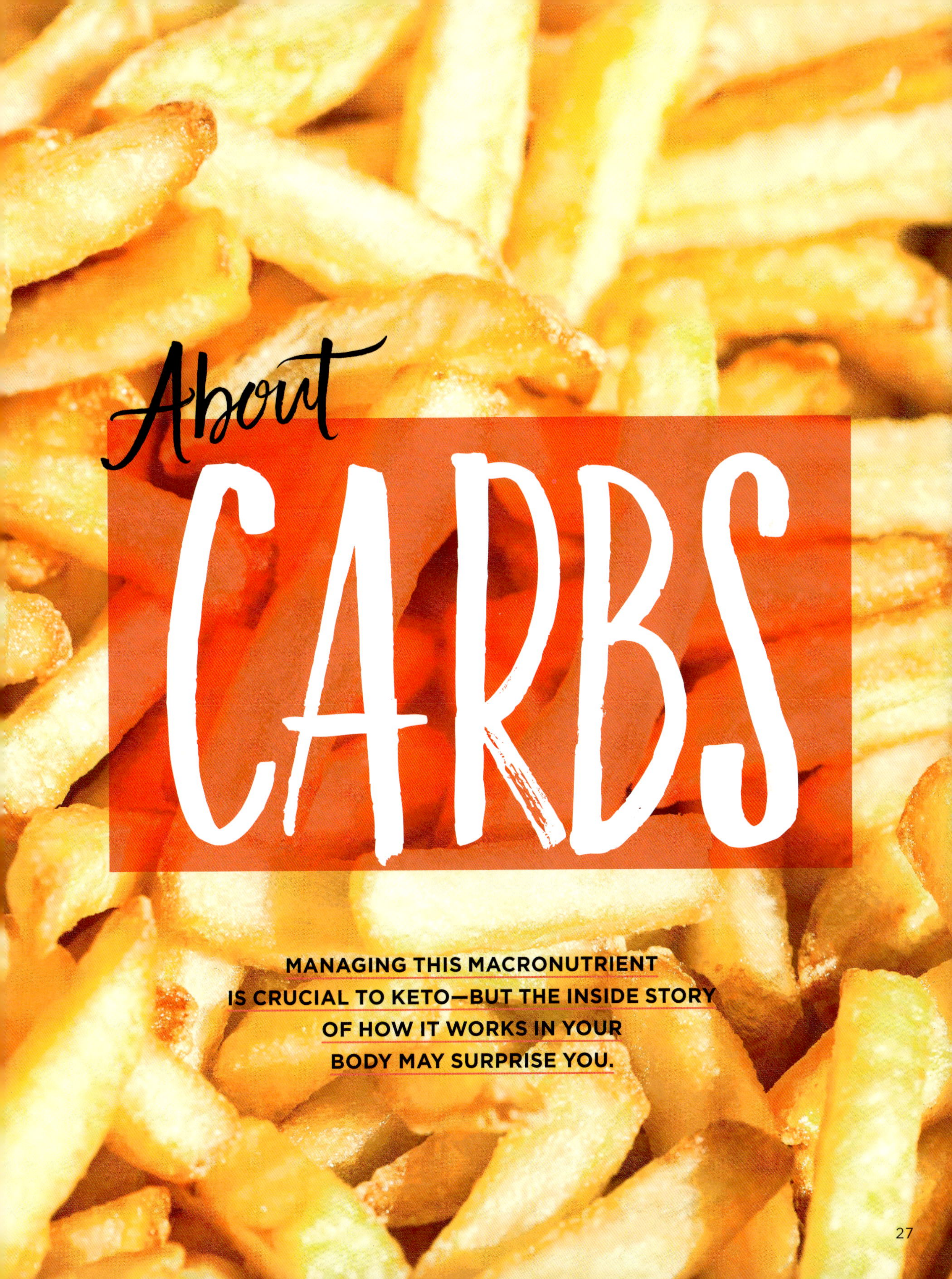

About CARBS

MANAGING THIS MACRONUTRIENT IS CRUCIAL TO KETO—BUT THE INSIDE STORY OF HOW IT WORKS IN YOUR BODY MAY SURPRISE YOU.

FATS ARE THE UNDISPUTED HERO OF the keto narrative. But carbohydrates? Their role is more complicated—sometimes the villain, sometimes an ally. Knowing how carbs work in a keto diet is key to following the plan in a healthy way.

First, a little history. Not long ago, carbs were celebrated as the base of an optimum diet. Remember the Food Pyramid, with its foundation of grains and starches, while fats and oils were in a tiny category at the top? Well, picture the pyramid turned upside down, and you have the paradigm of keto perfection. That shift is increasingly supported by science. For instance, a large decade-long epidemiological study, published in *The Lancet*, found that high carbohydrate intake was associated with a higher risk of total mortality, while a higher total-fat intake was related to lower mortality.

However, many of the healthiest foods on the planet are largely composed of carbs (think: broccoli, leafy greens, asparagus, tomatoes), so it's not as simple as making all carbohydrates the bad guy. "People are confused about how to manage carbs," says Maya Feller, MS, RD, a nutrition counselor specializing in chronic-disease prevention based in Brooklyn, New York. "The fact is that many whole foods that are largely carbohydrate are also rich in fiber, minerals and vitamins." While a ketogenic diet calls for reducing total carb intake to between 20 and 50 grams per day (depending on how strict a regimen you're following), the key to following it safely and healthfully lies in choosing the best carbs for your body.

BROCCOLI IS ONE OF THE "GOOD GUYS," DESPITE ITS CARB CONTENT. SAUTÉ IT IN OLIVE OIL FOR A KETO TREAT.

Are Net Carbs for Real?

You may have seen "**net carbs**" on food labels and in nutritional listings for recipes and wondered whether it's a gimmick or a reality. It's a simple formula—**the total grams of carbs in a food, minus the grams of fiber**—and it has science behind it, says nutritionist Kendra Whitmire. "Your body doesn't process fiber, so you don't break it down and use it as calories," she explains. "Instead, fiber is passed through to your colon and acts as a fuel source for bacteria, which helps move waste from your body." That's one reason that fiber-rich vegetables, for instance, are low in net carbs—and good for your whole system.

The "Bad" Carbs

A growing mountain of research is showing that one particular form of carbohydrates —the kind in highly processed and refined foods, like sweets and white bread—is not your body's friend. "All digestible carbohydrates are broken down into simple sugars in the intestines," explains Andreas Eenfeldt, MD, founder of dietdoctor.com. "That raises blood glucose levels, which increases production of insulin, our fat-storing hormone." With highly processed carbs, that happens even faster, leading to blood sugar spikes as your body gobbles up the easy fuel and ending with an equally quick drop.

The result: You're soon hungry again and craving quick energy in the form of more sugars and starches. "That starts the process again, and that vicious cycle leads to weight gain," says Eenfeldt. And because insulin

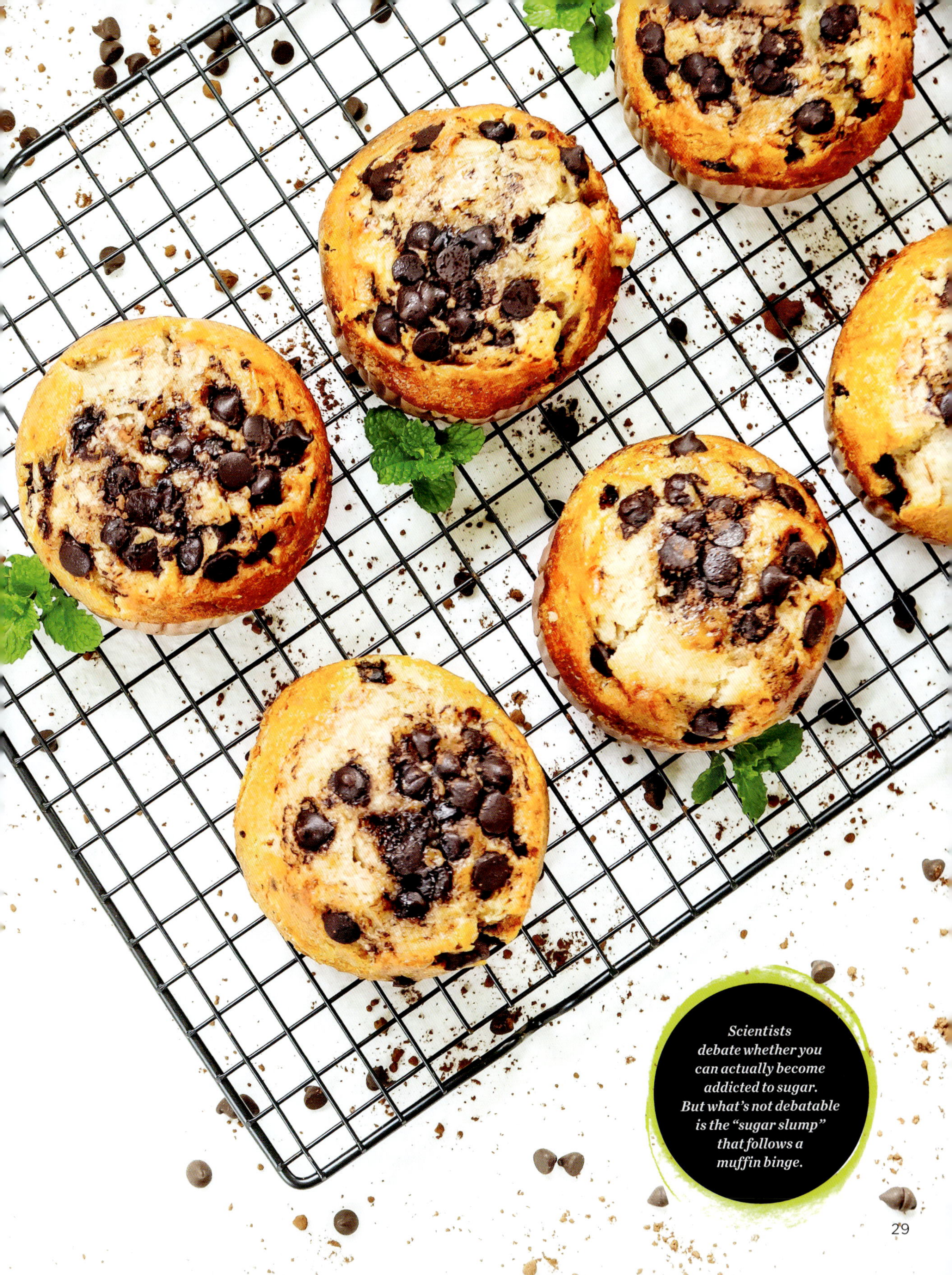
Scientists
debate whether you
can actually become
addicted to sugar.
But what's not debatable
is the "sugar slump"
that follows a
muffin binge.

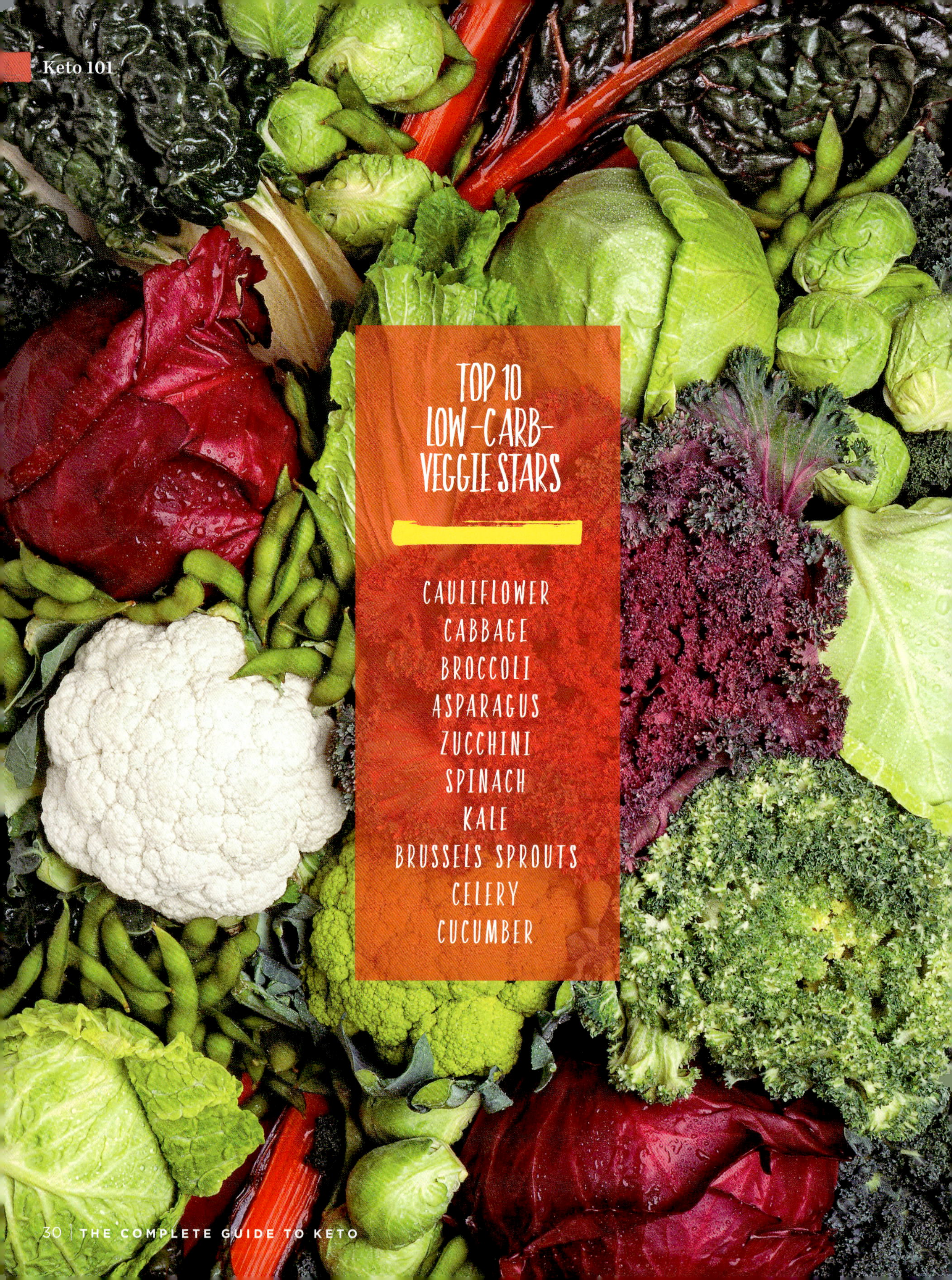

TOP 10 LOW-CARB-VEGGIE STARS

CAULIFLOWER
CABBAGE
BROCCOLI
ASPARAGUS
ZUCCHINI
SPINACH
KALE
BRUSSELS SPROUTS
CELERY
CUCUMBER

prevents fat burning and stores any surplus in fat cells, your body hangs onto those extra calories in the form of fat, he adds.

But weight gain isn't the only downside of consuming refined carbs. There is growing evidence that they increase inflammation throughout the body, which contributes to a host of illnesses, including cardiovascular disease, cancer, Alzheimer's and diabetes. Eating low-carb, on the other hand, helps lower inflammation. A study in *Annals of Medicine* compared a low-carbohydrate diet to a low-fat one for six months and found that inflammation was significantly reduced in the low-carb group—but not among the low-fat contingent.

Yet another drawback to simple carbs is that they are, as your mom used to say about candy and soft drinks, empty calories. "Carbohydrates like breads or cookies are highly processed, and are stripped of nutrients," notes Kendra Whitmire, a nutritionist and dietitian in Laguna Beach, California. So while they have plenty of calories—they're energy-dense—they aren't nutrient-dense. "A whole food that's largely carbs, though, like kale or cauliflower, still has all its vitamins, minerals, antioxidants and flavonoids—all the good nutrients in plant foods. So a hundred calories of white bread is not the same as a hundred calories of cauliflower rice," says Whitmire. One causes a quick energy spike and drop before getting stored as fat, and the other brings all kinds of healthy nutrients and fiber to the table, releasing its fuel more slowly into your system as your body breaks it down. Your blood glucose remains more stable, so you don't need to release a flood of insulin.

The "Good" Carbs

A healthy keto diet aims not only to limit carbs in general to induce ketosis, making your body burn fat instead of glucose, but also to maximize the bang for your buck that you get from the nutrient-dense carbs you *do* eat. So first, always opt for whole foods over processed ones, shopping in the produce section rather than the packaged-foods aisle. But even within the universe of carb-based whole fruits and vegetables, there are optimum choices.

"Here's a good rule," says Eenfeldt. "Vegetables growing above ground are usually low in carbs and can be eaten freely. Those growing below ground though, are higher in carbs, so be more careful with them on a low-carb or keto diet." Root vegetables, like potatoes, beets and carrots, are examples of relatively high-carb whole foods. Leafy greens, cabbage, zucchini and broccoli, which grow above ground, are a few of the many satisfying veggies that are very low in carbs and high in nutrients, vitamins and antioxidants. Other good choices are veggies with a high water content, says Whitmire, like cucumbers, celery and lettuce, all of which are 90 percent water. They're filling and very low-carb, and they can help replenish the water you may be losing on a keto diet (which can cause dehydration and constipation).

Fruits are a different story, because most are high in natural sugar. "Fruit is nature's candy," says Eenfeldt. "On a low-carb or keto diet, you'll have to be careful with it, because the carbs can quickly add up. If you want a taste of fruit, your best choice is berries, like raspberries and blackberries." Those have three or four net carbs per half-cup, compared to 21 in a medium apple and 24 in a banana. These foods have always been in our diet, of course, but not in the amounts on offer today. "For most of human history, fruit was available only for a limited time each year, in season," Eenfeldt explains. Now, you can eat a banana from the tropics anytime, which can add up to a lot of sugar. The flip side is that you can pick up bell peppers or asparagus from across the globe all year long and pair those veggies with fish or steak for a keto dinner.

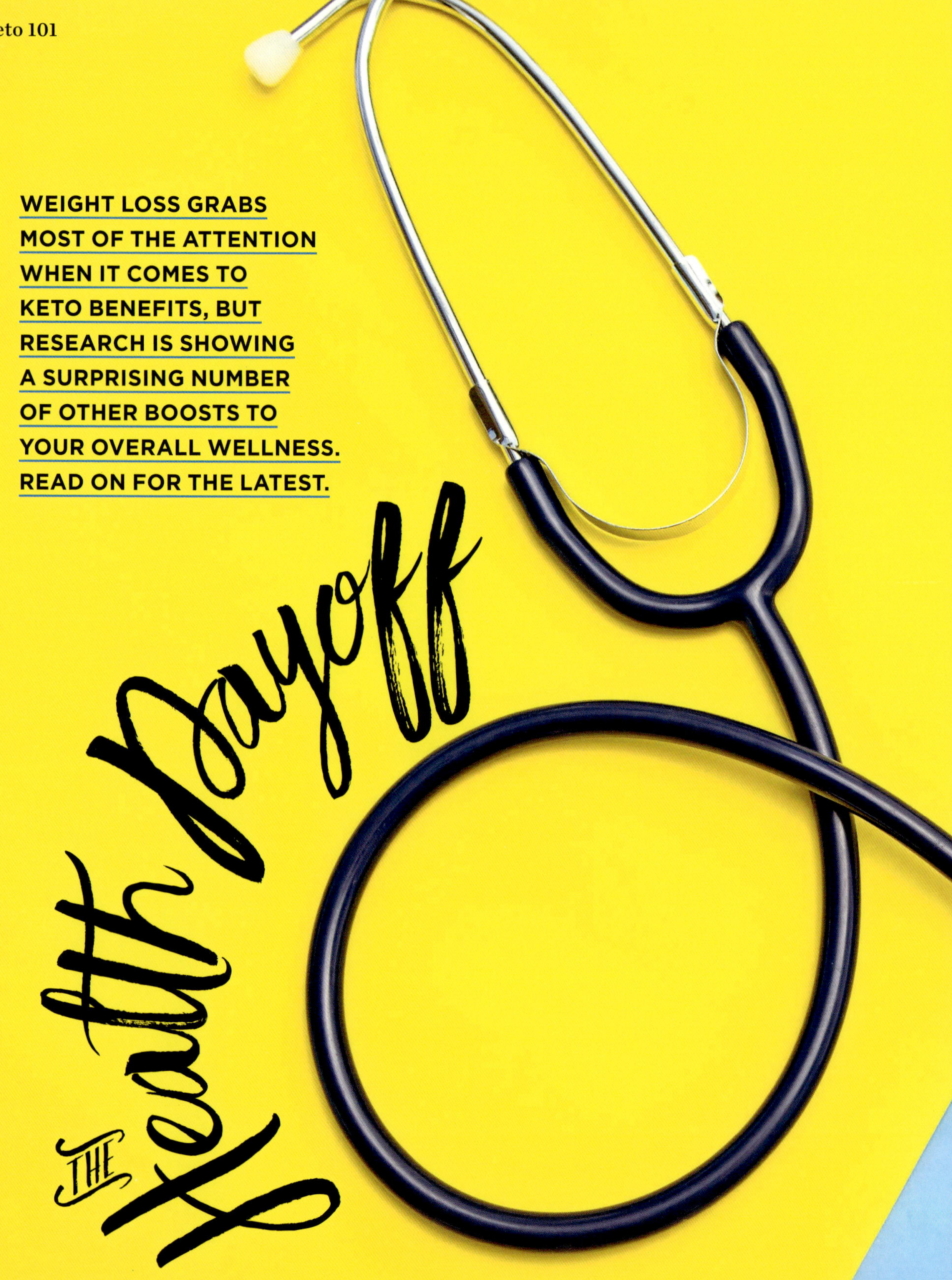

The Health Payoff

WEIGHT LOSS GRABS MOST OF THE ATTENTION WHEN IT COMES TO KETO BENEFITS, BUT RESEARCH IS SHOWING A SURPRISING NUMBER OF OTHER BOOSTS TO YOUR OVERALL WELLNESS. READ ON FOR THE LATEST.

KETO BRAGS AND "BEFORE/AFTER" photos on Instagram tend to focus on the diet's most visible effect: It helps most people lose weight, usually without feeling hungry or deprived. The Harvard T.H. Chan School of Public Health has posited several mechanisms for the weight loss, including the satiating effect of consuming so much fat; a decrease in appetite-stimulating hormones, like insulin and ghrelin; and a faster metabolism from the work of breaking down fats into a fuel source. That's beginning to look like the tip of the iceberg though, as doctors and researchers sit up and take notice of the other ways a ketogenic lifestyle may promote health. So far, evidence is pointing to keto's impact on the following issues and ailments.

HIGH BLOOD PRESSURE? BAD CHOLESTEROL NUMBERS? DISCOVER THE INTERNAL, LESS-VISIBLE REASONS FOR TRYING KETO.

Metabolic Syndrome and Type 2 Diabetes

Both of these related conditions have been surging in the U.S., and they appear to be countered by keto. Metabolic syndrome, or MetS, is a cluster of symptoms, including abdominal fat, high blood pressure, high cholesterol, and insulin resistance or high blood sugar. It is considered a precursor to type 2 diabetes and also increases your risk of heart disease and stroke. A growing number of studies have shown that keto can have a profound effect on both MetS and diabetes by replacing glucose with ketones as a fuel source. As a result, insulin release slows and blood sugar levels normalize.

A study in 2017 found that people with MetS who were put on a ketogenic diet for 10 weeks experienced significant weight loss and an improvement in their body-fat percentage and blood sugar numbers. When it comes to diabetes, a recent study showed that when adults with diabetes reduced their carb intake from 250 to 100 grams per day, they lost weight and their blood sugar levels stabilized. "The data in this area is pretty good," says Ethan Weiss, MD, a cardiologist at the University of California, San Francisco. "They've had success treating type 2 diabetes with keto, and often, people get so much better, they can stop taking their diabetes meds."

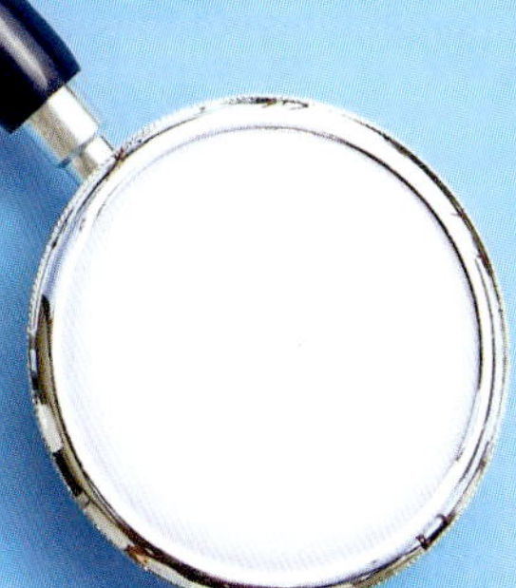

Heart Disease

While the cause-and-effect line from keto to cardiovascular health has not been definitively shown by long-term human studies, there's a wealth of evidence that keto can improve many risk factors for heart disease. "Researchers have looked at 30 different markers for heart risk, and except for a slight uptick in LDL cholesterol in some people, all of them went in the right direction," says Weiss. "That includes glucose blood levels, triglycerides, blood pressure and HDL cholesterol. It can be hard to tell whether some of those results are simply from the weight loss, but from my perspective as a cardiologist, if people drop extra weight and improve so many other factors—well, at the very least, it's neutral." And if your risk factors are trending the right way, you're likely to be lowering your chance of cardiovascular disease.

Cognitive Health

The brain is the fattiest organ, comprised of 60 percent fat. And studies have suggested that a high-fat keto diet offers neuroprotective benefits. In fact, the earliest and strongest

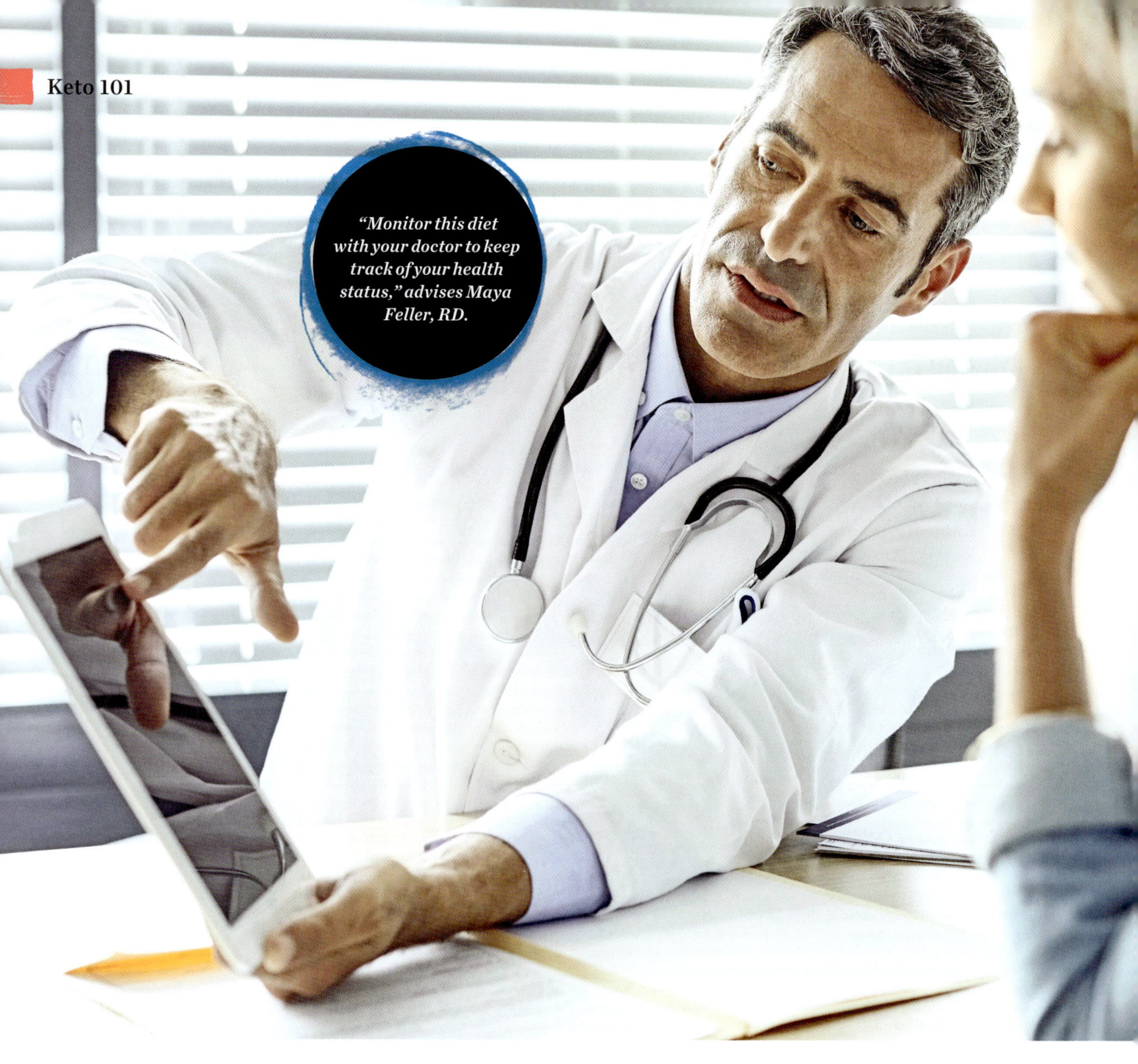

evidence in keto research emerged nearly a century ago, when it was found that a ketogenic diet reduced brain seizures in children with epilepsy. More recently, a study in the journal *Neurobiology of Aging* showed that older adults with mild cognitive impairment who were put on a keto diet experienced better memory function after just six weeks. (As a bonus, the subjects also showed reductions in weight, waist circumference, glucose and insulin, all of which are health-promoting.) Some researchers have surmised that ketones may be a more efficient and "clean-burning" fuel than glucose, providing more energy per unit of oxygen used.

"A ketogenic diet increases the number of mitochondria, the so-called 'energy factories' in brain cells," says Shelly Fan, PhD, a neuroscientist and the author of the book *Will AI Replace Us?* A recent study in rats on a keto diet showed genetic changes in their brains that prompted an increase in energy metabolism in the hippocampus—the part of the brain that's key to learning and memory. Another study, from the University

ONE FACTOR THAT MAY EXPLAIN KETO'S OTHER BENEFITS: LOWERED INFLAMMATION.

of California at San Francisco, also using rats, showed that a ketogenic diet reduced inflammation in the brain (inflammation can cause damage to neural circuits and increase your risk of dementia).

Yet another connection between keto and brain health: Researchers know that diabetes increases your chance of getting Alzheimer's, the most common form of dementia. But they've now begun to talk about another form of diabetes: type 3 diabetes, which is strongly associated with Alzheimer's disease. So if keto improves your glucose profile and reduces your chances of diabetes, it may be protecting your brain as well.

Cancer

The research about keto having an impact on cancer is in its early days—but it is intriguing. The new class of cancer drugs often leads to high levels of blood sugar, and according to a new study in mice, a ketogenic diet counteracts that effect and makes the therapy more effective. Another study in mice with malignant gliomas found that the animals who underwent radiation while they were being fed a keto diet lived much longer, most of them with no signs of tumor recurrence, compared to mice receiving radiation on a standard diet.

"Now they're lining up studies in humans, to see whether keto enhances chemotherapy," says Weiss. "There's really zero evidence in humans yet that keto itself is protective against cancer, but there's a lot of excitement about the mouse studies." Says nutritionist Maya Feller, MS, RD, CDN: "There's a lot of anecdotal evidence around people having a cancer diagnosis and then following a ketogenic diet. If I had a patient diagnosed with active malignancy, I wouldn't just give a blanket 'Do it'—it depends partly on where you are in your treatment. It's something to talk to your doctor about."

Polycystic Ovarian Syndrome (PCOS)

The evidence about keto and PCOS is also preliminary but promising. PCOS is an endocrine disorder that causes enlarged ovaries with cysts. It has been shown that a high-carb diet can negatively affect women with PCOS and that the condition can put them at risk for diabetes and obesity. A small pilot study found that overweight women with PCOS who limited their carb intake to less than 20 grams a day for six months showed reductions in weight and insulin as well as in levels of the hormones testosterone, LH and FSH, which may be factors in PCOS.

Experts agree that more research is needed, but some doctors now suggest keto to their patients as an adjunct therapy—partly because the diet helps with inflammation and insulin resistance, both of which play a large role in PCOS.

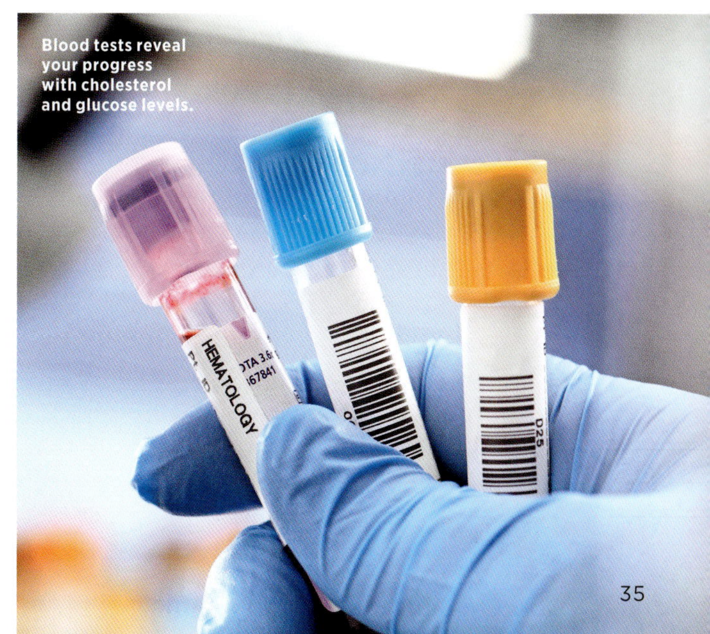

Blood tests reveal your progress with cholesterol and glucose levels.

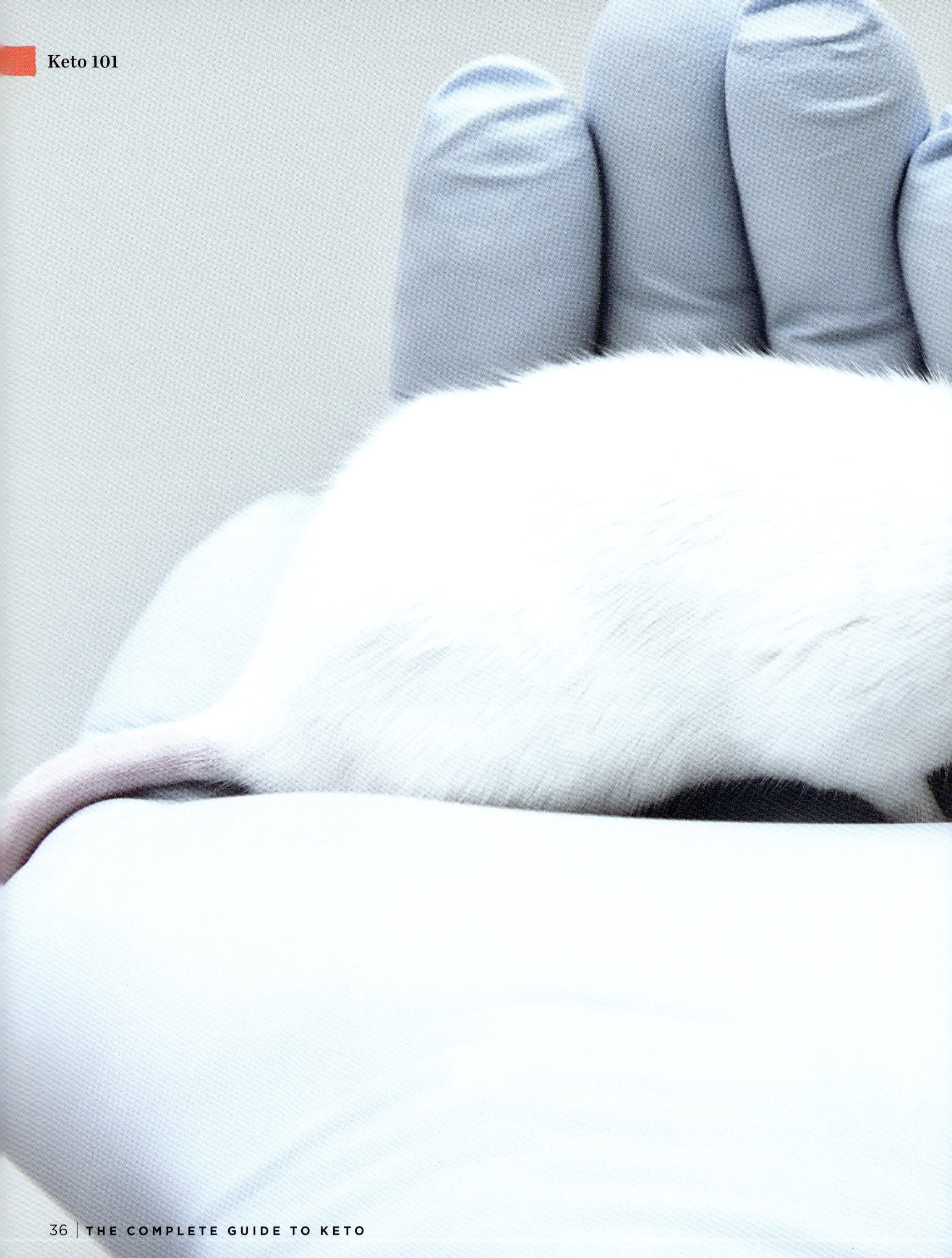

Of Mice and Men

Much—though not all—of the keto research thus far has been conducted in mice and rats. Does this mean we can apply those results to humans? Not exactly—or, at least, not yet. The results are suggestive rather than conclusive, says Ethan Weiss, MD. "Rodents are great tools for understanding biological pathways or unraveling single genes or molecules," he explains. "We've learned a lot from mouse models." Rodents are the most commonly tested animals for several reasons: They're easy to raise and control, and their genetic, biological and behavioral qualities closely resemble those of humans. Also, many symptoms of human conditions can be replicated in rodents, plus we've learned how to breed genetically altered mice that carry genes similar to those implicated in human ailments—giving us a jump start on studying a particular disease.

That being said, the resemblance only goes so far. "We've probably cured cancer 1,000 times in mice," says Weiss. "You can't automatically make the leap that any given therapy will be as effective in humans. But many studies done in mice have guided us to human trials. For instance, the appetite hormone leptin was first discovered in mice who became super obese from a spontaneous mutation, and it has become an important area for research in humans."

So those rodents? Be grateful to them for doing so much for science, but don't change the way you live because of one or two studies in mice, experts advise. Instead, look at that research as hope and inspiration for the human trials to follow.

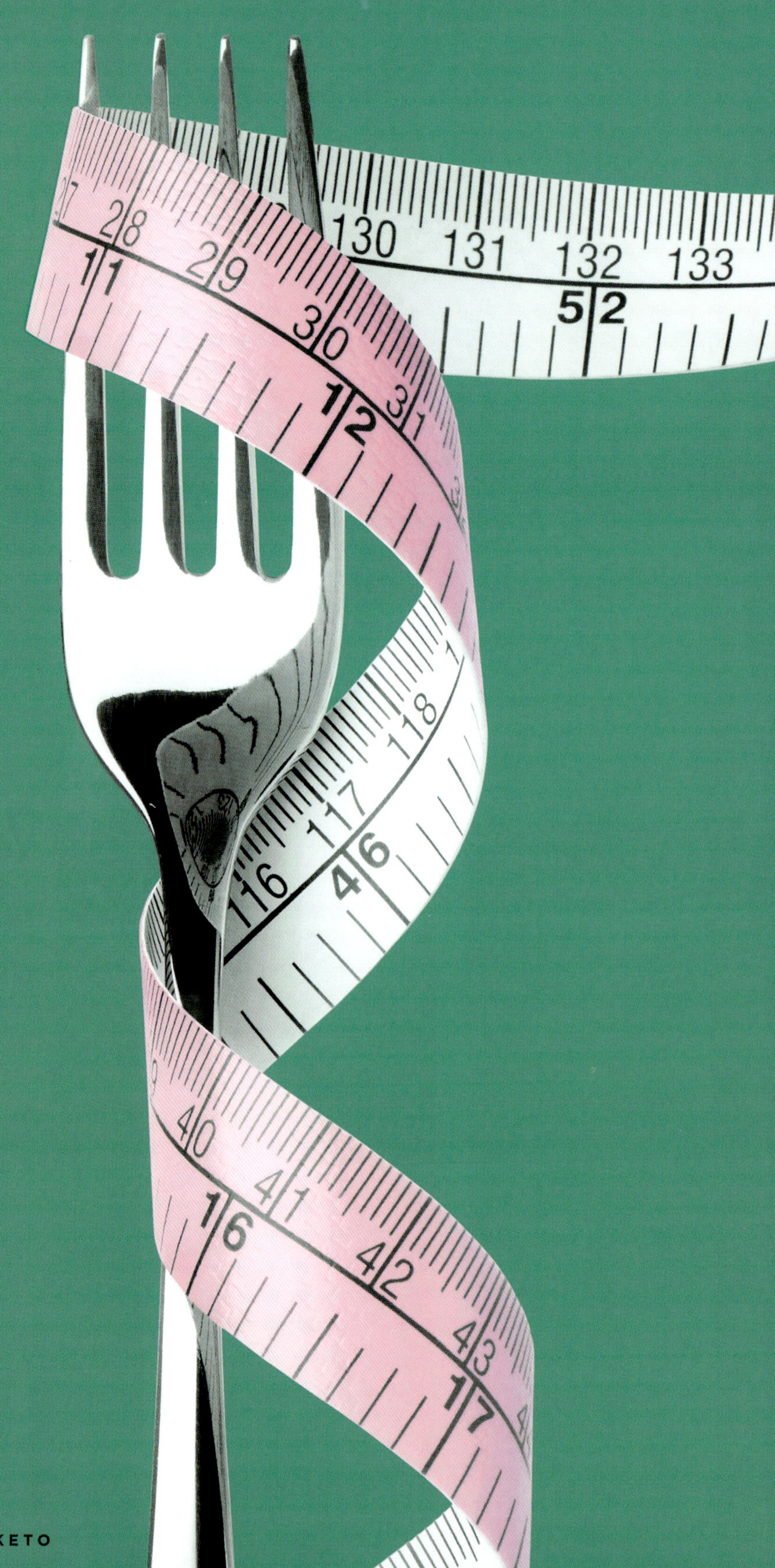
28
29
30
31
11
12
130
131
132
133
52
118
117
116
46
40
41
42
43
16
17

YOUR Body on Ketosis

ZOOM IN TO SEE THE CHANGES THAT KETO MAKES TO YOUR ENTIRE SYSTEM, FROM HEAD TO TOE.

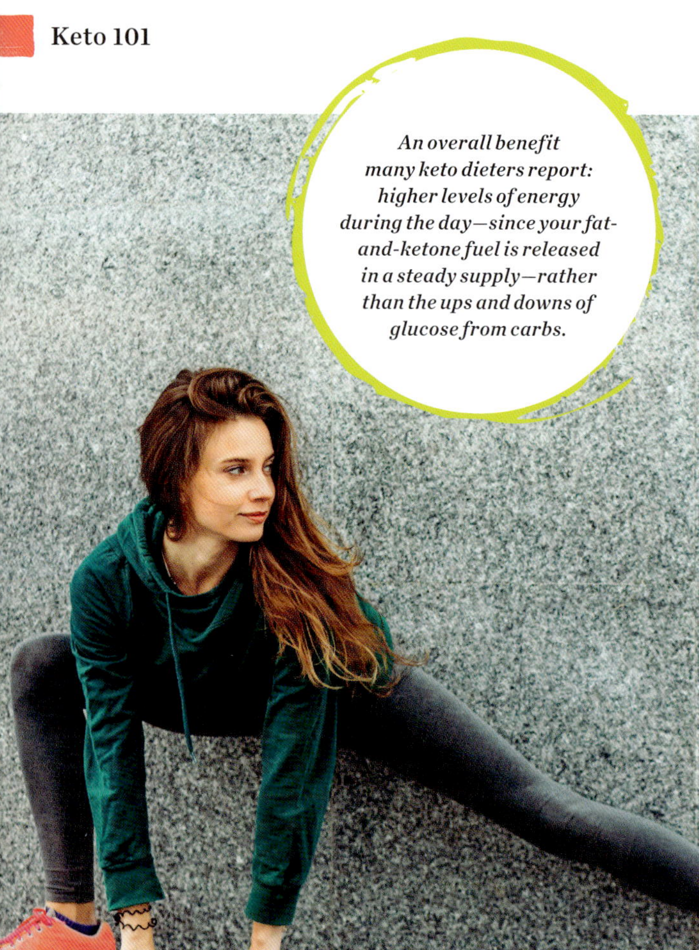

An overall benefit many keto dieters report: higher levels of energy during the day—since your fat-and-ketone fuel is released in a steady supply—rather than the ups and downs of glucose from carbs.

OF ALL THE WAYS THAT KETO CAN ALTER your anatomy, there's only one that's easy to see: weight loss. But under your skin, within your organs and bloodstream, research is showing that keto may transform how your body functions.

To be clear: The scientific research has yet to catch up to all the glowing reports from keto fans. Ethan Weiss, MD, associate professor at the Cardiovascular Research Institute at the University of California San Francisco, says he has been doing keto for a year and feels "terrific." He has lost weight, his borderline prediabetes is gone, and he feels a new kind of mental clarity. "And I'm skiing like I'm 25 years old again," Weiss adds. "It's like night and day. I haven't felt this way in ages." But, he concedes, a lot of the "softer claims" about keto—for instance cognitive boosts, or less joint pain—are anecdotal, rather than rigorously studied.

"A long-term ketogenic diet does not seem to be associated with significant side effects," says neuroscientist Shelly Fan, PhD. But she cautions that there are few long-term studies that have monitored all the possible side effects. "While it's too early to say that the diet is completely safe for everyone," for most people the risks seem minimal, and the benefits may be substantial.

Tracking Ketosis

How can you tell if you're getting to the promised land of ketosis? You have three choices:

KETO STICKS

Widely available, inexpensive and noninvasive, these test for ketones in urine. But it's a rough estimate—and they get less accurate as your body learns to use more ketones than it excretes.

FINGER PRICKS

The most accurate reading—but also expensive and invasive. You prick your finger and test a drop of blood to measure the major ketones.

BREATH ANALYZERS

The newest entry...and the costs end once you buy the device. Quick and easy, these measure ketones excreted in breath; but it's not yet known how accurate they are.

WHY THE WEIGHT LOSS?

Numerous studies have shown that many people drop pounds on keto—and also do better at keeping them off over time. Here's what we know, so far, about why.

Satiation

Studies have shown that people feel more satisfied on high-fat diets, and over more hours, so it takes them longer to feel hungry again. One study found that overweight adults with type 2 diabetes consumed one-third fewer calories when eating from a low-carb high-fat buffet than when eating from a standard buffet; they also said they felt more satiated. That may be due to slower "gastric emptying" when digesting fats: They stay in your stomach longer than carbs, dampening hunger.

Appetite Hormones

Several hormones, including ghrelin and insulin, work to stimulate appetite, and both hormones decrease on a keto diet. Insulin is released from the pancreas when you eat carbs to control blood sugar, so in the absence of carbs, you put out less. Ghrelin is released largely from the gut; it's called the "hunger hormone," because it is directly related to appetite. A study in *Nature* found less ghrelin (and lower appetite) in people who lost weight on keto—even though people who lose substantial weight usually have more ghrelin. The increase may be why many people who lose weight on a low-fat diet end up gaining it back.

Ketone Bodies

Ketones may also have a hunger-reducing effect. A 2017 study in *Obesity* gave people either a "ketone ester" drink or a glucose drink; those drinking ketones had less physical hunger and a reduced desire to eat. The key, again, may be ghrelin: The ketone drinkers had lower levels of it for hours afterward.

Metabolism

There may be a metabolic "boost" from keto, because eating fewer carbs makes your body work harder to turn fat into ketone fuel. It's the opposite for most low-fat dieters, who show a drop in metabolism, thus leading to regain. A higher metabolism means more calorie-burning, even at rest.

Fat Burning

On keto, your body has to dive into fat stores to get energy. Also, insulin stores fat, so when levels decrease on keto, your fat stores become accessible and your body starts firing up its fat-burning furnace.

The Inside Story

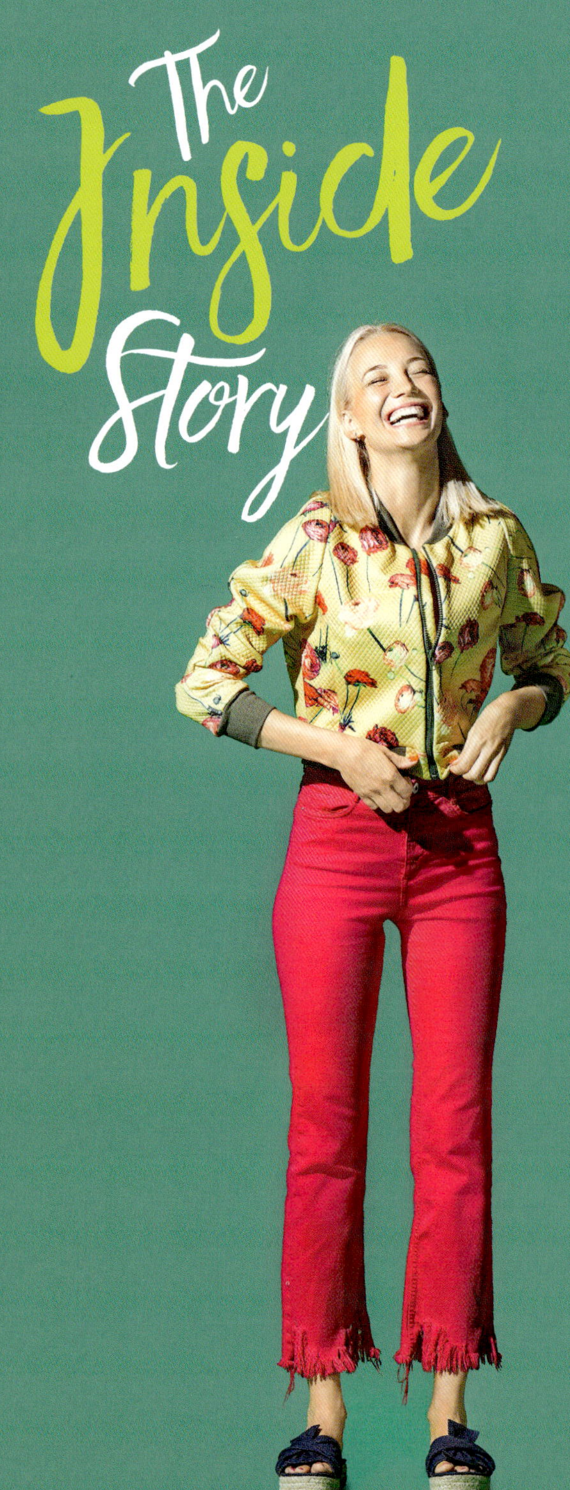

Abdominal Fat

Not only does keto encourage overall weight loss, but a study in the journal *Endocrine* found that the diet seems to target inflammatory visceral (belly) fat in particular. That isn't just a cosmetic issue: Belly fat is considered a risk factor for all kinds of conditions, including cardiovascular disease and cancer, because it wraps around key organs and leaks toxins into them.

Liver

This organ is where the action is with ketosis: Fatty acids are stored in the liver, and when your body runs out of glucose energy on the keto diet, your liver starts converting stored fat into ketone bodies. One ketone in particular, beta-hydroxybutyric acid, has been found to be key to cell signaling (the way cells communicate) and may play a key role in treating metabolic diseases, including type 2 diabetes.

Colon

You may have some adjustment issues here when you first go keto. Some people have either constipation or diarrhea in the first few weeks, due to changing over from high-carb to high-fat eating. For many people, that means a lack of fiber or changes in the gut microbiome, the intestinal bacteria that aid in many processes, including digestion. Drinking lots of water and eating leafy greens can help.

Muscles

Your muscles store carbs as glycogen, but once they run through their stores on keto, they can start burning body fat as fuel. Another benefit of keto compared to other diets is that it may help preserve lean body mass (aka muscle tissue) during weight loss, according to an article in the journal *Nutrition & Metabolism*. The benefit is twofold: You're burning fat rather than muscle—and the more muscle tissue you have, the stronger your metabolism becomes, because muscle takes more energy to "feed" than fat does.

Heart

Virtually every study looking at weight loss on keto finds improvements in numerous health indicators tied to cardiovascular disease. "While no one has done a 'hard outcome' trial looking at the rates of heart attack and keto, we've had studies that looked at 30 different markers for heart risk," says Ethan Weiss, MD. "Except for a slight uptick in LDL in some people, every other marker went in the right direction—blood glucose, HDL cholesterol, triglycerides, blood pressure and many more."

Pancreas

The pancreas is a key part of the digestive and endocrine systems: It regulates blood sugar by secreting hormones, including insulin, when you eat carbs. So when you cut carbs, the pancreas doesn't need to make as much insulin. That may help people with insulin resistance, in which your body gets "worn out" by insulin spikes and stops responding to the hormone's signals, resulting in rising blood sugar and potential diabetes.

Ovaries

There is preliminary evidence that keto may help women with polycystic ovarian syndrome (PCOS), an endocrine disorder that causes enlarged ovaries with cysts, often leading to infertility. PCOS is associated with obesity and insulin resistance, both of which can improve on keto. A pilot study followed women who ate 20 grams or less of carbs per day for six months and found significant weight loss and improved hormonal status. Two of the women even became pregnant after having previously been infertile.

Joints

Inflammation is behind the joint pain and swelling that can come from chronic conditions like rheumatoid arthritis or bursitis, and keto has been shown to lower systemic inflammation in all parts of the body. By contrast, high glucose levels in the blood from eating a high-carb diet increase inflammation.

Blood Pressure

Experts aren't sure whether the drop in blood pressure that occurs in many hypertensive people on keto is due to the weight loss itself or some other factor—but they all agree that a normalizing of blood pressure is a common benefit of keto. And since high blood pressure is a risk factor for many conditions, including cardiovascular disease, stroke, kidney damage and dementia,that's a win all around.

Brain

Your brain is 60 percent fat, but it can use only glucose or ketones for fuel (unlike muscles, which can burn fat directly). Some studies show that ketosis enhances memory in people with mild cognitive impairment, and researchers are looking at whether keto can protect against brain aging and neurodegenerative diseases, like Alzheimer's Studies in rodents show that keto diets reduce inflammation (a cause of neurodegeneration) and improve outcomes after brain injury.

Cancer Treatment

The evidence for a connection between keto and cancer treatment is preliminary but intriguing. Some studies have found that a ketogenic diet made chemotherapy and radiation more effective, possibly because it may reduce inflammation and edema around tumors. Another theory holds that glucose and insulin can drive tumor growth—and if you deprive cancer cells of their "food" by reducing both of those with a keto diet, you can weaken and "starve" cancer cells.

Four Degrees of Keto

KETO IS KETO, RIGHT? NOT EXACTLY. THERE'S A QUARTET OF CHOICES IN HOW YOU GO ABOUT IT. HERE'S THE TRICK TO FINDING THE RIGHT PLAN FOR YOU.

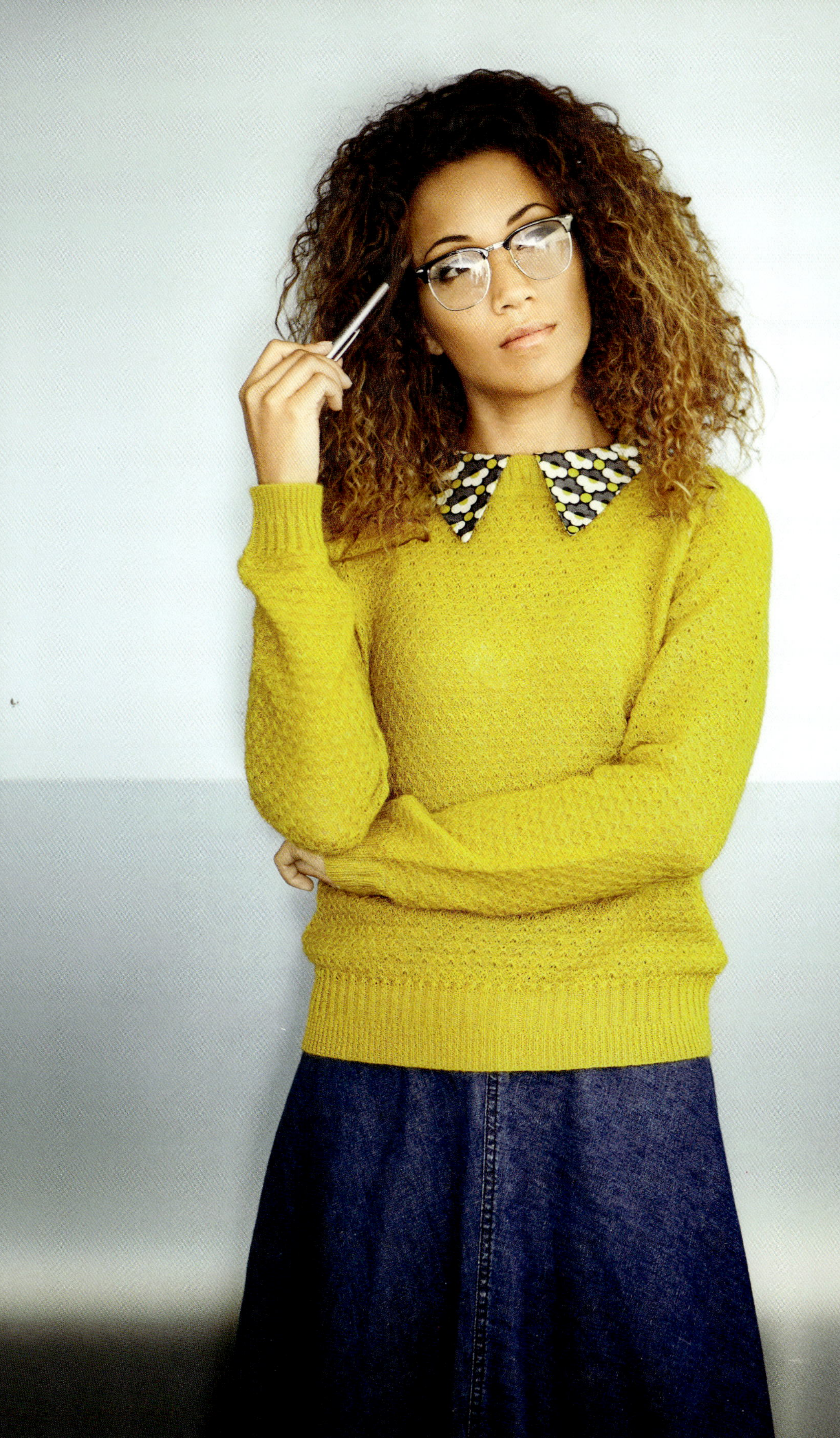

MANY PEOPLE TRYING A KETOGENIC diet have no problem upping their intake of butter, cream, meat and cheese. Letting go of not only processed and refined carbs (buh-bye, crackers!) but also starchy vegetables (see ya, baked potatoes and french fries) is often way more challenging. Not to mention that full-on keto relies heavily on cooking your own meals to ensure you're taking in the right kinds of fats and following a strict ban on carbs—but not everyone wants to, or is able to, spend that much time in the kitchen.

The good news is that there are several variations on keto that still confer benefits, including fat loss and metabolic results, but may be easier for some people to follow. The main distinction between these variations and standard keto, says Julie Upton, MS, RD, CSSD, is how steadily you stay in ketosis. "The traditional ketogenic diet aims to keep you in the metabolic state where you burn fat rather than carbs as your primary fuel source," she explains. "On a modified keto diet, in contrast, your body may go in and out of ketosis—but you still shed weight and body fat." Read on to discover your options.

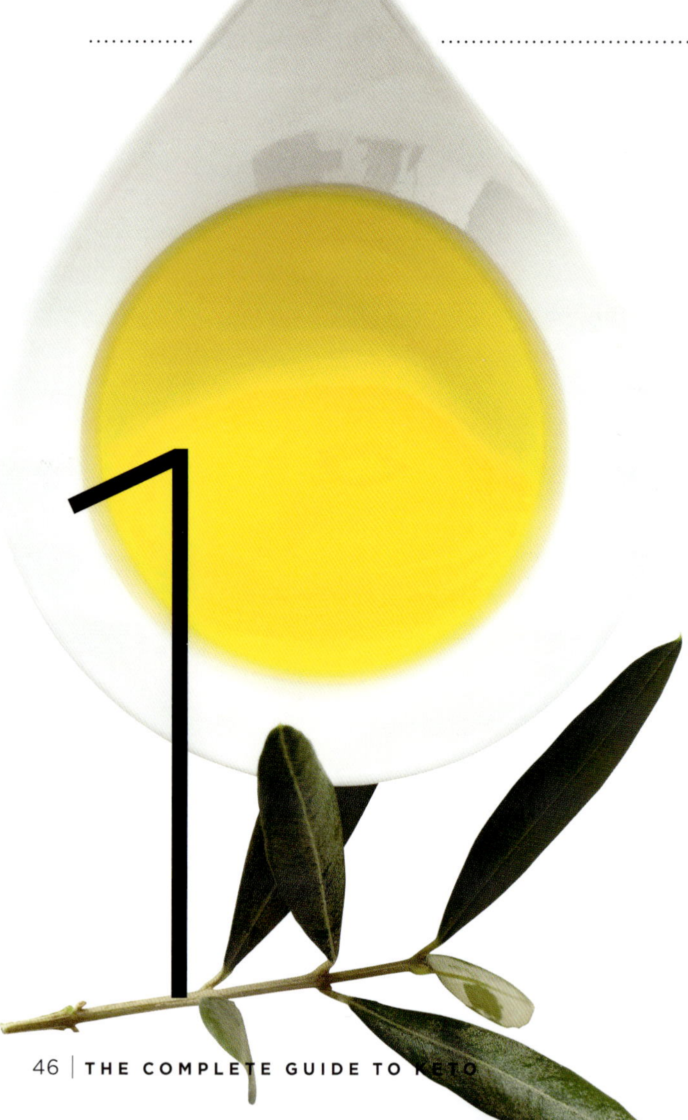

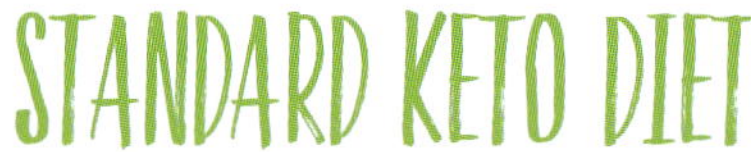

75% Fat, 15–20% Protein, 5–10% Carbs

The most demanding and strict of the four regimens, standard keto requires that you plan your meals around fats like avocados, butter, fatty fish and meats and olive oil. "You're aiming for about 150 grams of fat a day, which is probably around three times the amount of fat you were eating before," says Upton. Your protein intake is moderate, amounting to about 30 grams at each meal—about four ounces of meat, fish or poultry. The biggest change for most people, adds Upton, is carb intake, which goes from the average 300-plus grams a day that most Americans consume to 50 grams or less (the amount in one regular bagel or two bananas). On keto, most of the few carbs you take in will come from leafy greens and nonstarchy vegetables. This plan is quite a jolt to your system, and many people experience various side effects, such as digestive problems or "keto flu," in the first few days of following the diet.

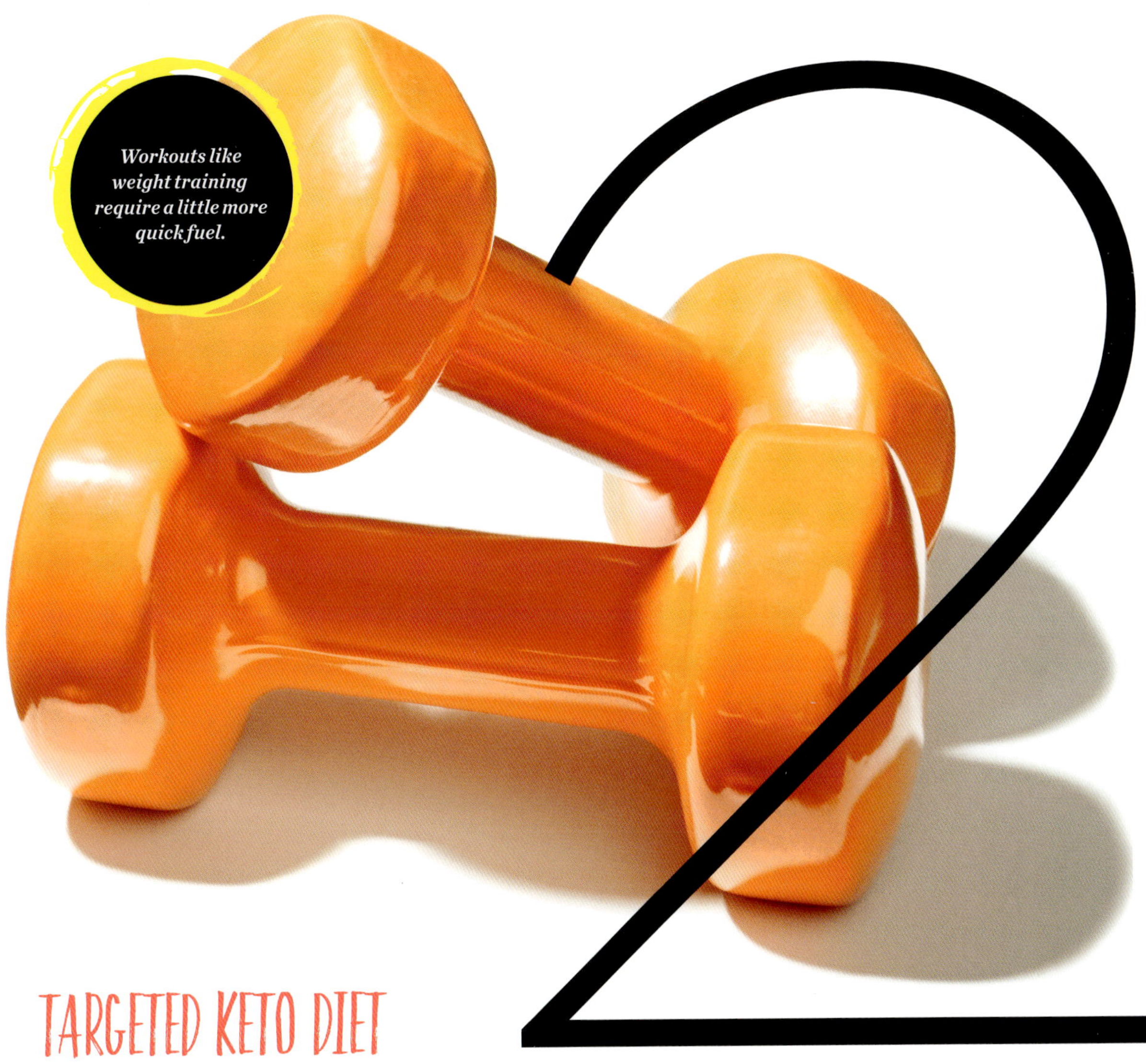

TARGETED KETO DIET

65–70% Fat, 20% Protein, 10–15% Carbs

Athletes or people who work out at high intensity can find themselves flagging while following standard keto. That's because when you're exercising at maximum effort, your muscles may run out of ketones and demand glycogen, which is a form of glucose stored for future use. Glycogen is usually your body's go-to fast fuel, but if your diet is very low-carb, you may be low on glycogen stores. The result: exhaustion rather than exhilaration during workouts.

That's why athletic folks may want to opt for the targeted keto plan, which ups the number of approved carbs. "Targeted keto allows athletes to have an additional 20 to 30 grams of carbs, bringing the daily total to between 70 and 80 grams," says Upton. "They should eat the extra carbs before, during and after exercise and then go back to keto for the rest of the day." Timing is key: The carbs you add in—preferably healthy options like fruit, dairy or whole-grain-based foods or sports-nutrition products—will get burned off by the exercise, so they won't be stored as body fat. And they allow you to work out harder, giving your muscles much-needed accessible fuel.

3

CYCLICAL KETO DIET

75% Fat, 15–20% Protein, 5–10% Carbs (On Keto Days); 25% Fat, 25% Protein, 50% Carbs (On Off Days)

Keto cycling is, for some, the best of both worlds. "A lot of people can't stay on keto every day, and need more flexibility," says Upton. When you cycle in and out of keto, rather than beating up on yourself if you cheat, you plan to go off in a measured way. "Say someone does three weeks on standard keto and plans for a few days off—knowing that the break is coming can power them through the keto phase," Upton says.

There's more than one way to cycle. Another approach is to spend five days of each week doing strict keto, followed by two non-keto days. You could, for instance, go keto during the workweek and take a break on the weekend, freeing you up to enjoy a non-keto meal or two out. But keep in mind two things. First, this isn't a pass to eat added sugars or processed foods; make sure the carbs you add are wholesome, like fruits, dairy, whole grains or sweet potato. Second, don't freak if you see temporary fluctuations on the scale. The added carbs may make your body hold on to more water, but once you're back on keto, that will quickly disappear. And you may have increased your odds of sticking with keto long-term by taking a break from the more strict protocol.

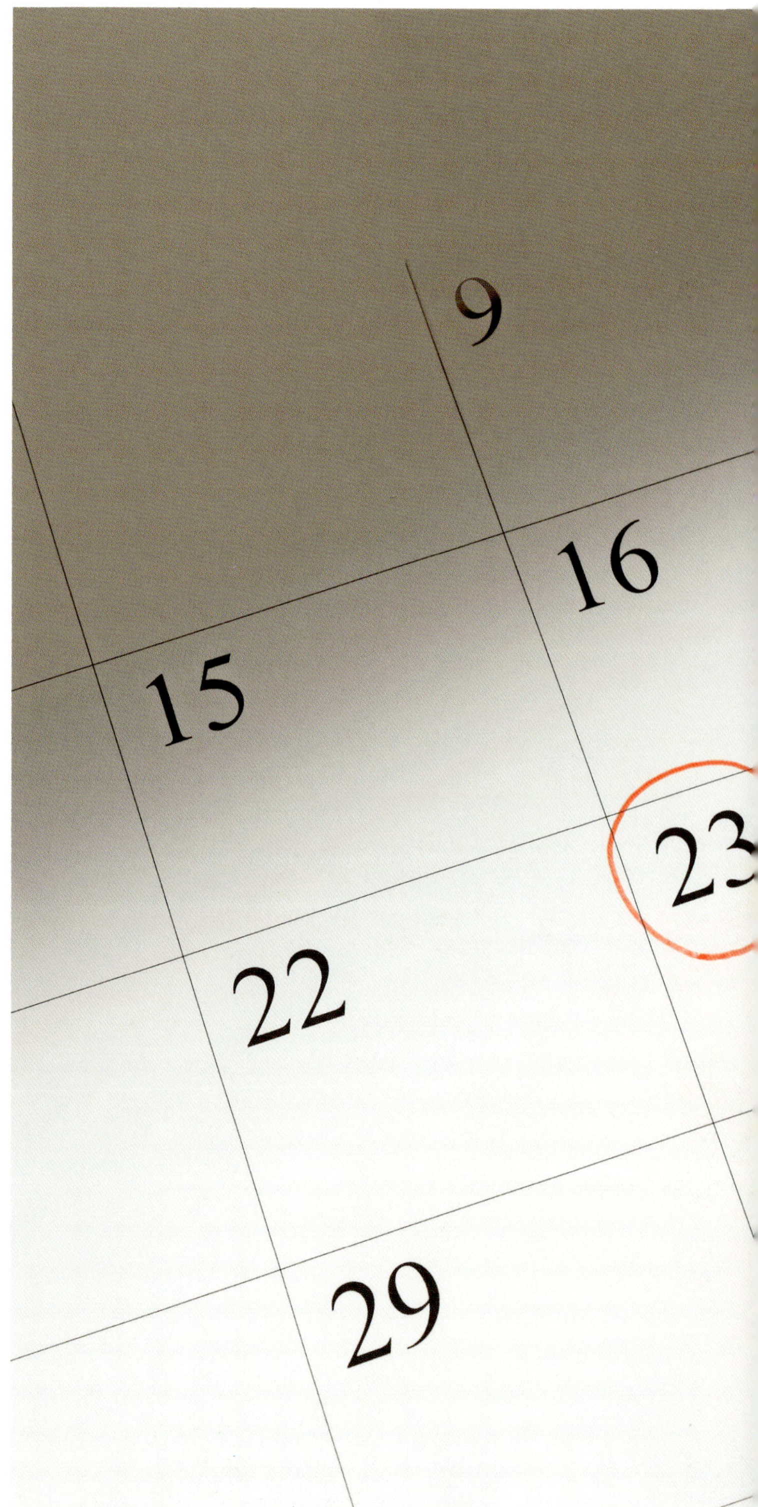

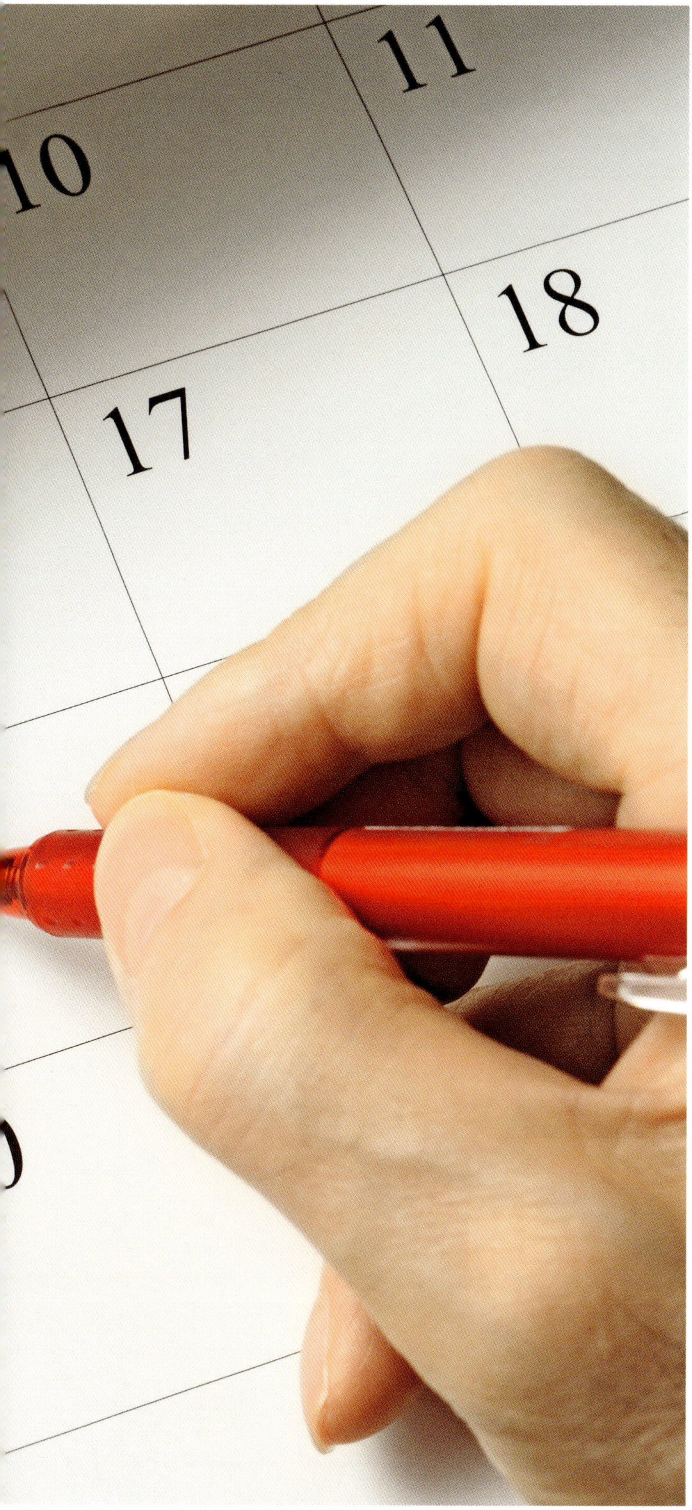

HIGH-PROTEIN KETO DIET

60–65% Fat, 30% Protein, 5–10% Carbs

This plan is an easy switch if you've already tried Paleo, making it a popular choice among people who have tried some form of low-carb diet before. And many high-fat foods are also fairly rich in protein, so high-protein keto is just a slight tweak of the standard plan. This diet boils down to eating about 120 grams of protein per day, or about four 4-ounce servings of meat, fish or poultry, and around 130 grams of fat. Those ratios can make it easier to plan meals, Upton points out, because it's a little closer to what most people are accustomed to putting on their plates.

Your carb level stays the same as on standard keto, so you are still likely to drop weight fairly quickly, says Upton. One key difference is that you may not always be in ketosis, because your body converts any excess protein into glucose for fuel. But because you're not increasing your consumption of carbs, you'll be able to continue to lose weight.

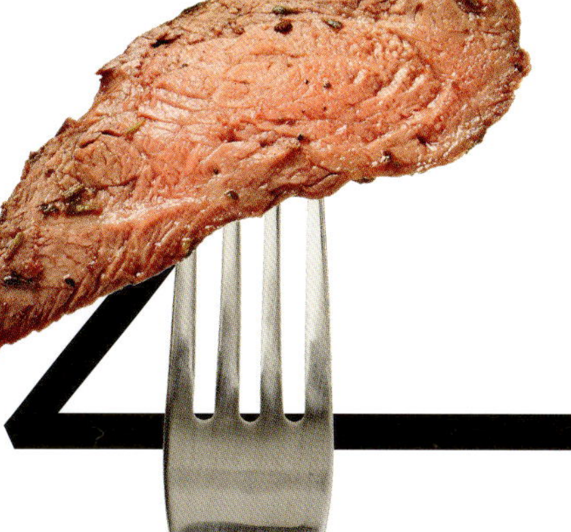

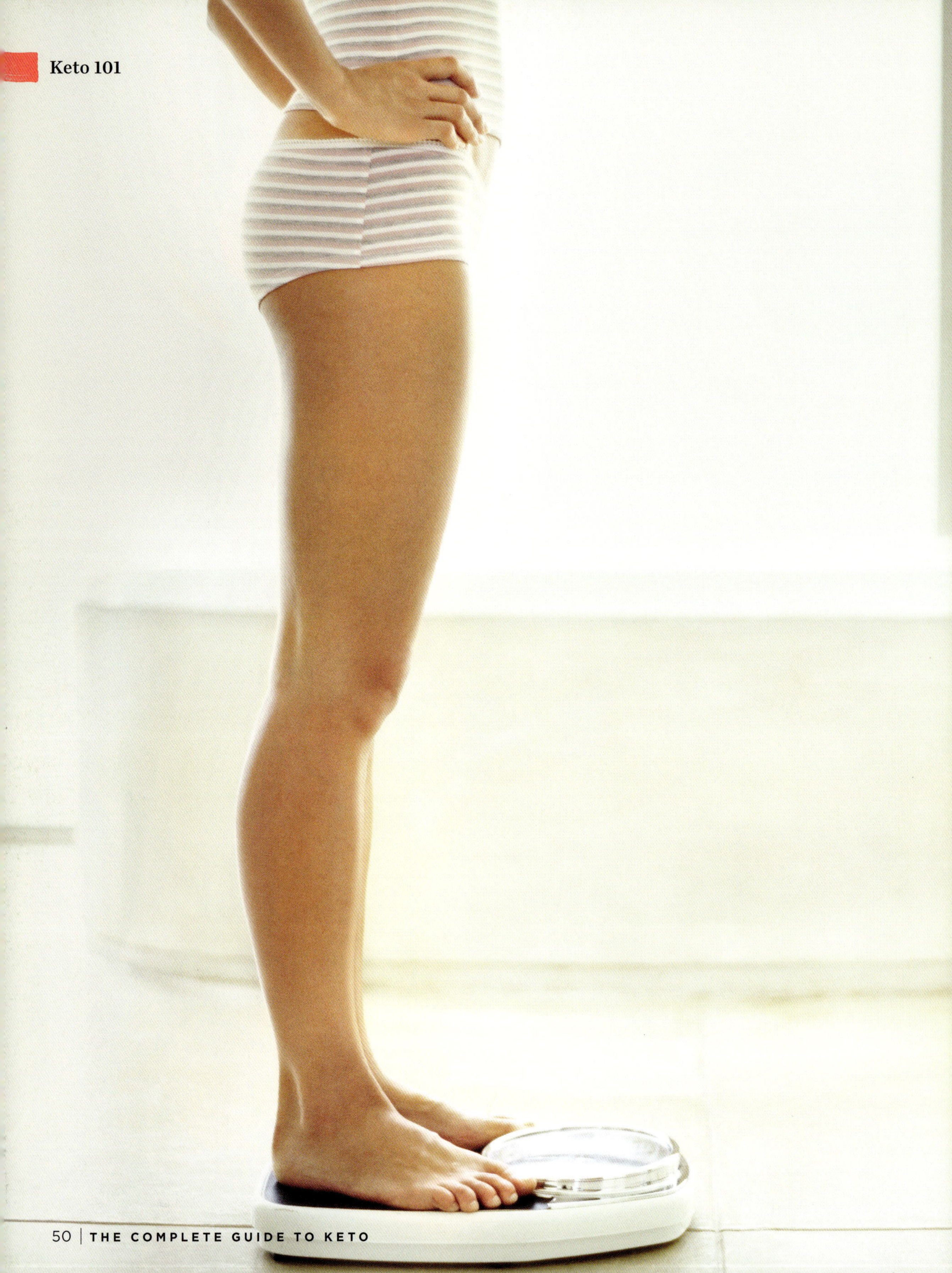

The Plateau Problem

"Plateaus always happen—period," says nutritionist Julie Upton. "As you lose weight, your metabolic rate declines, making it harder to keep losing weight." But the number on the scale isn't the only marker; there are times when you may stay the same weight for a few days or a week while the tape measure shows another story as you lose inches. If you're convinced you're on a true plateau, try these three strategies.

Start (or Resume) Counting

When you started on keto, you probably were careful to count up your total carbs for the day to make sure you were adhering to the plan. That tends to fall off as you settle into your keto lifestyle. If your body fights back, take another look at the carbs you might be taking in. "Carbs are sneaky," says Julia Sweet, a keto follower and contributor to the website Ketogasm. For instance, many food labels round nutrient amounts up or down. "All heavy cream has 0.4 grams of carbohydrate per tablespoon, but some brands round that up to 1 gram and others round down to zero," she says. "It adds up. There are also carbs in eggs—one large egg has 0.6 grams of carbs. So your breakfast, with cream in your coffee and three eggs, can easily bring you to 10 percent of your carb grams for the day—all while you're thinking you're eating carb-free." Another example: One ounce of cheddar cheese (which looks like a cube the size of four dice put together) also has 0.4 grams of carbs, and yet many keto guides say it has "zero" carbs. Cured meats and condiments, like hot sauce, are another source of hidden carbs, says Sweet.

Use Your Kitchen Scale

Another way you can kid yourself, says Sweet: eyeballing portions. "You may very well be taking in a lot more than you think," she says. "If you're picking the biggest strawberries and thinking you're gaming the system, it's time for a reality check—there really are more carbs in strawberries the size of your fist than in the ones half that size." Also, stop shaking a cup of sliced almonds until they settle into half their original volume. "Get a keto calculator," Sweet advises. "Then recalculate what you should be taking in, based on your new weight. If you're still eating for your old weight, you're overdoing it." A scale keeps you honest.

Amp Up Your Workouts

Especially strength training. At the beginning of eating keto, you may have felt a bit too keto flu-ish to work out a lot. But after a few weeks, you should be energetic enough to get back to the gym—and your focus should be on weightlifting. "The more muscle mass you build or maintain, the more you boost your metabolic rate, helping you combat the drop in metabolism that always comes with weight loss," says Upton.

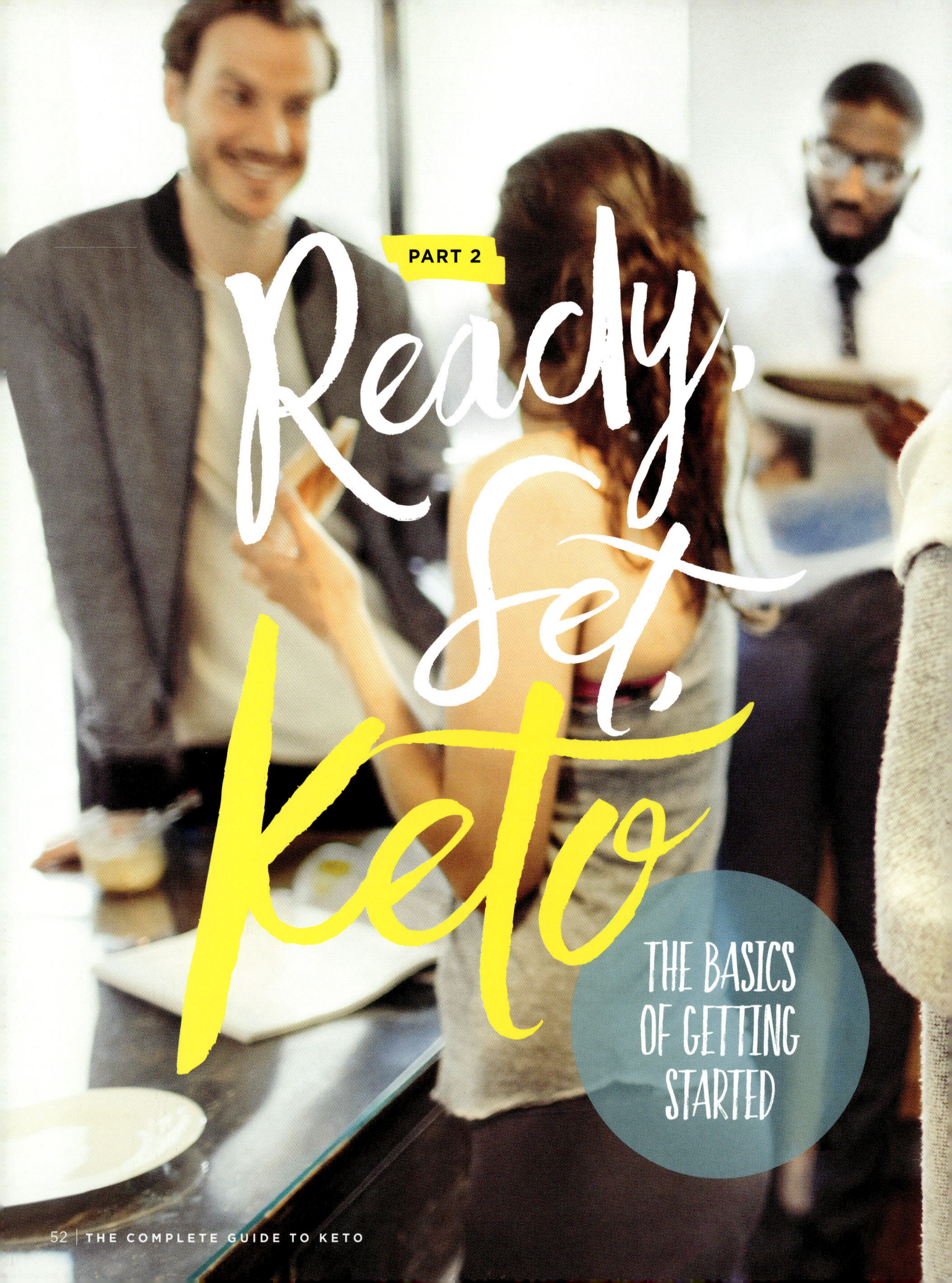

PART 2

Ready, Set, Keto

THE BASICS OF GETTING STARTED

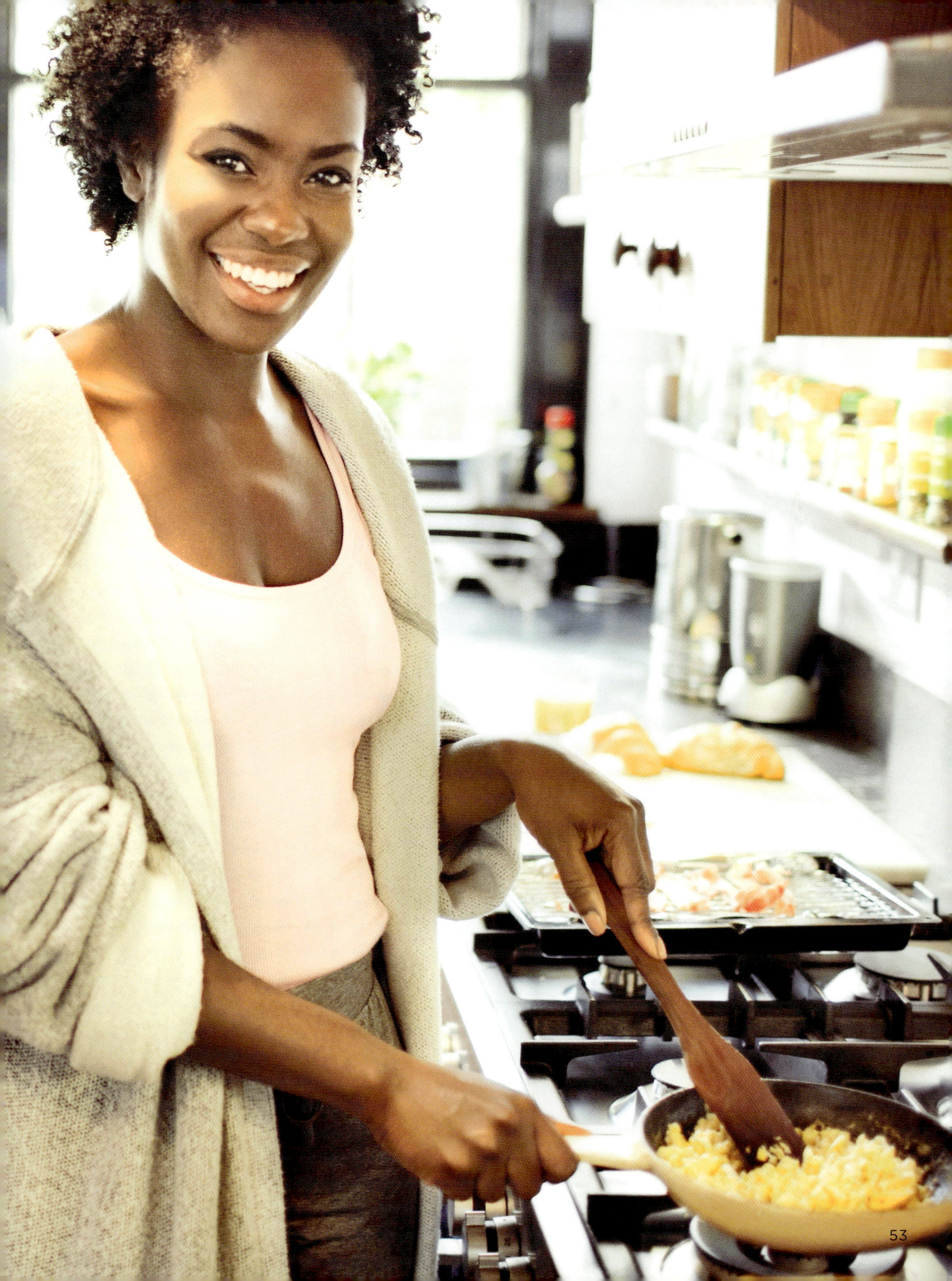

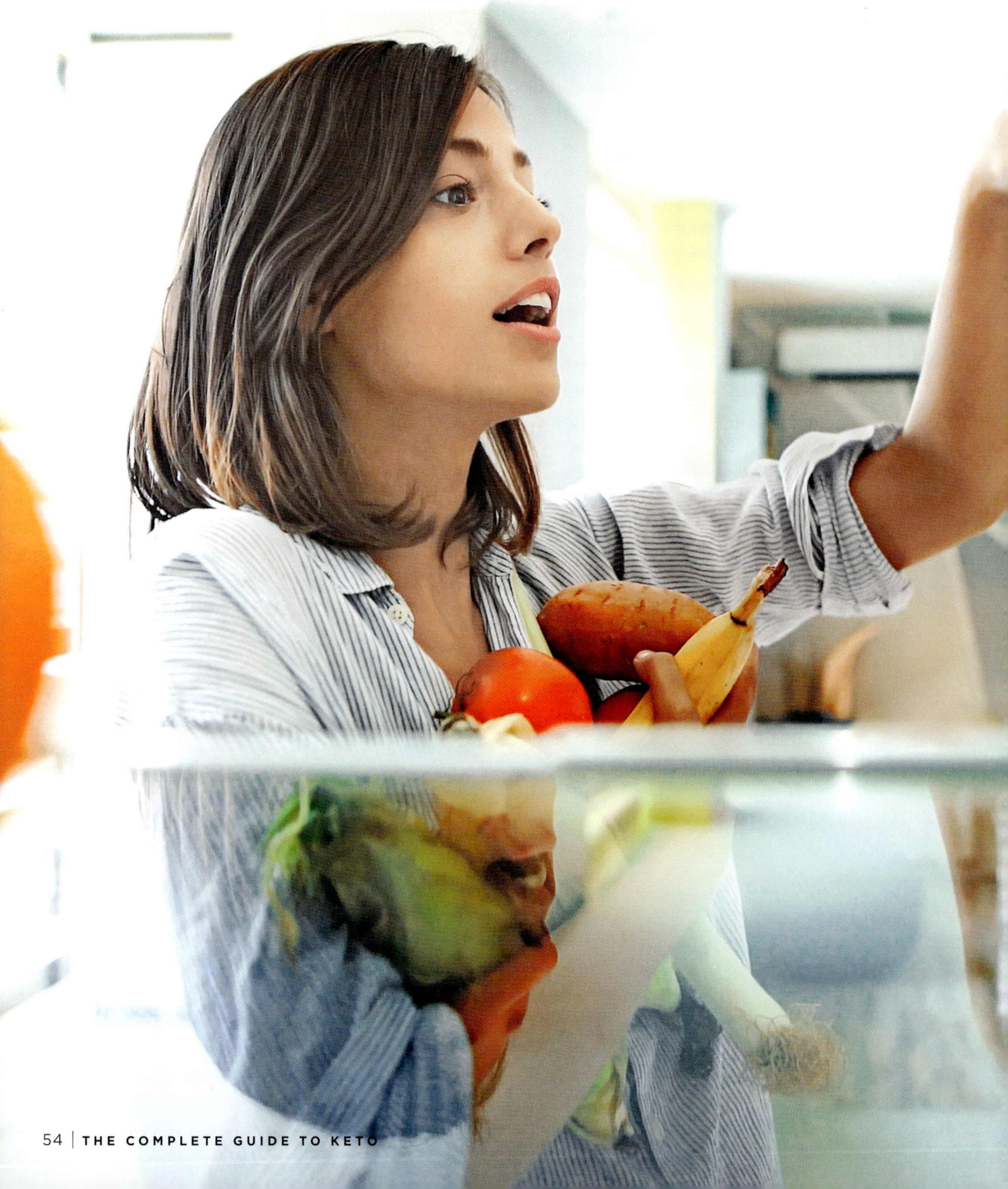

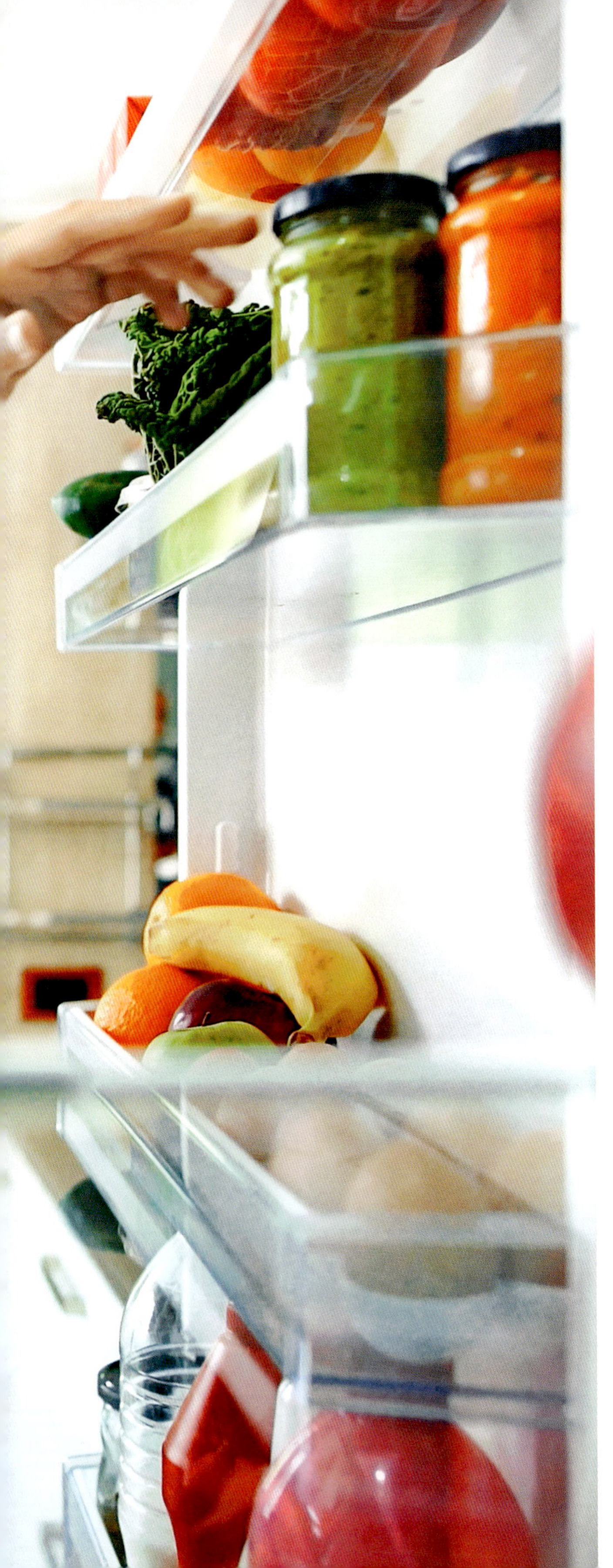

Before You Begin

WHEN YOU'RE READY TO GO KETO, PREPARATION CAN MAKE ALL THE DIFFERENCE! LAY THE NECESSARY GROUNDWORK TO BECOME A KETO WINNER.

NOW THAT YOU KNOW WHAT YOU'RE signing up for, it's time to take the plunge. Well...almost: Before you dive in, there's some essential preparation to be done to successfully kick off your diet makeover.

Think of this as an exotic trip (Thailand? Bali?). To get the most out of your journey, you research the country and make an itinerary of what you want to see. You plan what you need to bring, and go shopping for essentials. You pack and organize. And finally, you open your mind to all the wonderful things you'll experience.

Going keto works best with a similar plan. For most of us, a fat-driven weight-loss program is completely new territory, one that takes some getting to know. You'll need to understand the parameters and decide on your method; to get rid of inappropriate foods and buy new pantry staples; and to adopt a positive mind-set for the good things to come.

Here's a checklist to facilitate your keto countdown.

Cold Turkey or Gradual?

No two people do keto exactly the same—especially when starting the plan. One of the first decisions you'll need to make is whether to ease in or jump in. If you want the fastest results, you'll have to slash carbs drastically, down to 20 grams a day or less—and that sudden change in diet is often what triggers the so-called keto flu, a range of unpleasant symptoms from headaches to lethargy that fortunately dissipate over time. If you can tough it out, great. But if personal obligations or health concerns are an issue, it's also possible to taper off carbs, starting by limiting to 100 grams a day and cutting back slowly, while increasing fat intake. This usually staves off the side effects while slowly working toward ketosis. "I suggest starting at a pace that works for you," says certified nutrition counselor Naomi Whittel. "You might choose to eat keto in the morning but have a small serving of carbs with dinner. For some people, a gentle transition feels more comfortable than diving in all at once."

TAKE A "BEFORE" PICTURE AND WEIGH AND MEASURE YOURSELF. THESE MARKERS WILL MOTIVATE YOU AS TIME PROGRESSES.

Get Friends and Family on Board

Not everyone will "get" the keto concept at first. After all, we've been indoctrinated to avoid fat for 50-plus years, and many people—even some in the medical community—aren't up-to-date on the new science regarding healthy superfats. But experts say that social support is vital to reaching health goals, and it's best to share your aspirations, needs and plans when starting keto. Ideally, you'll convince a family member or friend to take the keto adventure with you. If not, broadcast your commitment. Consider writing down your reasons for going on the program, specifically: "I want more energy so we can have more fun together" or "I want less joint pain so we can travel again." Share this with your people and promise not to nag or fuss about what they choose to eat. They'll likely rally around you, once they see the value of your intentions.

Adopt a Positive Mind-Set

Visualize the new you, and make a pact to be kind to yourself. Whether you lose weight or not, you are about to make a healthy change and are moving toward a more empowering lifestyle. Doing nothing would make things worse. Remember, 0.2 pounds lost is 0.2 pounds less than the day before—and 50 days of 0.2 pounds adds up to 10 pounds lost! "When you think about how you want to behave in situations that have always broken your resolve in the past, you can create new go-to behaviors," trainer Bob Harper writes in *Skinny Habits: The 6 Secrets of Thin People*. "When you train your brain to go to a happier place instead of a negative and unproductive one, when you set up your environment to support your goals, you reach them."

Clean Out Your Pantry

"The spirit is willing, but the flesh is weak," the Bible cautions. But sometimes just removing temptation works as well as willpower. When there are no potato chips on hand, are you actually going to get dressed and go to the store when you're already in your pajamas watching

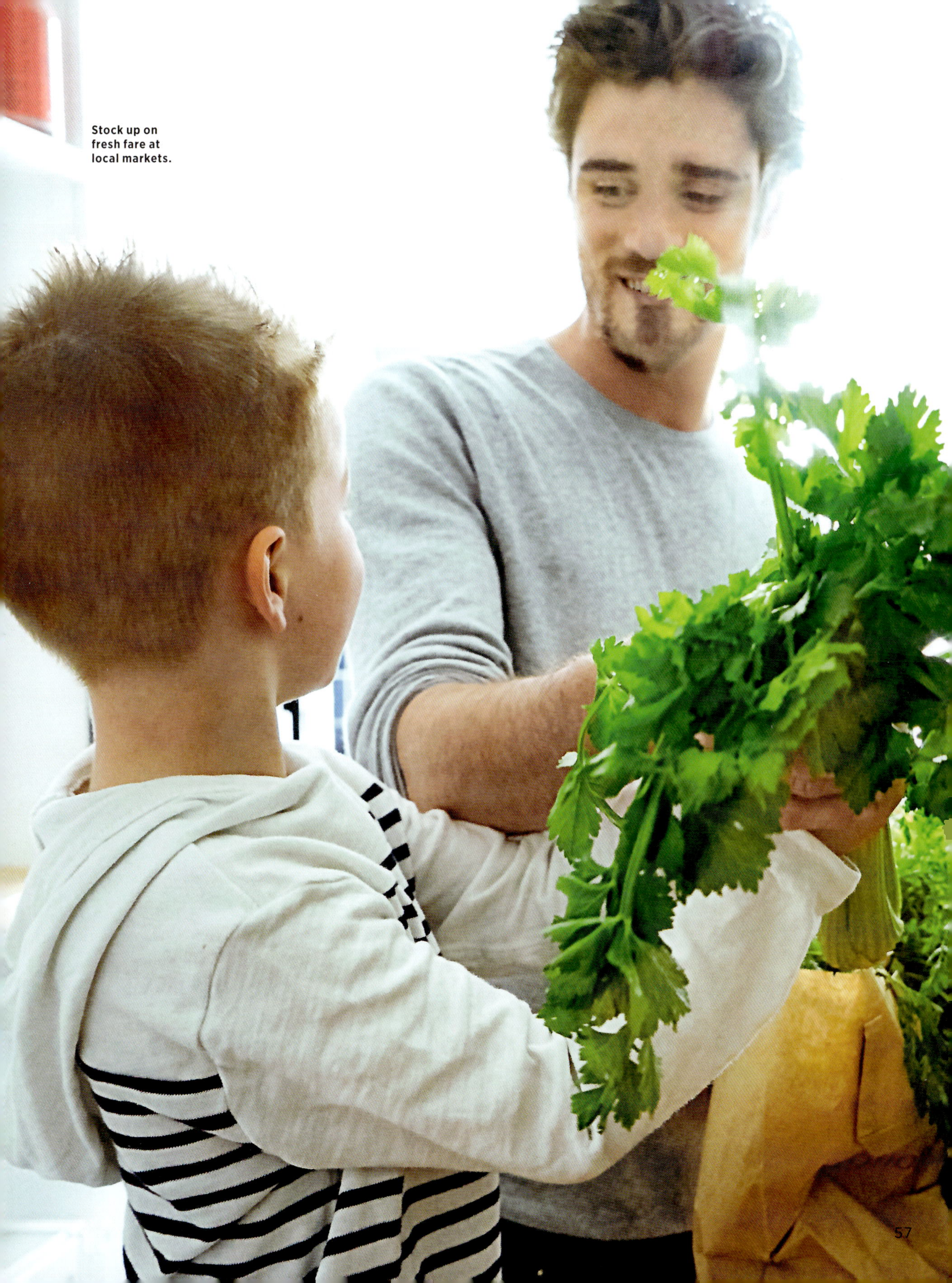

Stock up on fresh fare at local markets.

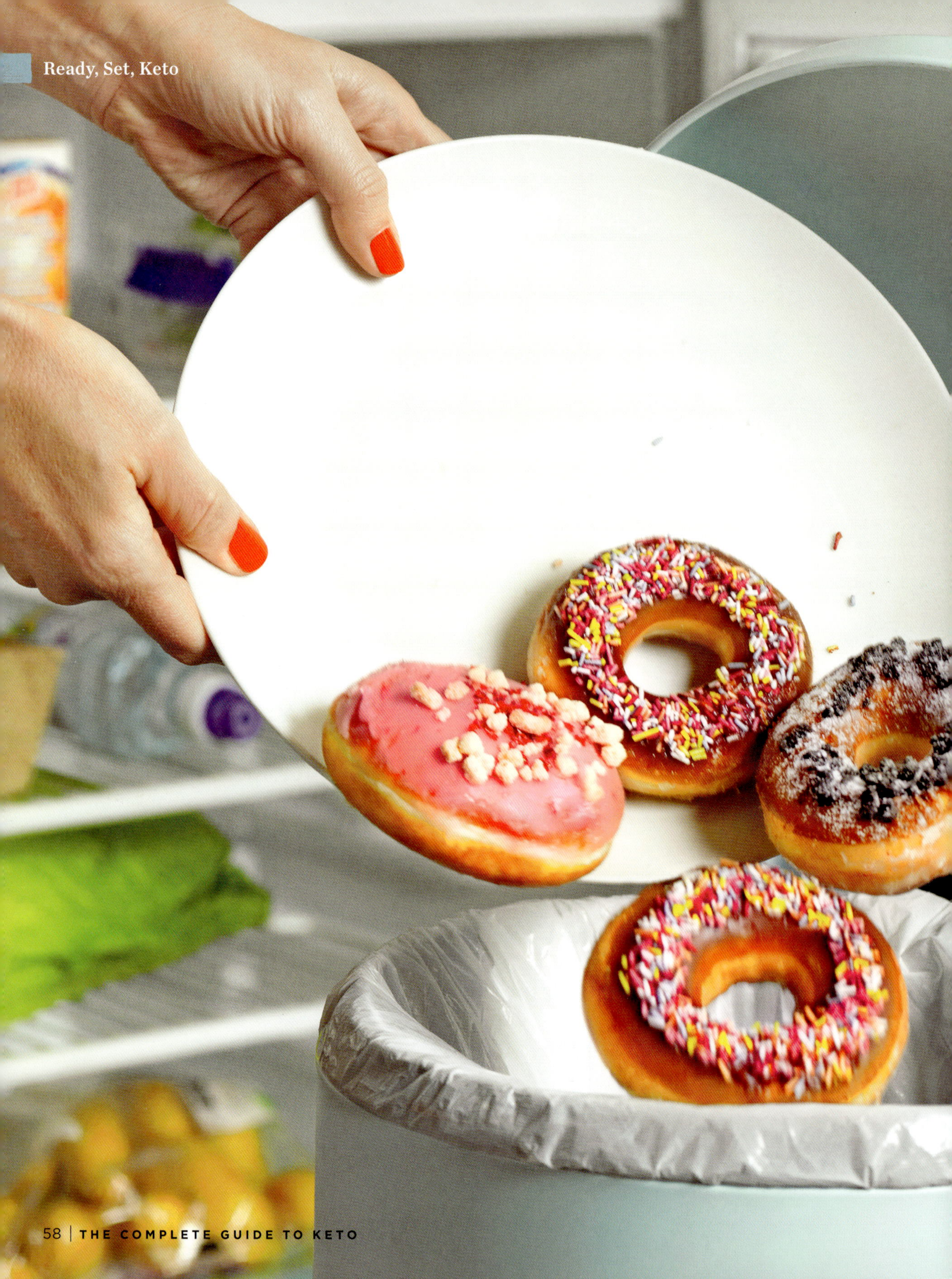

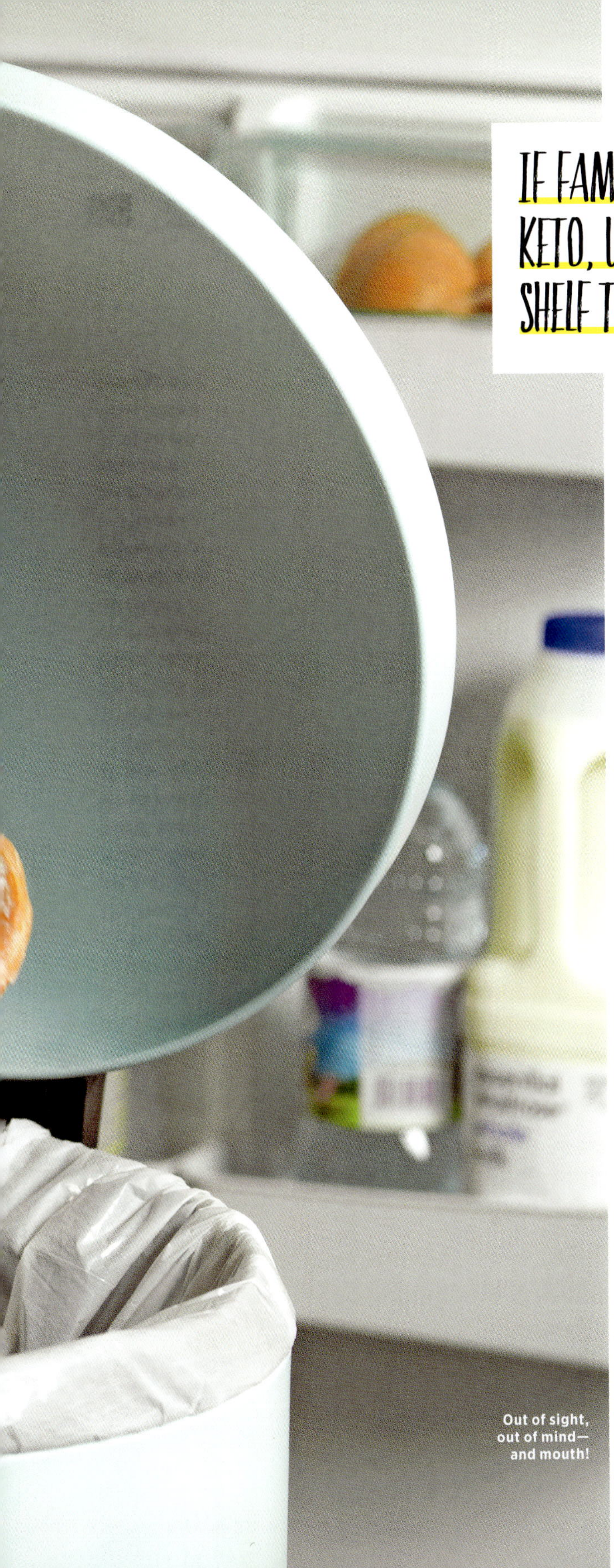
Out of sight, out of mind—and mouth!

IF FAMILY MEMBERS AREN'T DOING KETO, USE A SEPARATE CABINET OR SHELF TO STORE THEIR FOOD.

Jimmy Fallon? Before embarking on the keto plan, purge your cupboards and fridge. You may want to give non-keto food to neighbors or donate it to a local food bank or shelter.

Toss These

Grains and starches Cereal, pasta, rice, potatoes, corn, oats, quinoa, flour, bread, bagels, wraps, rolls and high-carb snacks (popcorn, pretzels, chips)
Sugary foods and drinks Refined sugar, soda, fruit juices, milk, desserts, pastries, milk chocolate, candy, cookies, ice cream and low-fat or fat-free anything
Fruit High-carb fruits, including bananas, dates, grapes, apples, mangos and dried fruits
Legumes Beans, lentils, peas
Processed polyunsaturated fats and oils Vegetable oils and most seed oils, including sunflower, safflower, canola, soybean, corn and grapeseed. Trans fats, such as shortening and margarine (anything that says "hydrogenated")

Set Up the Kitchen

There's lots of cooking involved in keto—so arm yourself with these helpful tools.
Spiralizer to make vegetables like zucchini into noodles ("zoodles") as pasta substitutes
Food processor to prepare fat bombs (high-fat treats), shakes and sliced veggies. Some blenders can't handle tougher fare, like cauliflower and nuts.
Food scale to measure solids or liquids when you're trying to hit your macro goals. Use with an app, like MyFitnessPal, for easy tracking.
Hand mixer When whipping up eggs and sauces, it's a lot quicker and less messy than dealing with the heavy-duty stand type.

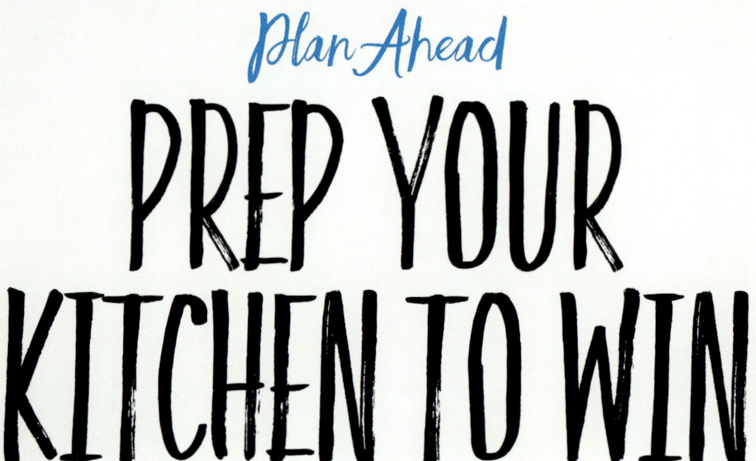

Plan Ahead

PREP YOUR KITCHEN TO WIN

THE KEY TO SUCCESS ON THIS DIET? STOCK UP ON THE RIGHT FOODS, THEN FIND EASY WAYS TO GET THEM PREPARED AND READY TO EAT.

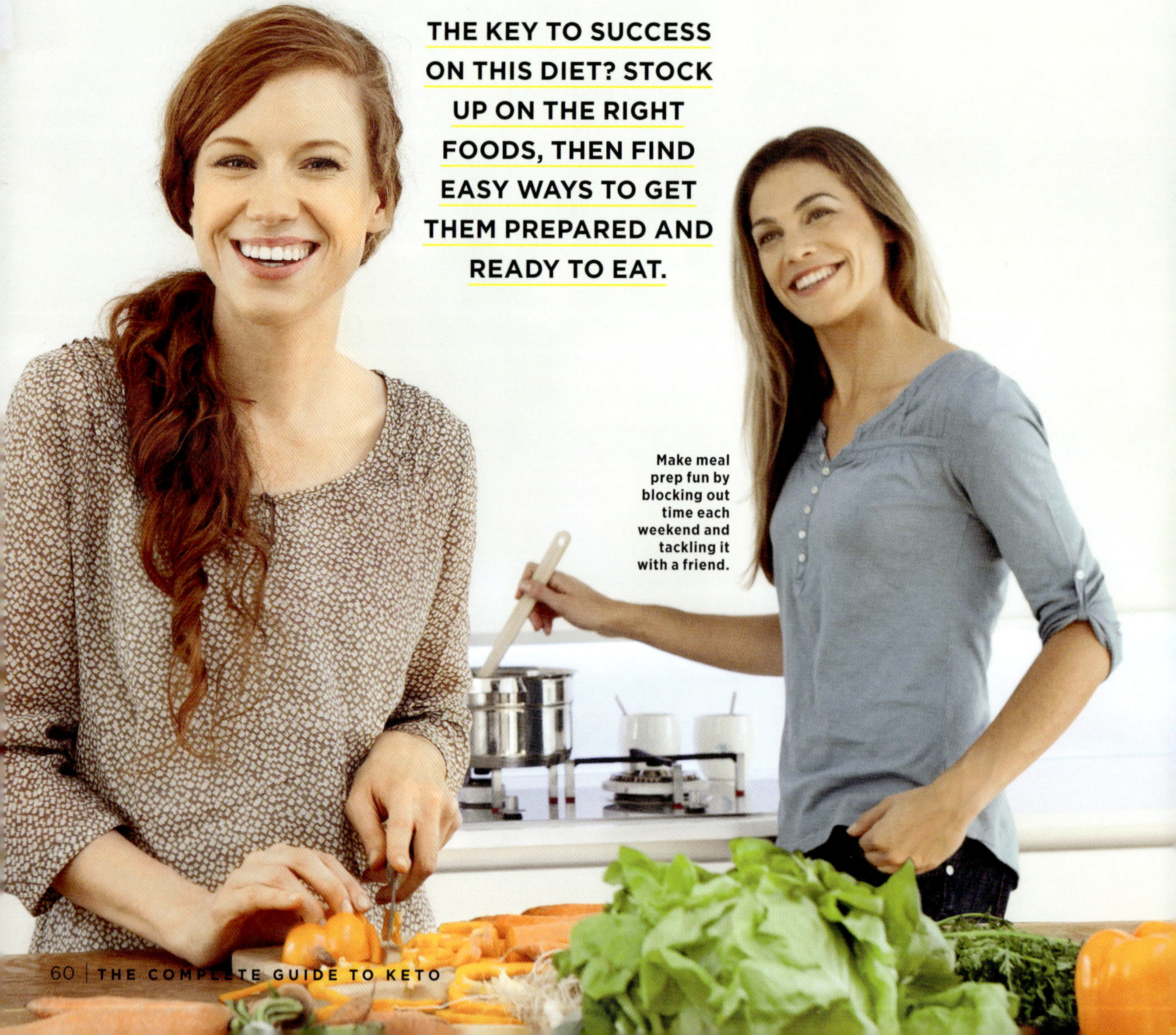

Make meal prep fun by blocking out time each weekend and tackling it with a friend.

USE THESE KITCHEN TOOLS
Spiralizer, to make things like zoodles (zucchini noodles) • Kitchen scale • Measuring spoons • Measuring cups • Vegetable peeler • Good knives • Food processor, for chopping veggies • Sheet pans, for roasting and baking • Slow cooker

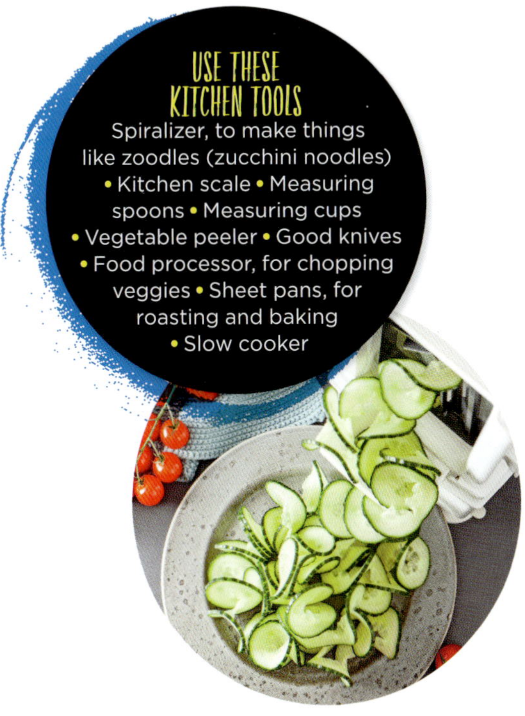

ANYONE FOLLOWING KETO successfully will tell you that it requires a lot of cooking and prep time.

"Doing keto was like a full-time job," says Liz Josefsberg, CPT., weight-loss expert and author of *Target 100: The World's Simplest Weight Loss Program in 6 Easy Steps*. Josefsberg followed the ketogenic diet for about two months as an experiment, losing 15 pounds (after putting on 12 to prepare)—and she saw her body fat drop from 36 percent to 29 percent. "Especially as you get started, there's a lot of stuff that you need to think about, including stocking up and getting all the correct foods into your house. I already cook often, but I had to cook a lot more and do a lot of meal prepping and bringing my own food places when I would be away from home."

Here's a starter list to follow as you clean out your kitchen for keto. Have family members who aren't following the plan? Keep their food on different shelves in the fridge and in a separate cabinet so you won't be tempted to indulge when reaching for a keto meal or snack.

Keep These Foods Front and Center

In Your Pantry

Nuts • Seeds • Keto protein powder • Sunflower-seed butter • Almond butter • Almond flour • MCT oil • Brain octane oil • Coffee • Coconut oil • Avocado oil • Olive oil • Macadamia nuts • Pistachios • Cocoa • Chia seeds • Flaxseeds • Pumpkin seeds • Dark chocolate • Shirataki noodles • Nutritional yeast • Chicken bouillon cubes (to help replenish electrolytes lost) • Bone broth • Seaweed snacks

Alcohol

Clear liquors • Low-carb wines: cabernet sauvignon, pinot noir, merlot, pinot grigio, sauvignon blanc, Champagne • Low-carb beer (look for beers with fewer than 5 grams of carbs)

NOTE You probably shouldn't start drinking alcohol until your body is in ketosis and you're losing fat. Keep in mind that drinking can slow your weight loss. Alcohol will also hit you harder without carbs in your system.

In Your Refrigerator

Unsweetened almond milk, hemp milk, coconut milk • Seafood • Greek yogurt (full-fat) • Cottage cheese (full-fat) • Ricotta cheese • Cheese • Grass-fed ghee • Grass-fed beef • Salmon • Poultry • Eggs • Ranch dressing • Bacon • Green, leafy vegetables • Cauliflower • Eggplant • Mushrooms • Spaghetti squash • Celery • Berries (any kind) • Avocados

Check out keto-friendly snacks on page 74.

What To Toss

Bananas • Apples • Pineapple • Ice cream • Packaged sweets • Cookies • Pretzels • Popcorn • Fat-free anything • Low-fat anything • Soda • Sugary beverages (Basically, anything that isn't healthy or on the other lists)

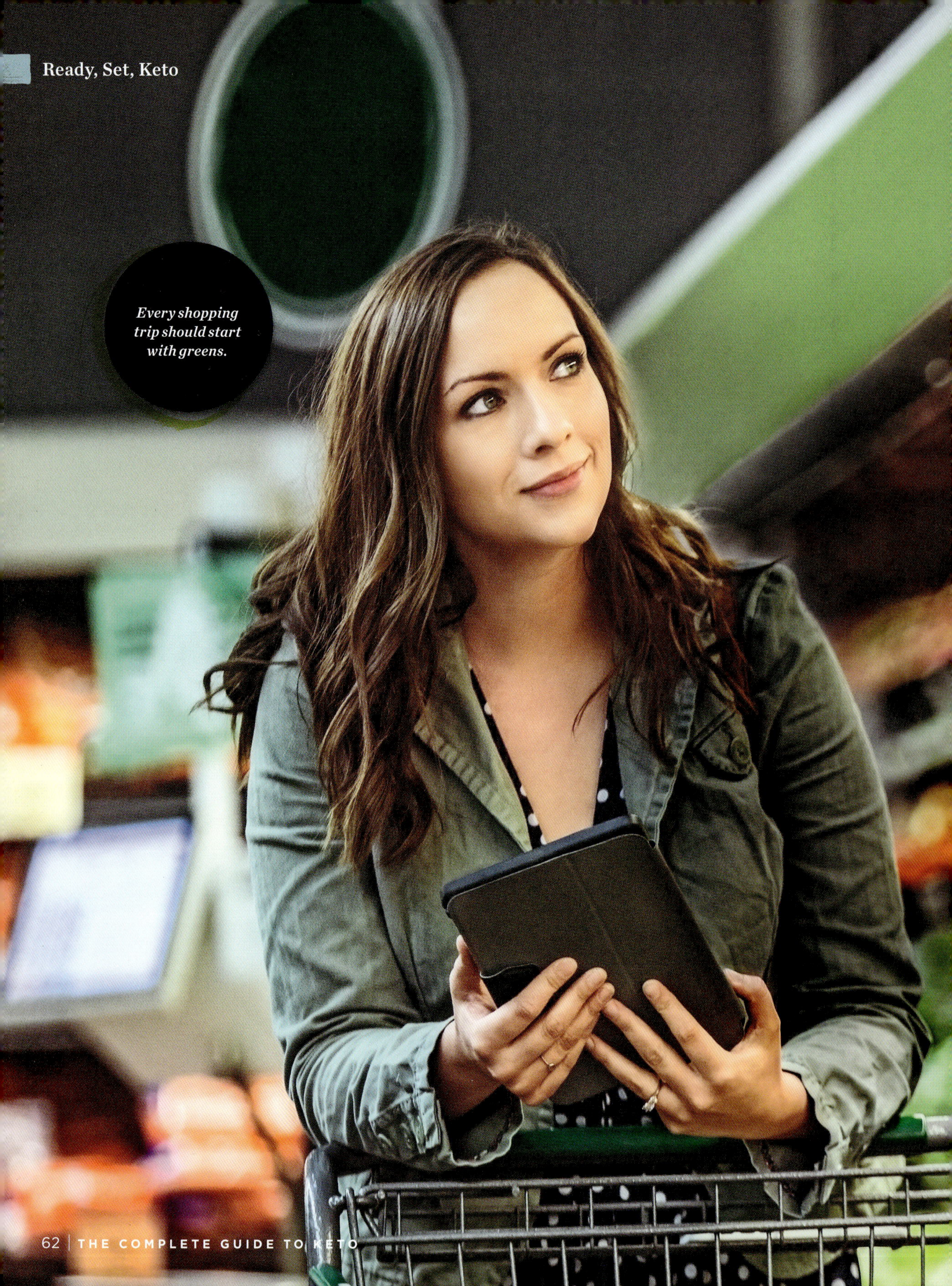

Every shopping trip should start with greens.

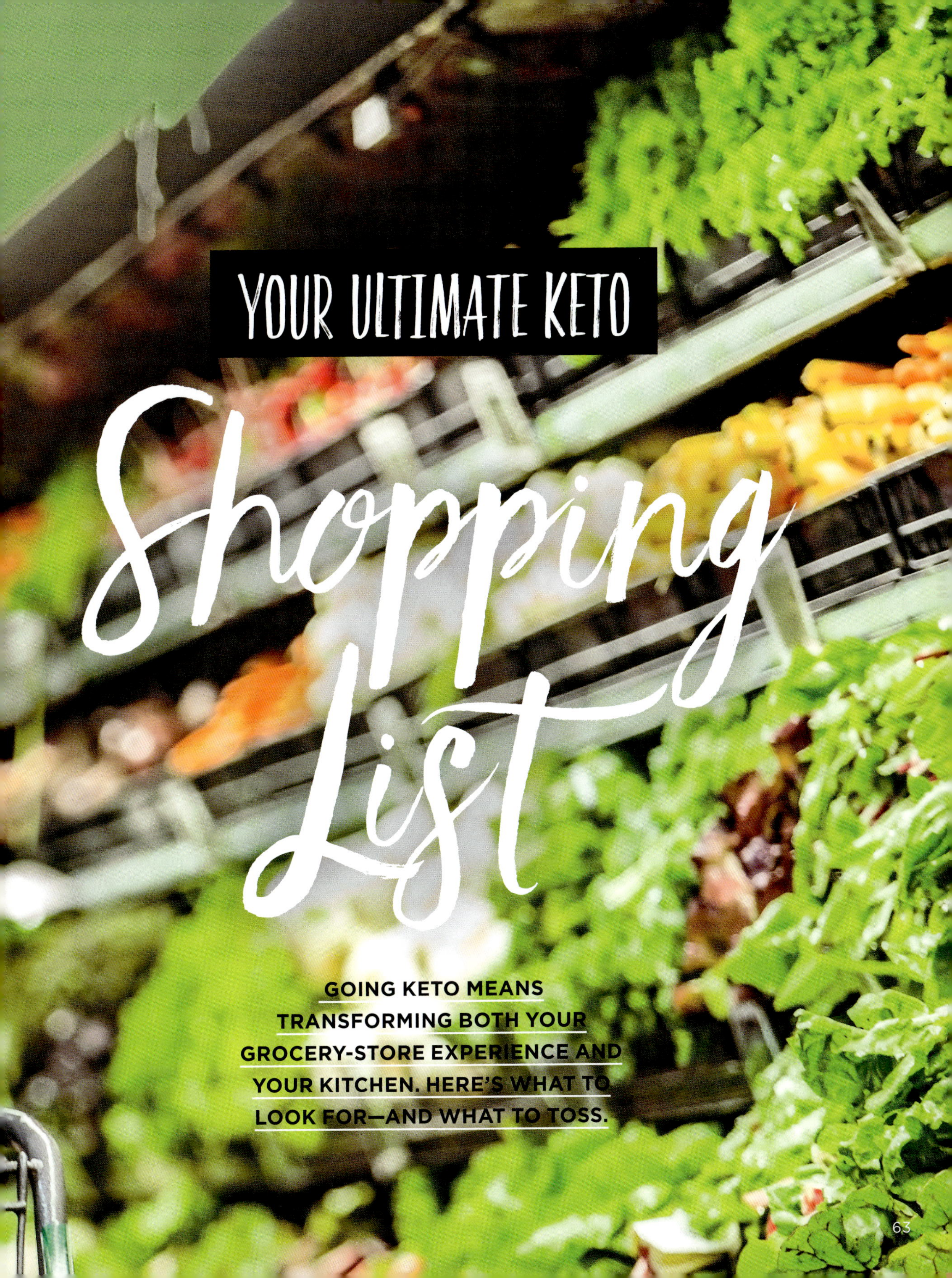

YOUR ULTIMATE KETO Shopping List

GOING KETO MEANS TRANSFORMING BOTH YOUR GROCERY-STORE EXPERIENCE AND YOUR KITCHEN. HERE'S WHAT TO LOOK FOR—AND WHAT TO TOSS.

ONE OF THE FIRST THINGS YOU'LL notice when you switch from a typical American diet to a ketogenic plan is a total "recalculating" of your supermarket GPS route. That's because grocery stores are designed to put all the boxed, packaged, processed foods—along with goodies like chips and soft drinks—right smack in the heart of the store, where you can't help but be tempted. The more basic, unadorned, whole foods, the kind you'll be looking for on keto, are relegated to the far corners. "You're going to end up walking around the perimeter of the store," says Craig Emmerich of Keto-Adapted, "because that's where you'll find high-quality meats and low-carb vegetables. Those are your mainstays." We took a stroll through the supermarket aisles with Emmerich to create a road map to your new eating plan.

Produce

This colorful section is one place you'll spend a lot of time. First stop: butter lettuce. "It's a great tool to use as a replacement for buns or wraps," says Emmerich. It's soft and flexible yet strong enough to hold an Asian chicken filling, burgers, tacos or deli meats. As a bonus, butter lettuce contains vitamins A and C along with folate.

Stay in the greens section for other leafy friends, like romaine lettuce, spinach, Swiss chard, kale, collard and beet greens, and arugula. All are packed with vitamins—including A, B, C and K—fiber and antioxidants, along with other nutrients. Then stop by the cruciferous area and pick up broccoli, cabbage, bok choy, Brussels sprouts or cauliflower, which is particularly versatile as a stand-in for rice and as mashed "potatoes." Other good choices: asparagus, cucumber, bell peppers and green beans. Plus, summer squash, like zucchini, makes a great pasta impersonator. Give a pass to starchy veggies, such as potatoes, beets, parsnips, rutabagas and carrots.

When it comes to fruit, most are off the keto menu, but there are three notable exceptions. Berries, especially blackberries and raspberries, are fine as an occasional treat. And two things we tend to think of as vegetables but are actually fruits—tomatoes and avocados—are a keto yes. Avocados, in fact, are so high in healthy fats that they're an undisputed star.

All these foods can provide you with a laundry list of vitamins, minerals and nutrients—health boosters like magnesium, potassium and calcium, as well as a wide array of antioxidants that help your cells resist damage and fight inflammation.

Meats and Fish

These foods give you a double whammy on keto: fats plus protein. When shopping for fish, look for wild-caught, which has the best nutrient profile. For meats and poultry, grass-fed, pasture-raised and organic are ideal. Organic is especially important, says Emmerich, because all animals' bodies store toxins in fat cells—so when you're eating a lot of fat, you want the source to have been raised as free of chemicals as possible. "It is more expensive, and you do have to shop according to your budget," he points out. "If you can't always afford grass-fed, regular will be OK. What we've found though, after helping thousands of clients switch to keto over the past 16-plus years, is that the majority who budget and track grocery bills find that month to month, they end up spending less than they did when they were non-keto. That's because you're eating far fewer processed foods, and those tend to be considerably more expensive than buying whole foods. That makes spending five dollars for a dozen organic eggs not as big a deal."

Dairy

Some keto eaters decide to avoid dairy, and a number of people are lactose intolerant. If you do want to go for cheese and cream, keep in mind that lower-fat dairy does have some carbs. For instance, whole milk is not a good bet, but heavy cream is keto-friendly. As a substitute for whole milk, Emmerich recommends unsweetened almond milk, which has few to no carbs. Don't go too crazy with soy milk though. "It's very high in phytoestrogens, which mimic estrogen in your body, and that can mess with your hormonal balance," he adds. Most high-fat cheeses, like Swiss, brie, Gouda and Parmesan, are fine. As with meats, organic and grass-fed are key when buying cheese, butter and cream, because you don't want to load up on toxins from the animal fat.

Pantry items

Here, you take a turn into the center of the store for various essential and keto-approved products. First, the oils: Again, organic is best. Avocado oil is a star, because it has a very high smoke point, making it ideal for high-temp frying or sautéing. Olive oil is a versatile choice, excellent in salad dressings and good for cooking at a slightly lower temperature. Look for certain nut and seed oils as well—walnut, hazelnut and sesame are all good. Organic lard, long banned under "healthy eating," is also back on the menu with keto.

THIS WEEK'S LIST

Asparagus
Broccoli
Celery
Wild-Caught Salmon
Cucumber
Garlic
Grass-Fed Butter
Heavy Cream
Parmesan Cheese
Zucchini

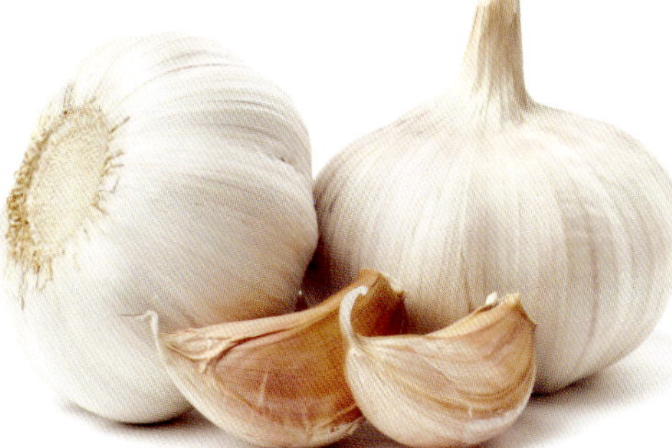

You'll want to stock various shelf-stable basics for recipes, including a good-quality, no-sugar-added tomato sauce that can be used for zoodle-pasta recipes and to make your own sugar-free ketchup. "Good bone broth is another must," says Emmerich. "We like Kettle & Fire, which is made in the traditional way and has lots of collagen and nutrients. Most important, it doesn't have added sugar—a lot of broths do. Use it for healing and in soup and stew recipes."

Heading to the baking aisle—yes, you can bake on keto!—there are several good choices for sugar substitutes to use in recipes, says Emmerich. One is Lakanto brand Classic Monkfruit 1:1 Sugar Substitute, which combines monk fruit extract with erythritol, a sugar alcohol that contains only 6 percent of the calories of table sugar. The sugar-alcohol molecules stimulate the sweet-taste receptors on your tongue, but your body can't digest them—so they pass through your body essentially calorie- and carb-free. Another erythritol-based brand is Swerve, which is called for in many keto recipes. A third option is stevia, which is mixed with erythritol to give it the bulk of regular sugar (stevia alone is many times sweeter than table sugar).

Keto-friendly, low-carb flours include almond and coconut, and you'll also want to stop by the spices. Not only do they add tons of flavor, says Emmerich, but "they have lots of nutrients, vitamins, minerals and antioxidants. Pick up things like oregano, dried parsley, tarragon, rosemary, ginger and cinnamon."

WATCH OUT FOR PROCESSED FOODS THAT ARE LABELED "KETO" BUT ARE FULL OF CHEMICALS.

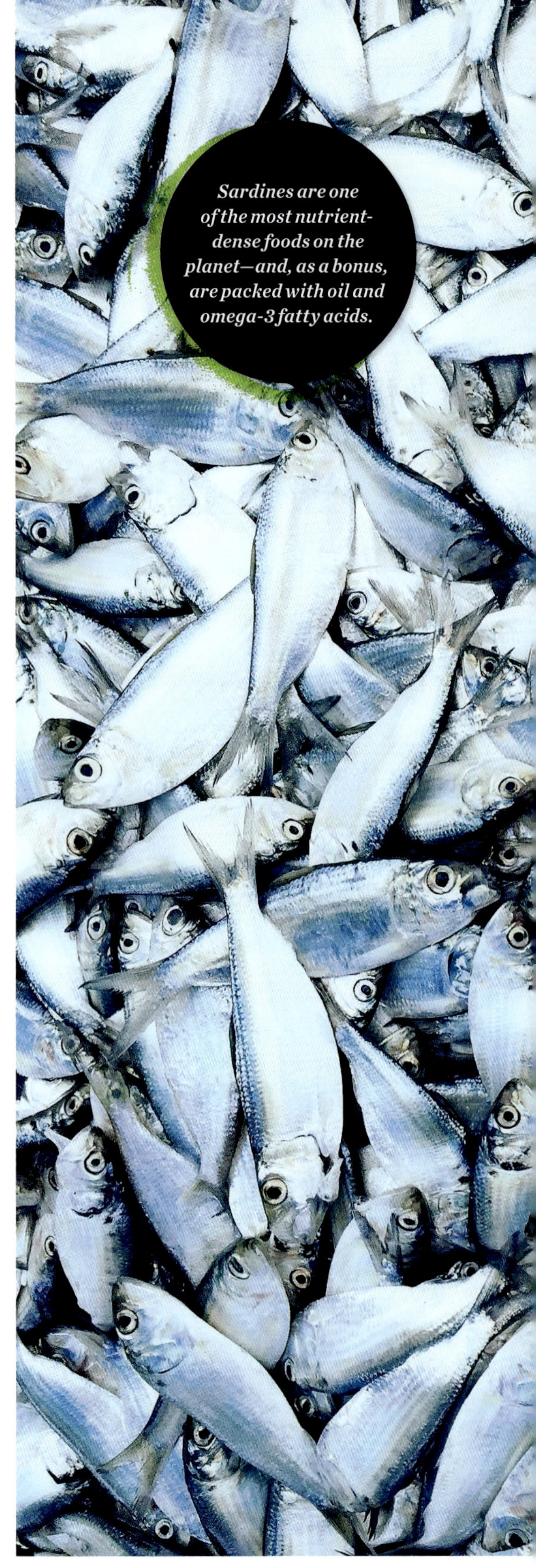

Sardines are one of the most nutrient-dense foods on the planet—and, as a bonus, are packed with oil and omega-3 fatty acids.

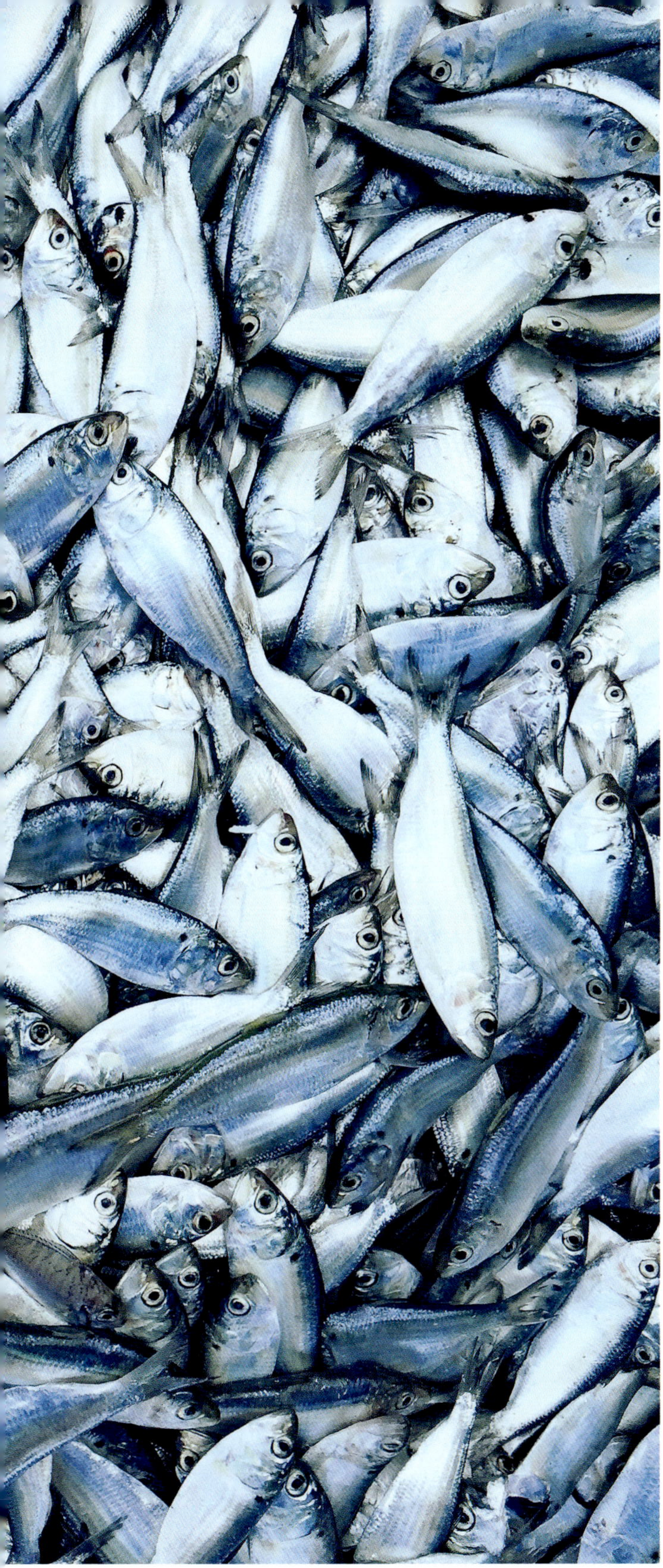

THE "OUT" LIST

Toss these from your larder.

Now that you're filling your shopping cart—and your kitchen—with the raw ingredients for your keto life, it's time to clear out the bad actors that might tempt you to fall off the keto wagon. Nix the following:

ANY TRADITIONAL BAKING PRODUCTS

White or whole-wheat flour, brown or white sugar, corn syrup, molasses

ALL SUGARY DRINKS

Not just soft drinks but also fruit juice (packed with sugar), energy drinks, bottled iced teas...anything with sugar on the label

NATURAL SUGAR SOURCES

Fruits are healthy foods, but on keto they simply have too many carbs—so most of them have to go. The same goes for honey, agave nectar and maple syrup, as well as starchy vegetables, like potatoes, beets, butternut squash and corn

GRAINS

Rice, couscous, oatmeal and other cereals, polenta

LEGUMES

Beans like kidney, garbanzos, lentils and cannellini are too carb-filled for keto.

AND, OF COURSE...

Cookies, ice cream, potato or corn chips, breads, crackers, popcorn, pretzels

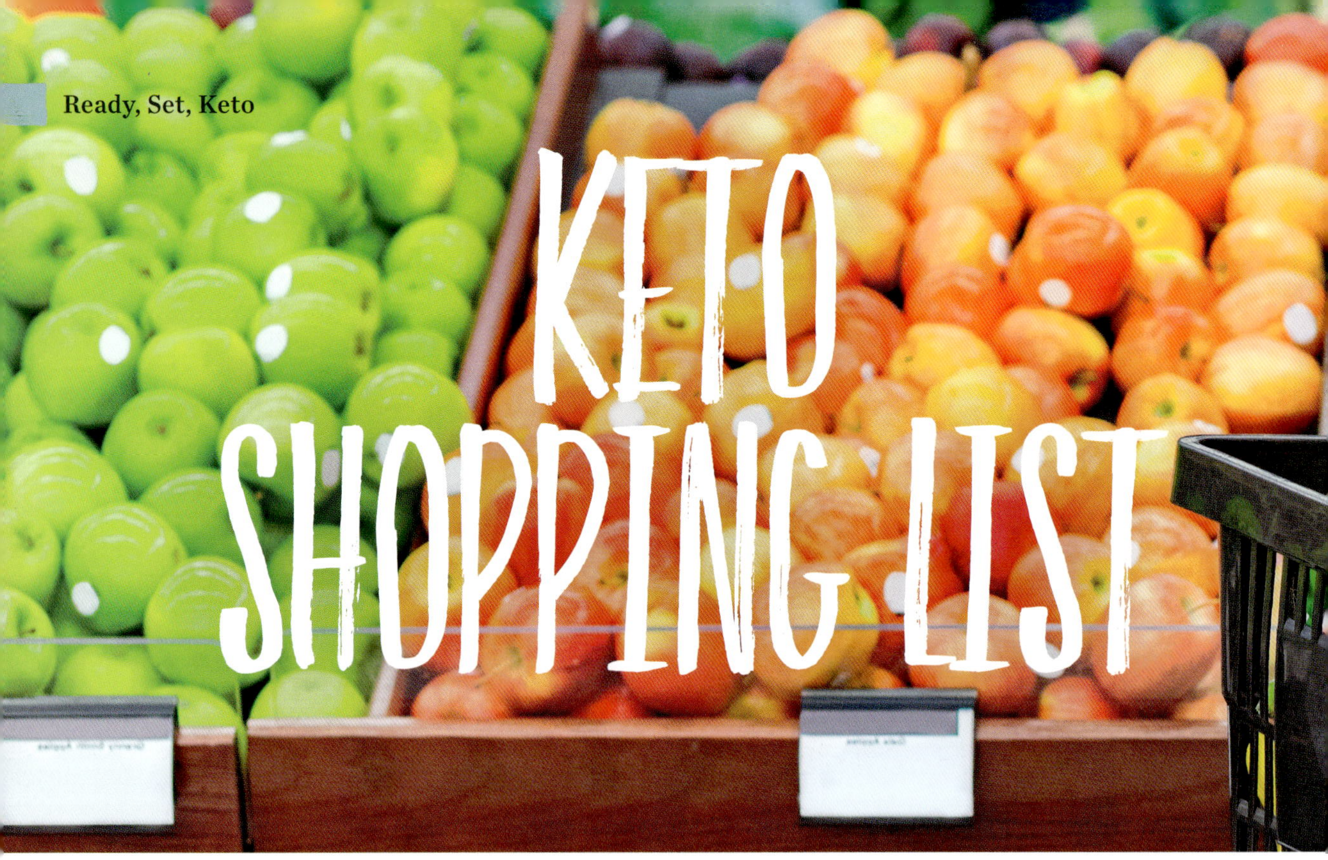

KETO SHOPPING LIST

Fats and Oils

ORGANIC

- ○ Avocado Oil
- ○ Butter (Grass-Fed)
- ○ Coconut Butter
- ○ Coconut Oil
- ○ Extra-Virgin Olive Oil
- ○ Flaxseed Oil
- ○ Ghee
- ○ MCT Oil
- ○ Sesame Oil

Proteins

ORGANIC, PASTURED, GRASS-FED

Poultry

- ○ Chicken, with Skin
- ○ Duck
- ○ Turkey

Meat

- ○ Bison
- ○ Ground Beef
- ○ Lamb
- ○ Steak (Well-Marbled)
- ○ Veal

Pork

- ○ Bacon (Nitrate-Free)
- ○ Ham (No Sugar)
- ○ Pork Chops
- ○ Pork Loin
- ○ Sausage

More Proteins

- ○ Anchovy, Mackerel and Sardine Fillets
- ○ Bone Broth
- ○ Canned Tuna and Salmon
- ○ Eggs
- ○ Fresh and Smoked Fish

Dairy

ORGANIC, FULL-FAT

- ○ Cheese (Firm) (Cheddar, Colby, Jack, Manchego, Parmesan)
- ○ Cottage Cheese
- ○ Cream Cheese
- ○ Feta Cheese
- ○ Goat's Milk Cheese
- ○ Heavy Cream
- ○ Sour Cream
- ○ Yogurt

Fruits

ORGANIC

- ○ Avocados
- ○ Blackberries
- ○ Blueberries
- ○ Lemons and Limes
- ○ Olives
- ○ Raspberries
- ○ Strawberries

Vegetables

ORGANIC

- ○ Arugula
- ○ Asparagus
- ○ Bell Peppers
- ○ Broccoli

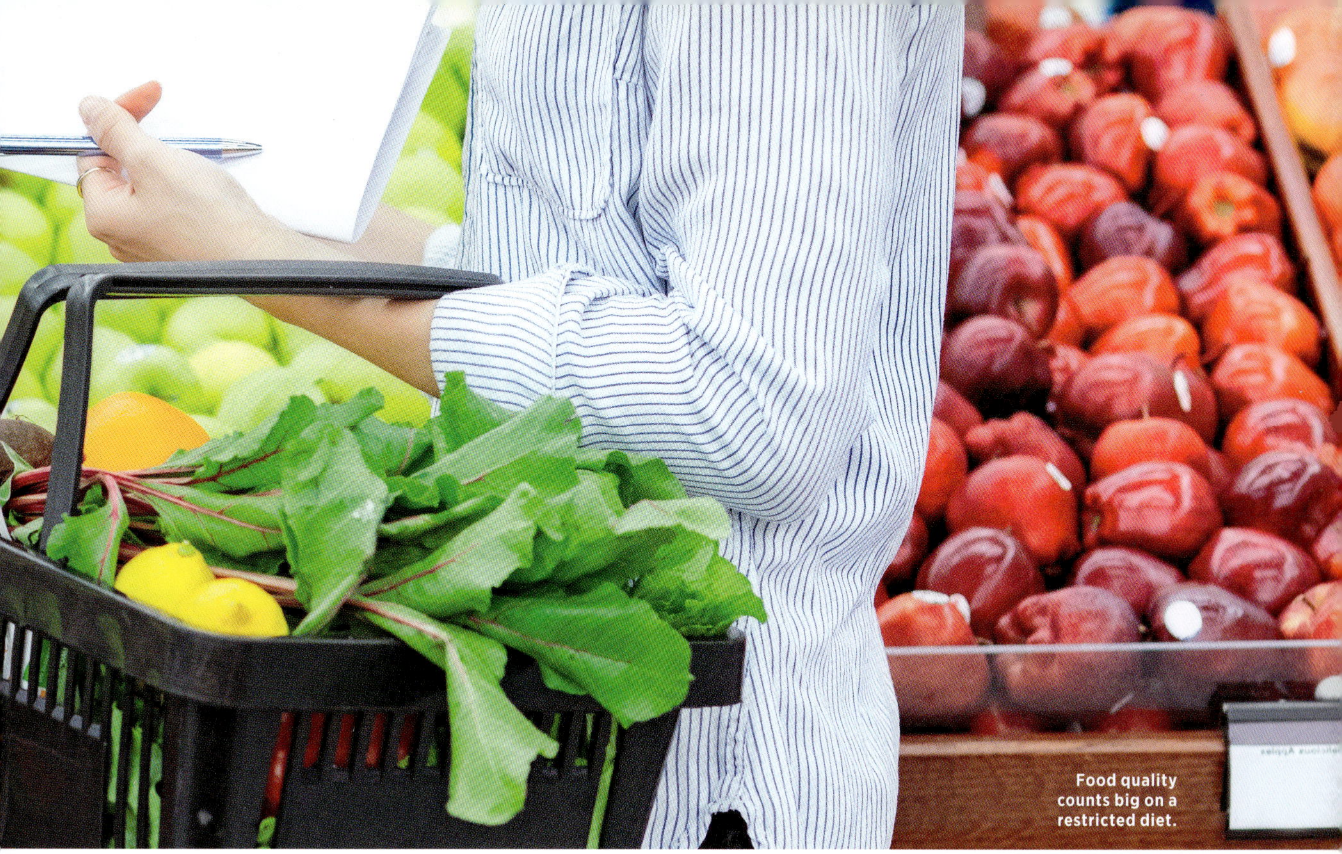

Food quality counts big on a restricted diet.

- ◯ Brussels Sprouts
- ◯ Cabbage
- ◯ Cauliflower
- ◯ Celery
- ◯ Cucumbers
- ◯ Garlic
- ◯ Greens
- ◯ Kale
- ◯ Lettuce (All Types)
- ◯ Mushrooms (All Types)
- ◯ Onions
- ◯ Radishes
- ◯ Shallots
- ◯ Spaghetti Squash
- ◯ Spinach
- ◯ Strawberries
- ◯ Tomatoes (Fresh and Canned Whole)
- ◯ Zucchini

Nuts, Nut Butters and Seeds

- ◯ Almond Butter
- ◯ Almond Flour
- ◯ Almonds
- ◯ Brazil Nuts
- ◯ Cashews
- ◯ Chia Seeds
- ◯ Coconut Flakes
- ◯ Coconut Flour
- ◯ Flaxseeds
- ◯ Hemp Seeds
- ◯ Macadamia Nuts
- ◯ Pecans
- ◯ Pine Nuts
- ◯ Pistachios
- ◯ Pumpkin Seeds
- ◯ Sesame Seeds
- ◯ Sunflower Seeds
- ◯ Tahini
- ◯ Walnuts

Condiments

- ◯ Apple Cider Vinegar
- ◯ Balsamic Vinegar
- ◯ Coconut Aminos
- ◯ Dill Pickles (No Sugar Added)
- ◯ Hot Sauce
- ◯ Kimchi
- ◯ Mustard
- ◯ Salsa
- ◯ Sauerkraut
- ◯ White Vinegar

Sweeteners

- ◯ Erythritol
- ◯ Monk Fruit
- ◯ Stevia
- ◯ Swerve

Miscellaneous

- ◯ Cacao Nibs (Unsweetened)
- ◯ Cacao Powder
- ◯ Cinnamon
- ◯ Collagen Protein Powder
- ◯ Dark Chocolate (80 Percent and up)
- ◯ Flaxseed Crackers
- ◯ Parmesan Crisps
- ◯ Vanilla Extract

Keto Cheat Sheet

WHEN YOU'RE CRAVING ONE OF YOUR HIGH-CARB FAVORITES (PANCAKES! PIZZA! BURGERS!), TRY ONE OF THESE DELICIOUS AND EASY SUBSTITUTES.

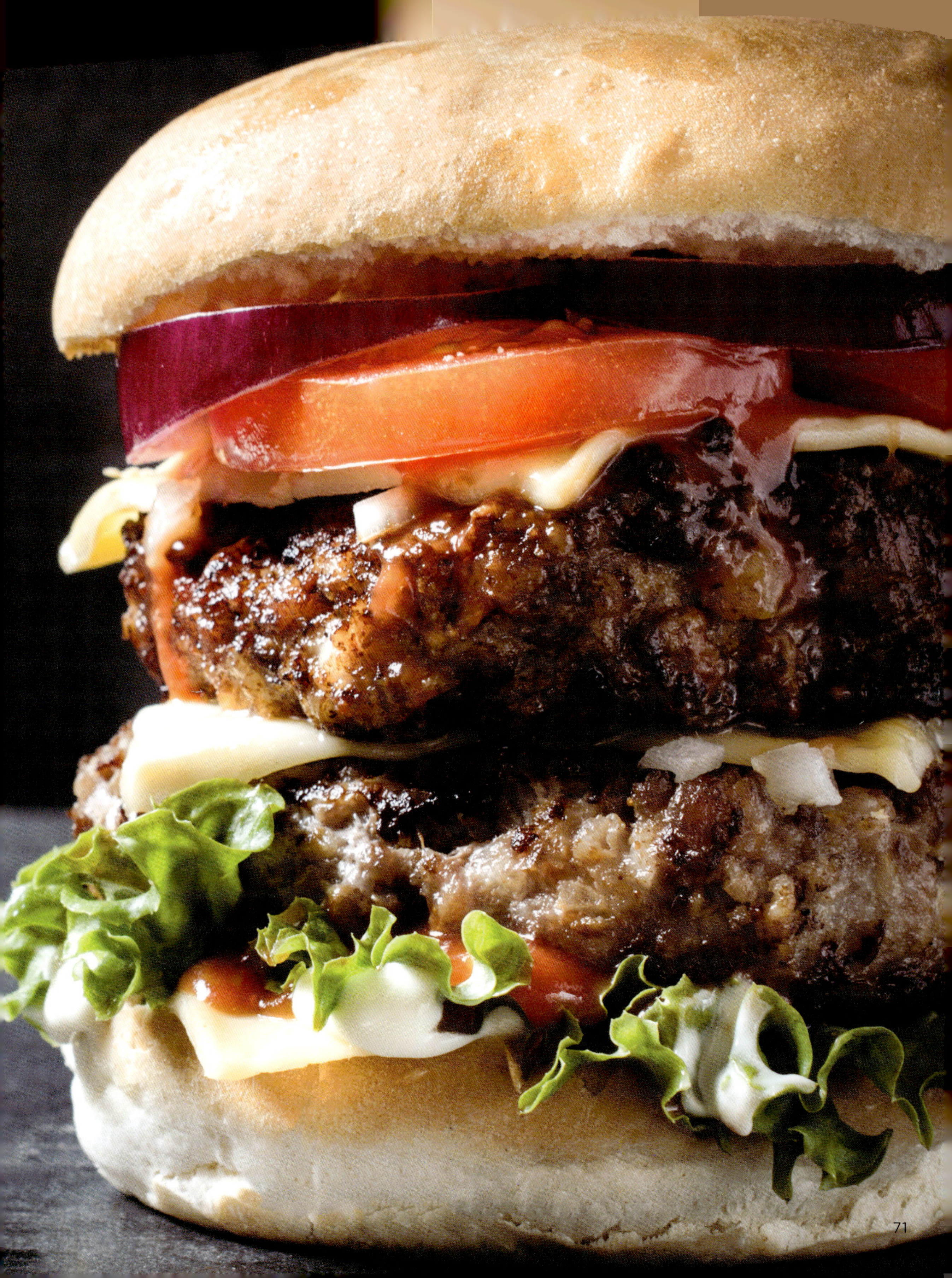

BREAKFAST

TRADE OUT THE CONVENTIONAL CARBS IN THESE.

Bacon, Egg and Cheese on a Bagel

KETO FIX

Bacon and Egg Cups Line a greased muffin tin with cooked bacon, crack eggs into each portion (or scramble them all, if you want), top with salt and pepper and bake in a preheated oven at 375°F for 12–15 minutes.

Muffins

KETO FIX

Blueberry Basil Smoothie Get the recipe on page 132.

Pancakes With Syrup

KETO FIX

Make **Almond Pancakes** instead, using the recipe on page 127.

LUNCH

IMPROVE YOUR MIDDAY MEALS WITH THESE VARIATIONS.

Deli Turkey, Lettuce and Tomato Sandwich With Low-Fat Mayo

↓

KETO FIX

Turkey wrap Deli turkey, bacon, full-fat mayo, onion slices and full-fat cheese, wrapped in large Iceberg or bibb lettuce leaves

Tacos in the Shell

↓

KETO FIX

Taco bowl Top salad greens with cooked ground beef made with taco seasoning; add cheese, full-fat sour cream or guacamole, hot sauce and your favorite toppings

Fast Food Burger and Fries

↓

KETO FIX

Have a **bunless burger**, topped with cheese, guacamole, bacon and hot sauce or salsa, paired with a salad and full-fat dressing

SNACKS

UPGRADE NOSHES WITH KETO ADJUSTMENTS.

Crunchy Carbs: Chips, Popcorn, Pretzels

There's room for snacks on keto, but ask yourself if you're truly hungry or simply eating out of habit.

Smoothie Made With Fruit and Milk

KETO FIX

Cheese Snacks
Try Whisps cheese crisps snacks or make your own by placing 1 tablespoon portions of grated Parmesan cheese 2–3 inches apart on a parchment-paper-lined pan and bake in a 350°F oven for 12–15 minutes.

Chips With Guacamole or Salsa

KETO FIX

Keto Smoothie, made with full-fat canned coconut milk and ½ cup strawberries, raspberries or blackberries.

KETO FIX

Celery sticks or jicama leaves, dunked in guacamole.

DINNER

SWAP OUT COMMON CARB-HEAVY SUPPERS.

Steak and Potatoes

↓

KETO FIX

Rib-eye or New York strip (the fattiest cuts), topped with sautéed mushrooms and served with **garlic mashed turnips** and asparagus

Chicken, Rice and Mixed Vegetables

↓

KETO FIX

Top **baked chicken** with bacon and avocado and serve with **cauliflower rice** and **steamed spinach**

Pizza Slices With the Works

↓

KETO FIX

Keto pizza made with **cauliflower crust**, no-sugar-added tomato sauce and mozzarella cheese, topped with sausage and pepperoni

QUICK-FIX: Keto Snacks to Buy

SAVORY

Pork Rinds (Chicharrones)

These puffy bites may seem unhealthy because they're fried. But a 1-ounce serving contains 0 carbs, 17 grams of protein and 9 grams of fat. That's nine times the protein—and less fat—than you'll find in one serving of carb-loaded potato chips.

Moon Cheese

Cheetos lovers rejoice! These crunchy all-cheese balls contain just 70 calories per serving, with 5 grams of protein, 5 grams of fat and 0 carbs. Bonus: They don't have that orange "cheese" coloring that stains your fingers!

Beef, Chicken or Salmon Jerky

Another no-carb snack that's high in protein, jerky makes an ideal between-meals pick-me-up. While some brands are packed with high-sodium ingredients, such as MSG and sodium nitrate, you can opt for the grass-fed, pastured or wild-caught versions. Research has shown that, unlike grain-fed meat, grass-fed beef contains the same healthy omega-3 fats that are found in fish.

SWEET

Shredded Coconut

Even though coconut is packed with saturated fat, it appears to have a beneficial effect on heart-disease risk factors. Even better, its natural sweetness will tame a sugar jones without spiking insulin. Have a handful of shredded, unsweetened coconut anytime, straight from the bag. But don't gorge; it's still high in calories.

Dark Chocolate

Chocolate is rich in flavonoids—the heart-healthy compounds in red wine and green tea. To stay keto-friendly, choose bars with 85 to 99 percent cocoa. (Note: Their more bitter taste may take some getting used to if you're a milk chocolate fan.) But at just 2.5 net carbs per square, you'll soon come to appreciate its delicious taste. Cacao nibs sprinkled on yogurt are another way to get a chocolate fix.

Strawberries and Cream

For a blast of antioxidants along with natural sweetness, just pop some frozen berries into a dessert bowl and top with ¼ cup heavy cream. The berries will chill the cream to a soft freeze...and voilà! Ice cream cravings calmed, at just 8 net carbs.

About Those Sweeteners

SUGAR IS VERBOTEN ON THE keto diet—but thanks to modern science, you can still enjoy plenty of sweet goodness. Just try to stick with natural products, as opposed to artificial substitutes (aspartame, sucralose, Splenda): In some people, these chemicals can affect blood sugar, lead to more cravings and even disrupt hormones and ketosis. On the other hand, the four natural sweeteners here have few side effects.

MONK FRUIT

Made from a fruit native to Asia, this sweetener provides low-calorie sweetness without the insulin spikes of sugar. **Unlike stevia, monk-fruit sweetener never has a bitter aftertaste,** yet it still scores a zero on the glycemic index—and may even have a stabilizing effect on blood sugar. The only downside? It costs more than stevia or erythritol and is not as widely available. But it's 300 times sweeter than table sugar, so a little goes a long way!

ERYTHRITOL

This keto favorite is a powdered or granulated form of sugar alcohol, which is found naturally in fruits and vegetables and does not appear to have negative side effects when used in moderation. The structure of its molecules gives it a sweet taste without the side effects of sugar. Calorie-wise, it has just 0 to 0.2 calories per gram, while sugar has 4 calories per gram. Like stevia, it ranks zero on the glycemic index. Erythritol is not quite as sweet as sugar, so you might need to use a little more of it to get the same taste. It's now available at most specialty markets.

SWERVE

Swerve is an all-natural, no-calorie, zero-glycemic-index sweetener that is actually a combination of erythritol, natural citrus flavor and oligosaccharides, which come from starchy root vegetables. Sounds off-limits, right? Don't worry. The body doesn't digest oligosaccharides—so they don't affect blood sugar. Swerve is great for baking, because it can be browned and caramelized like cane sugar—so it's useful for making keto desserts.

STEVIA

The earlier forms of this extract of the herb *Stevia rebaudiana* tended to have a bitter aftertaste, but that has been greatly improved in most brands. **Pure stevia contains no calories or carbs and ranks zero on the glycemic index.** It is also 200 to 300 times sweeter than table sugar—meaning you need to use only a little. It's available in powder or liquid form.

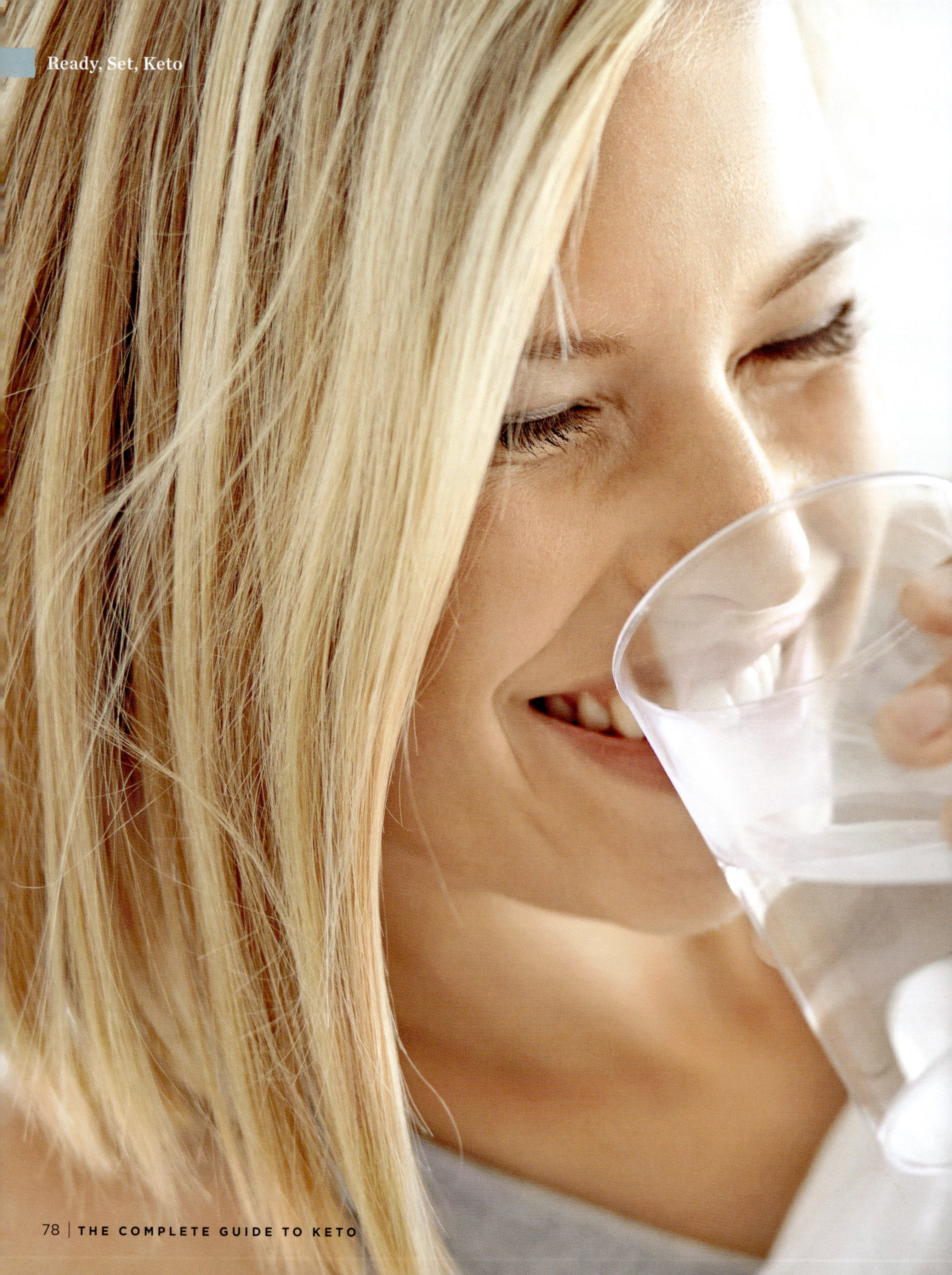

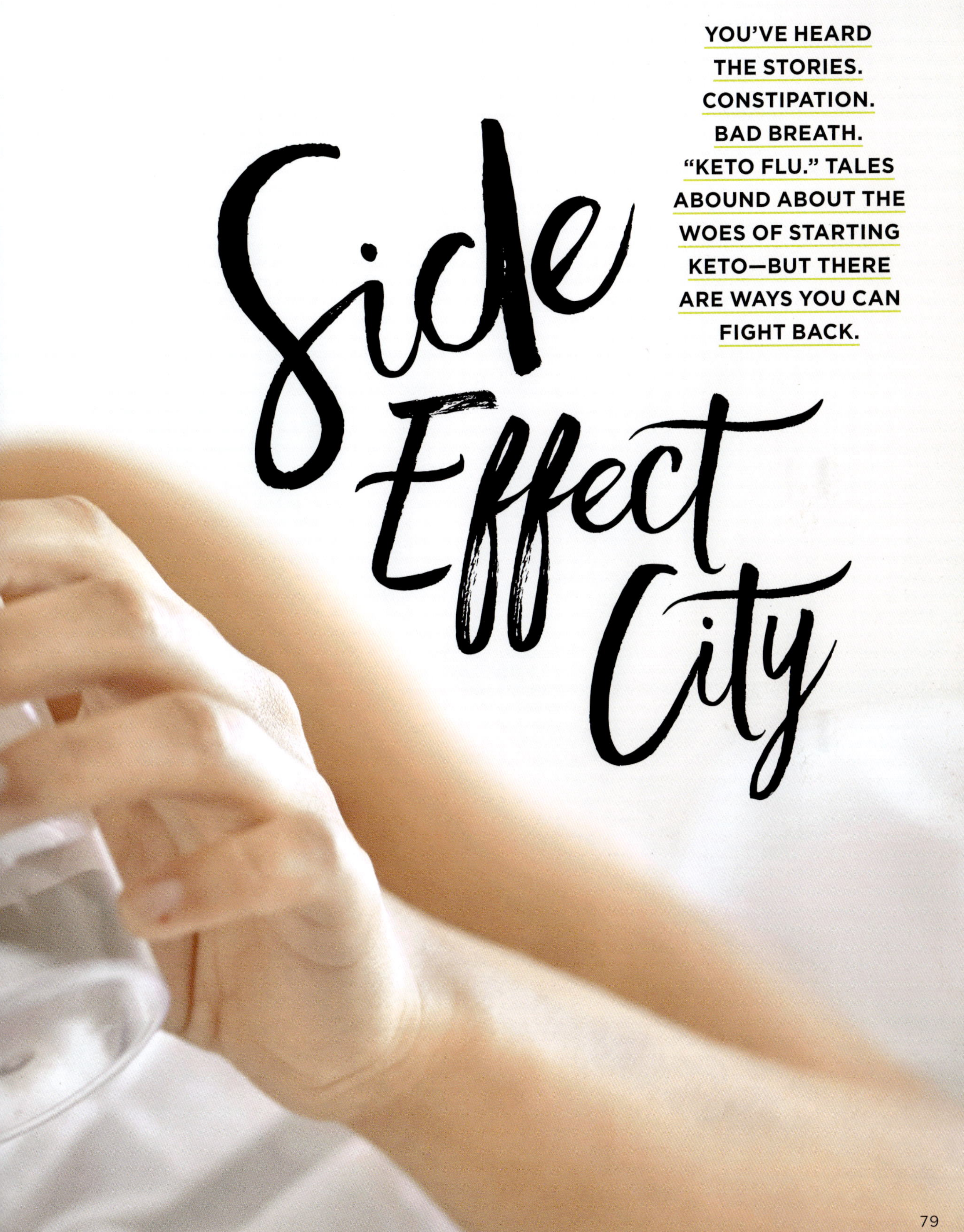

Side Effect City

YOU'VE HEARD THE STORIES. CONSTIPATION. BAD BREATH. "KETO FLU." TALES ABOUND ABOUT THE WOES OF STARTING KETO—BUT THERE ARE WAYS YOU CAN FIGHT BACK.

FOR MOST PEOPLE, KETO IS A JOLT to the system. That's because the standard American diet relies heavily on carbs of all kinds—from bread and pizza to hidden carbs in "healthy" foods, like granola and low-calorie frozen entrées. So it's often a big change to switch to mostly homemade foods, especially if you were getting the bulk of your fiber from grains, which are outlawed on keto. Often, the side effects are short-term, as your body adjusts to an entirely different system. But while they're happening, they're no fun. "It's important, if you've never been on a ketogenic diet, to talk to your doctor first," cautions Julie Stefanski, RD, a specialist in ketogenic dieting. "Plan to start the diet when you don't have a lot of social events and can be low-activity," she adds. Here, Stefanski walks us through what to expect when you start keto—and how to weather the storm.

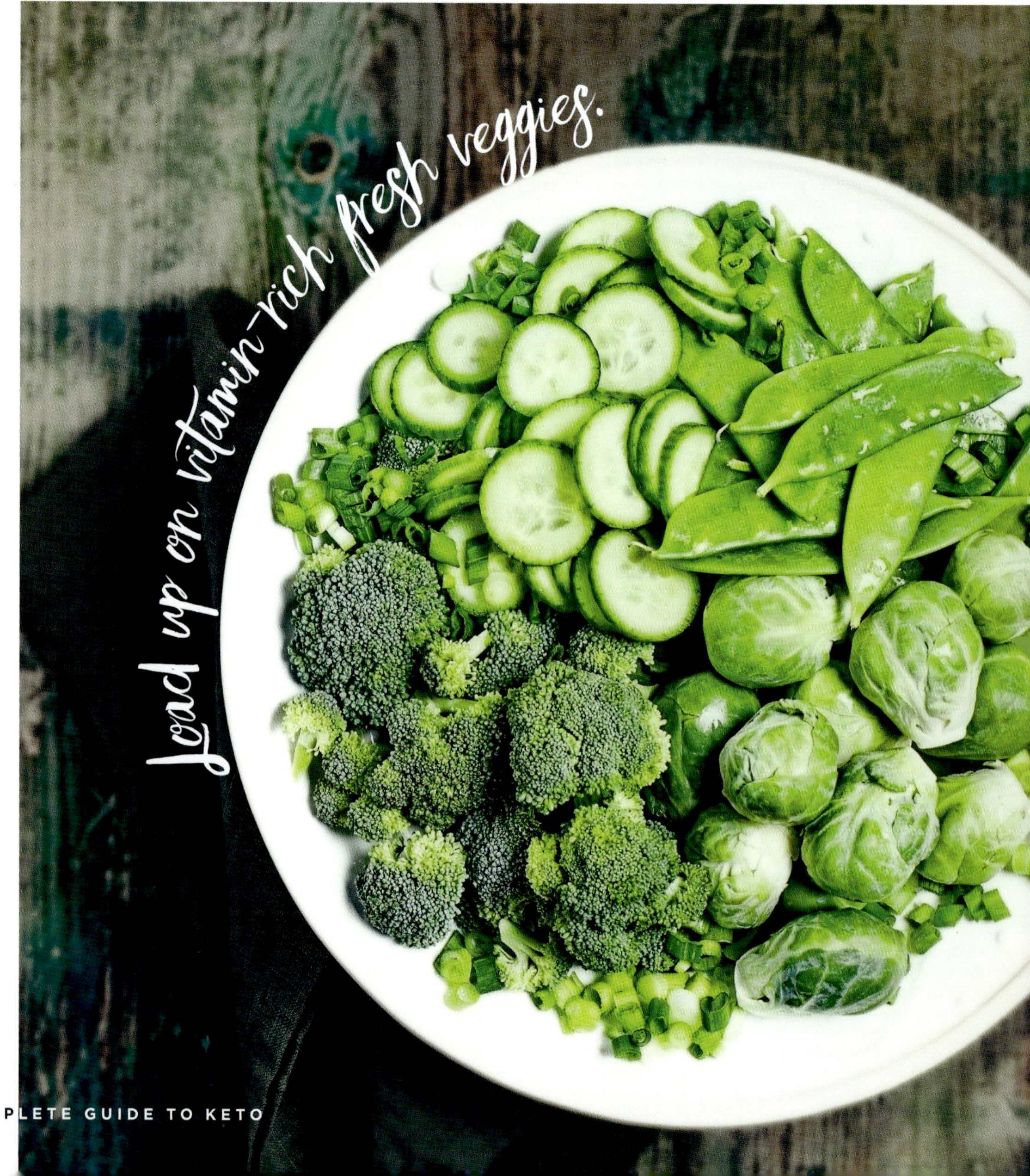

"Keto Flu"

"Just like no one sleeps the same way, shifting from typical metabolism to a state of ketosis is different for everyone," says Stefanski. For some—an estimated 25 percent—that process makes them feel crappy for a few days, if not a week. Symptoms include fatigue, dizziness and mood swings. If that sounds like substance-abuse withdrawal, it's not a coincidence. Research has shown similarities between the effects of sugar on the body and brain to the effects of drugs and suggests that, at the neurobiological level, the "rewards" to your brain from taking in sugar are "more robust than those of cocaine," according to one study.

So if you've been loving your candy bars, it's no surprise that you feel bad when they're suddenly taken away. Your brain is reeling from losing its "drug," and your body has become accustomed to getting easy energy from carbs and sugars. "Glucose is your body's preferred fuel, because it's so easily accessed," explains Stefanski. "There may be an interim period where you're not getting that quick fuel and it takes a little while for your body to process enough fat to give you ketones for energy."

THE TREATMENT

Don't push yourself the first few days. "You'll have plenty of time later to do hard workouts," says Stefanski. "For now, your body is adjusting." Drink lots of fluids and work to get enough vitamins from fresh vegetables, especially high-potassium leafy greens. "After a few days, your body should adapt so you feel more energetic, although for some people it will take longer."

Digestive Issues

The most common keto problem is constipation —usually from a lack of fiber—but diarrhea can be an issue for some people as well, says Stefanski. The bottom line is that changing your dietary intake so drastically has a profound effect on your gut flora, or microbiome, and that can cause both constipation and its opposite, diarrhea. The job of your microbiome, which is essentially a universe of helpful bacteria, is to keep things moving through your system in a healthy way. When that gets thrown off by a big change—especially if you're suddenly taking in much more fat—the result can be diarrhea. The microbiome is fed by fiber and many plant foods, and both of those may decrease when you're switching to keto.

THE TREATMENT

As with "keto flu," one of the major antidotes to constipation and diarrhea is hydration. "Make sure you're drinking a lot of water and also concentrate on adding keto-friendly sources of fiber to your daily meals," says Stefanski. "Some examples are chia seeds, flaxseed, nuts and seeds, all of which can help with regulating your system." Some people opt to take a gentle fiber supplement when starting keto, to help the body adjust. Others have found relief by drinking a mixture of hot water with lemon, along with a teaspoon of apple cider vinegar, every morning, which can help boost digestive function.

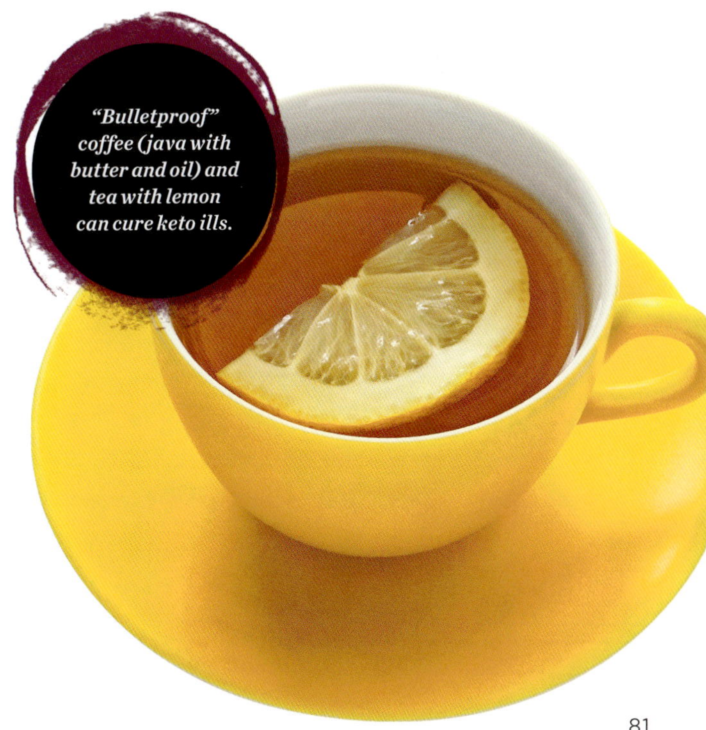

"Bulletproof" coffee (java with butter and oil) and tea with lemon can cure keto ills.

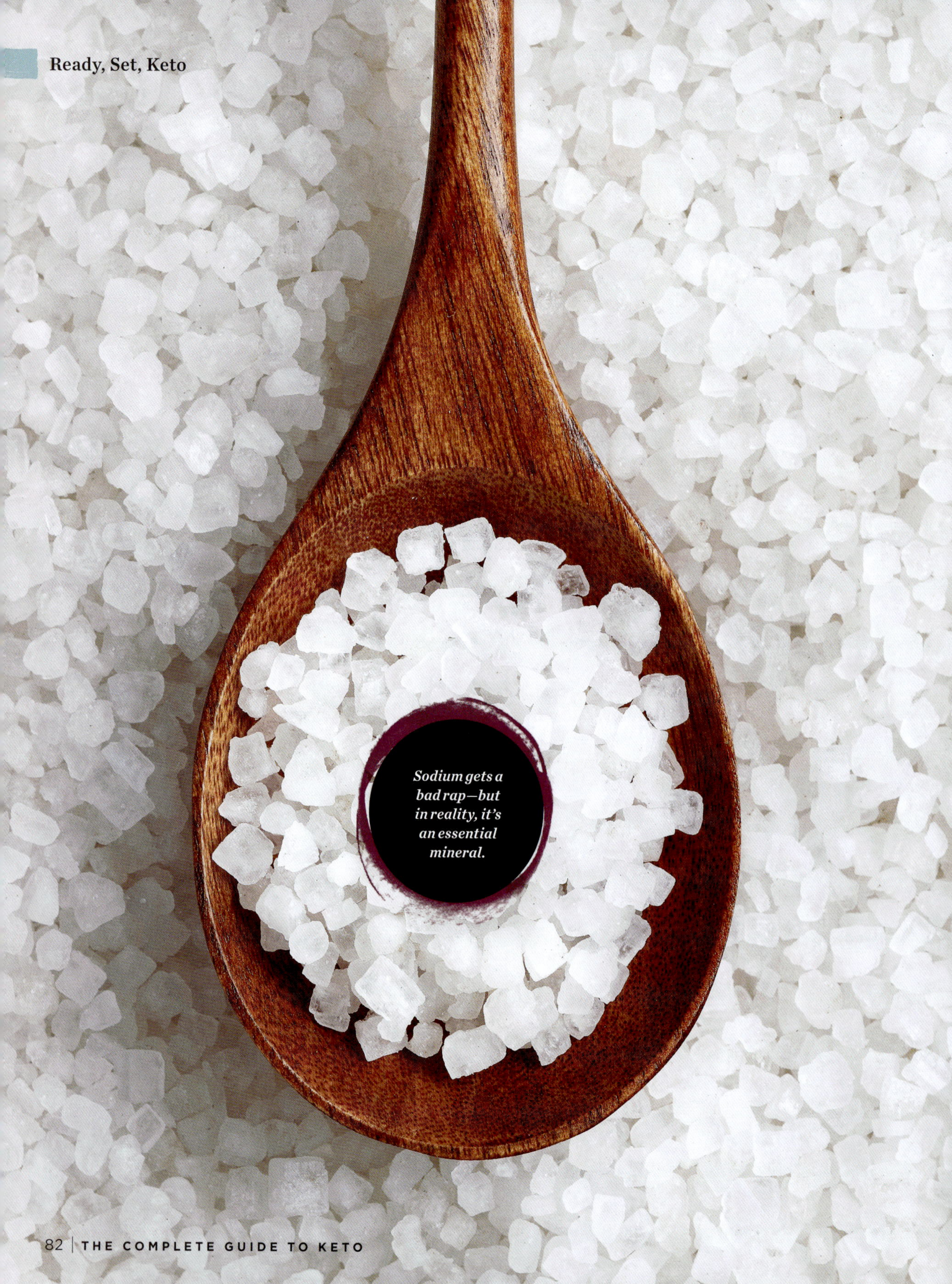

Sodium gets a bad rap—but in reality, it's an essential mineral.

Muscle Cramps

When you're in the early days of keto, you may suddenly find yourself experiencing charley horses—that sudden painful knotting of your calf muscle, often at night or the first thing in the morning. This usually is caused by a mineral imbalance as you adjust to keto, as well as with dehydration. Minerals like sodium, potassium and magnesium, which are known as electrolytes, are key to regulating nerve and muscle function and maintaining blood acidity: It's all a delicate balance that starts with making sure you're getting enough water. Carbohydrates hold on to water in the cells, so when you withdraw most of the carbs that your body is accustomed to, you can also get low on the minerals in that water. The result? Painful muscle cramps.

THE TREATMENT

Again, drinking a lot of water is at the heart of the matter. But you may also want to take potassium and magnesium supplements, at least at the beginning, says Stefanski. Don't be afraid to salt your food, as sodium will help you retain enough water to hydrate your cells—and relieve your cramps.

Bad Breath

It's infamous: that strangely sweet or pungent breath odor that happens when you're in ketosis. And it's a real thing; one researcher even created a version of keto sticks that measures ketones by breath rather than urine, because it's completely quantifiable. You are literally exhaling ketones, and one of the ketone bodies produced by your liver is acetone (yes, acetone as in nail-polish remover), an odor that some are alarmed to find themselves breathing out through their mouths. Most people, though, find that any kind of "ketone breath" fades with time—often within a few weeks, if not days.

THE TREATMENT

While you're dealing with "keto breath," you may be tempted to use sugar-free mints or gum, says Stefanski, but these are often not carb-free and may interfere with ketosis. Instead, your best bet is old-fashioned remedies, like being vigilant with flossing and brushing and, especially, making sure to drink enough water. Dehydration is a major cause of bad breath, and when you're just starting keto you may be more prone to dehydration in general.

Headaches

While some people find themselves afflicted with headaches when starting keto, on the opposite end, "a growing body of research is focusing on the benefits of the keto diet on headaches, specifically migraines," says Stefanski. "We're not sure yet whether the improvement is due to the elimination of certain foods that trigger migraines or a change in the way the brain is fueled," she adds. It's intriguing to note, though, that the first use found for ketogenic diets, almost a century ago, was in children with epilepsy that was resistant to treatment. There may be some not-yet-understood way in which a keto diet alters brain chemistry.

THE TREATMENT

For the run-of-the-mill headache, drinking more water and also making sure you're getting enough potassium and sodium may be the key, Stefanski says. That could be as easy as sprinkling a bit of "lite salt" (a high-potassium salt substitute) on your food. If you're afflicted with migraines, consult with your doctor or a neurologist about whether keto might help.

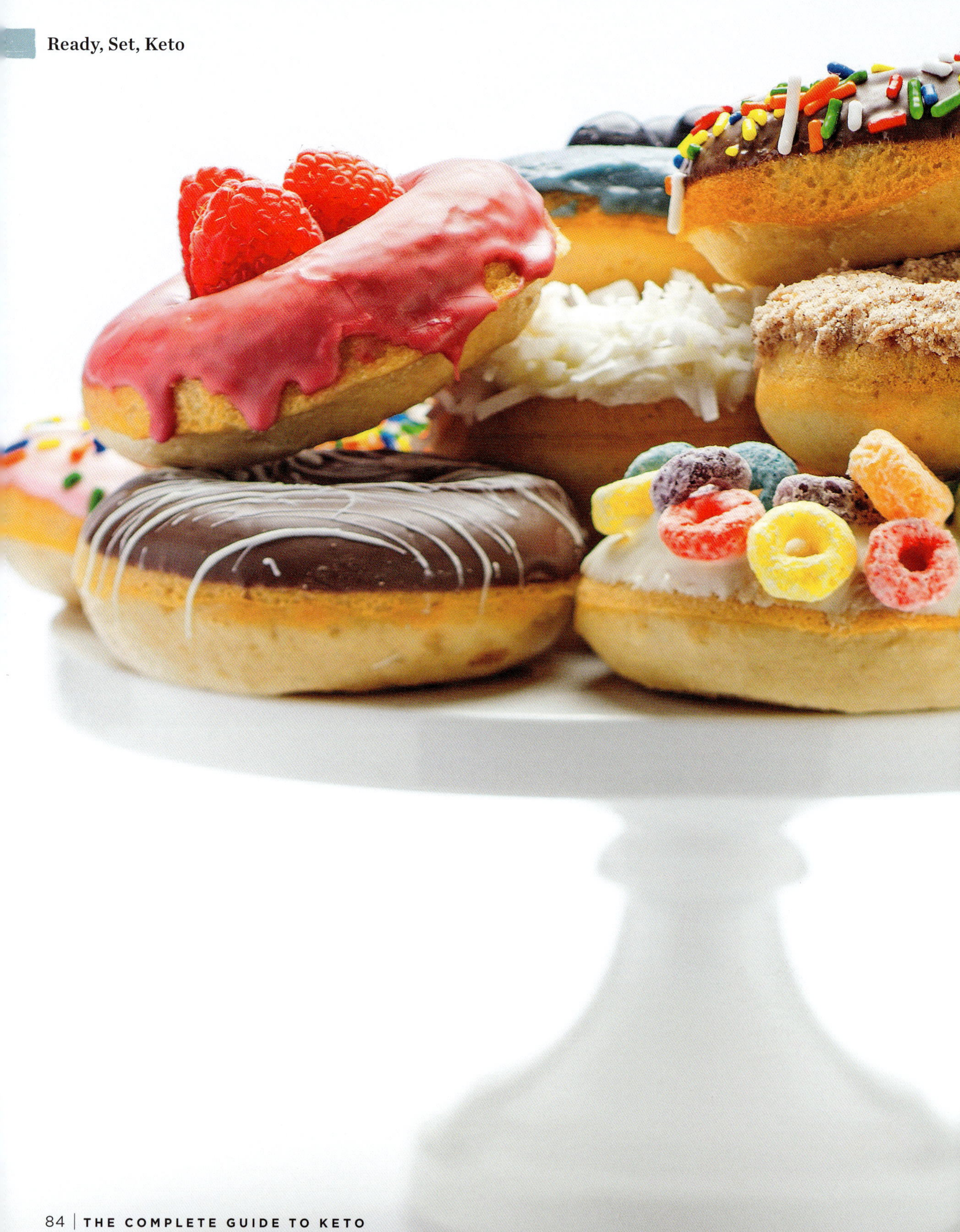

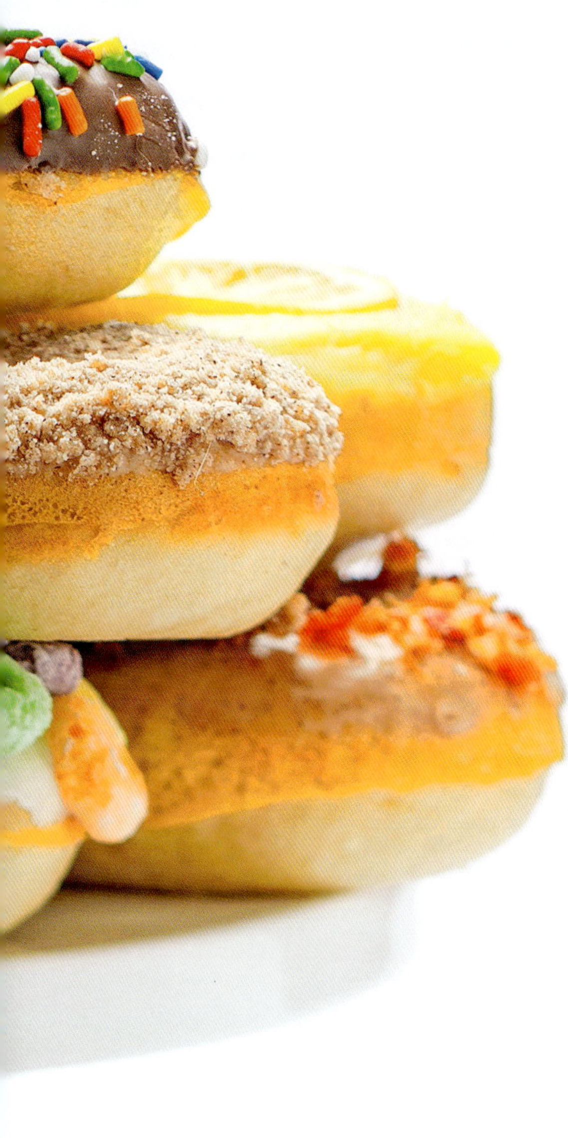

How to Own It

TEMPTATIONS, MISSTEPS, CRAVINGS.... GOING KETO CALLS FOR A NEW MIND-SET, NOT JUST A NEW MEAL PLAN. HERE'S HOW TO GET YOUR HEAD IN THE GAME.

STICKING TO A KETO DIET DEFINITELY involves a learning curve—and not only about what the heck "macronutrients" are. You're most likely taking a big step away from the typical American diet, which relies heavily on carb-based foods, like bagels and pizza, and on the convenience that comes with them. At first, you may be dealing with constant temptation on every street corner (or every strip-mall fast food joint) you pass. There will be ups and downs, triumphs and roadblocks. Here are six ways to power through.

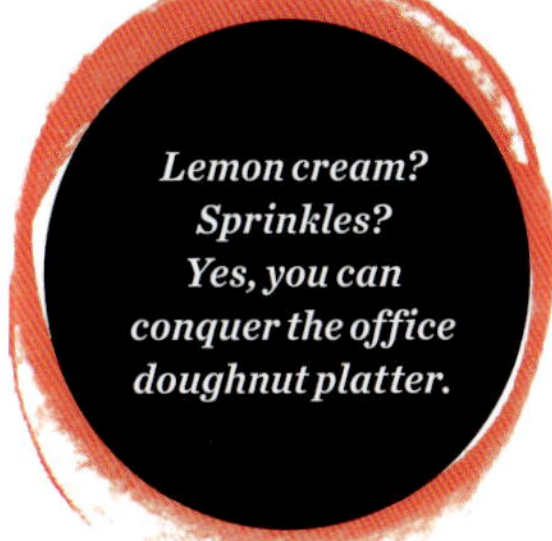

Lemon cream? Sprinkles? Yes, you can conquer the office doughnut platter.

Focus on the Big Picture

Think of keto as a lifestyle change, not as a "diet," advises Josh Axe, DNM, CNS, DC, founder of Ancient Nutrition. "When you commit to living in a healthy way long-term, you're more likely to bounce back after any setbacks." If you're hit with a craving, think about the payoffs down the road in terms of health and weight, and contrast them with the short-term, immediate gratification you would get from eating the "forbidden" food.

Celebrate the Small Victories

One huge plus to the keto diet is that most people see some weight-loss results quickly. "That can be highly motivating to help you stick with it," says Axe, so play up the good news. Lost 3 pounds in the first week? Pat yourself on the back. Down a dress size? Go shopping! Some people also find that celebrating (as well as commiserating) with fellow ketoers online in Facebook groups or on Instagram can help them keep the emphasis on the positive.

Don't Despair at Mistakes

On the flip side...if you do, perchance, have a slice of that colleague's birthday cake at the office party, don't beat yourself up. "You don't have to be perfect on the keto diet to experience real change and improvements in your health," says Axe. "A temporary slip here or there doesn't mean you won't make progress or that you should just give up. The best thing to do if it happens is to forgive yourself, move on and get back on track as quickly as possible, starting with the very next meal."

Get Your Beauty Sleep

Especially when you're just starting keto, the plan puts a little extra strain on your body as it learns to break down fatty acids into ketones for fuel. So give yourself a break and catch some extra shut-eye. Not only will this boost your immune system, but studies show that being sleep-deprived can lead to overeating. According to the National Sleep Foundation, when you don't get adequate rest, the level of the hunger hormone ghrelin in your blood spikes and the level of the appetite-suppressing hormone leptin falls. The result: It becomes harder to resist temptation and stay on the plan.

Visualize Your Goals

Give your imagination a workout, Axe suggests. "Write down a list of concrete goals and reasons that you want to make changes," he says. "It could be keeping excess weight off—or losing weight—for heart health, feeling consistent energy, boosting your mental clarity." Really picture what those results will look like and feel like, then tuck your list somewhere safe so that you can look at it often.

Reduce Stress

Lowering your stress levels helps you stick to keto in several ways. For one, you're less likely

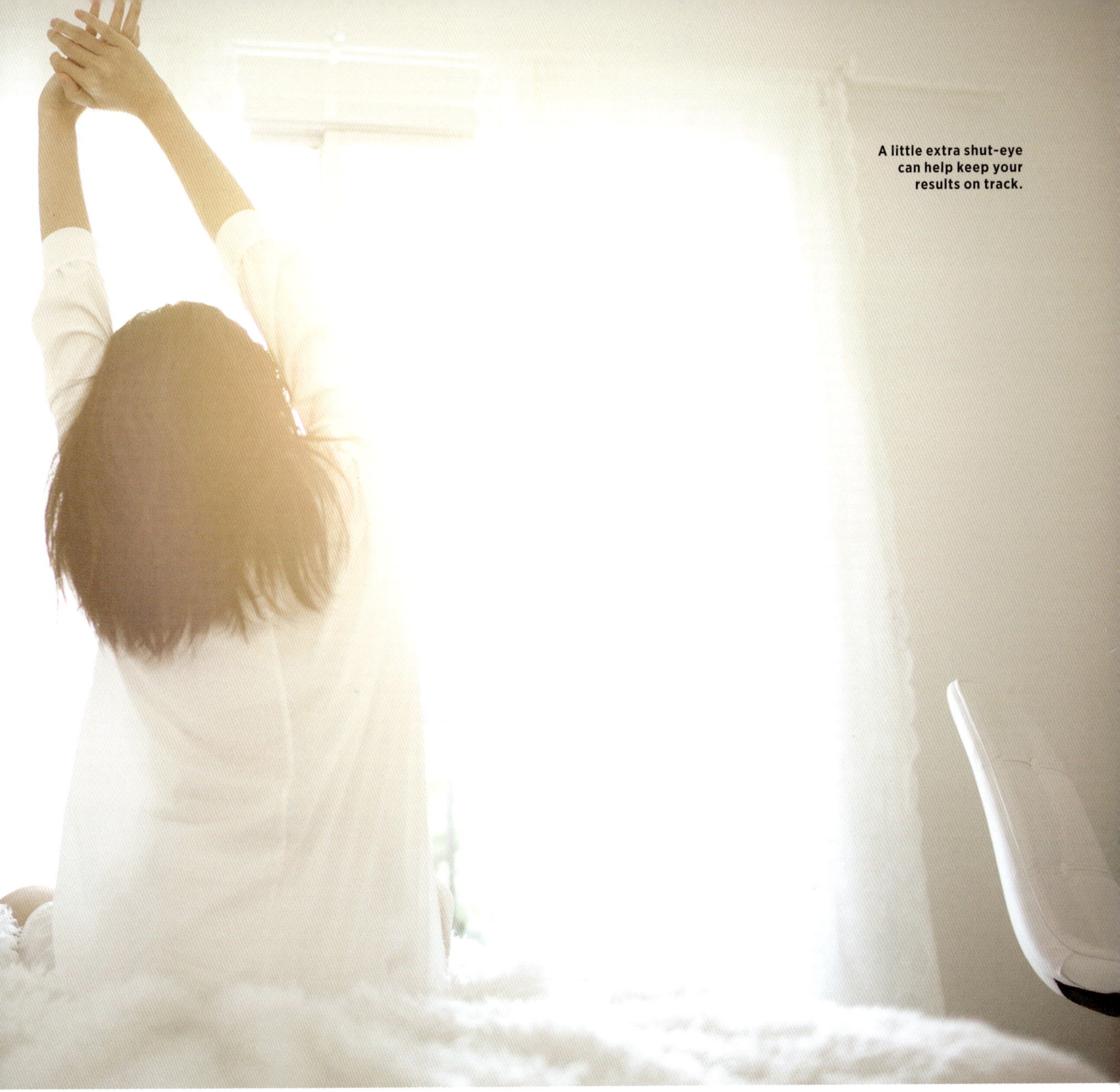

A little extra shut-eye can help keep your results on track.

to give in to emotional eating and dive into a pint of ice cream to relieve tension. Also, chronic stress raises levels of the hormone cortisol, which tells your body to store fat —a useful survival tactic in caveman days but counterproductive today. One approach is to use a meditation app (or join a meditation group) to learn mindfulness, which has been shown to strengthen emotional self-control. A 2013 study found that just two weeks of regular meditation practice helped smokers reduce their cigarette use by 60 percent. Brain scans of the participants revealed that meditation increased activity in areas related to self-control; experts believe the practice would have the same effect for dieters. Another stress-buster that packs a double punch: moderate exercise. Going for a half-hour walk daily is good for your mind and spirit, and will also help speed weight loss.

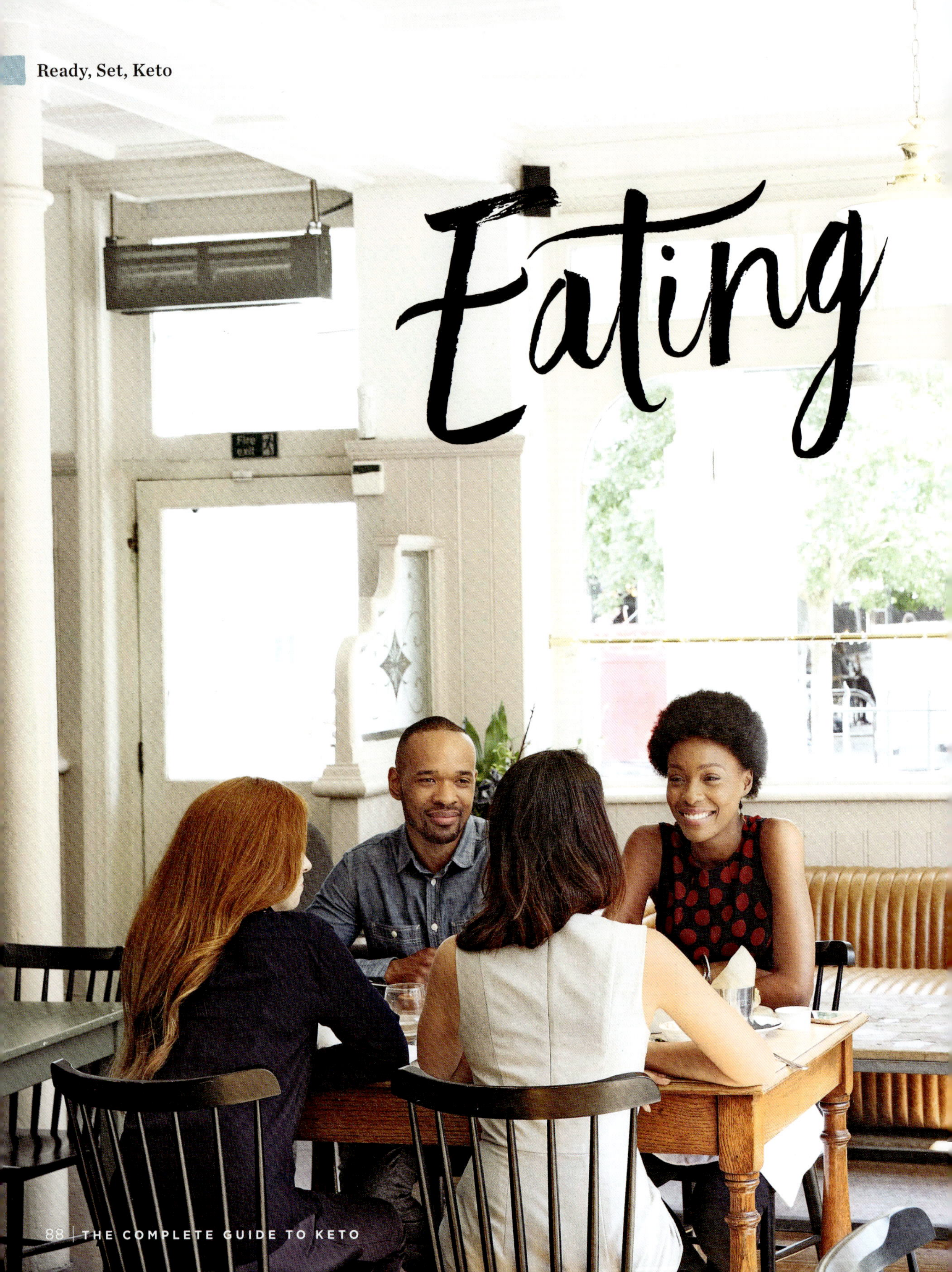

Eating

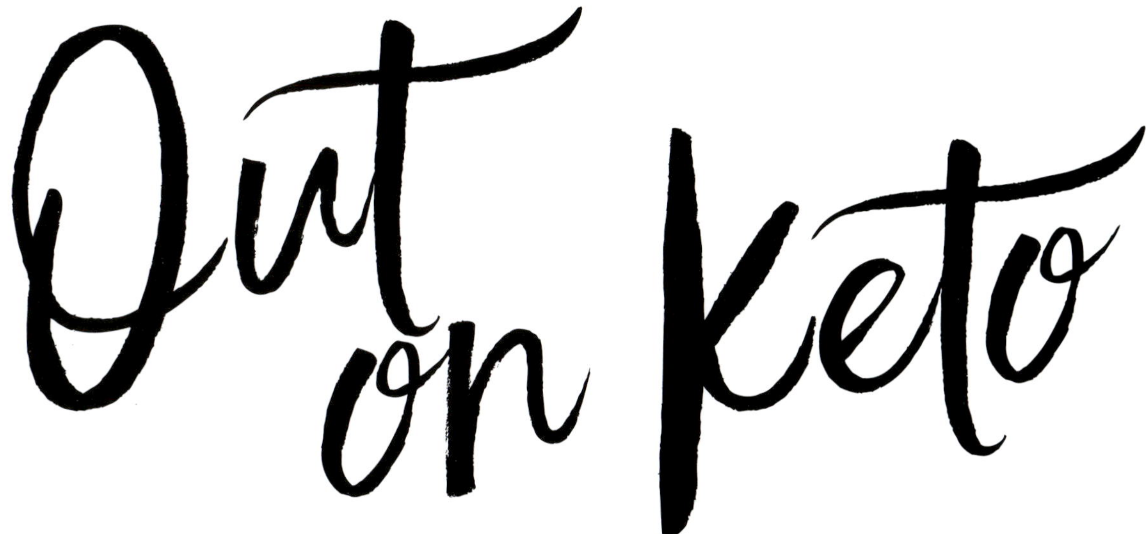

Out on Keto

EVERYONE NEEDS A SOCIAL LIFE, BUT RESTAURANTS CAN BE A CHALLENGE WHEN YOU'RE STICKING TO A KETO PLAN. WE BREAK DOWN HOW TO NAVIGATE YOUR MEALS OUT WITH FRIENDS OR FAMILY.

A GOOD (READ: HEALTHY) KETO PLAN IS founded on lots of homemade food—but everyone deserves to be treated to a restaurant meal occasionally. Yes, there are hurdles, but with this menu cheat sheet, you can dine out and totally stay on track.

First, some guidelines. "The easiest thing, always, is to stick with protein and vegetables," says Katherine Brooking, MS, RD, "for instance, a grilled chicken breast or a piece of salmon with a side of asparagus or spinach." Heavy sauces are always suspect, she adds. Although some—like béarnaise—are mostly fat, many have hidden starches used to add bulk or smoothness. And as for the infamous breadbasket: If the waiter insists on bringing one to the table, ask on the down-low if he can instead serve bread individually so you're not facing down a collection of carbs.

Pro Tips

Go Local Nonchain, locally owned restaurants are more likely to be flexible and make requested changes in dishes—especially if you pick a few favorite spots and become a known quantity (and good tipper).

Be Careful With Chinese Food
This delicious cuisine presents a particular challenge, for two reasons. Virtually everything is served with rice, and many sauces have hidden sugars and starches. Order grilled entrées and steamed vegetables—and say no to the rice.

Choose Sashimi Going for sushi? Sashimi is perfect—but avoid items with white rice, like sushi rolls, or anything fried, such as tempura.

Plan Ahead Most restaurants put their menus online, so you can look up your choices and avoid any last-minute temptations.

Get Creative Consider ordering outside the box and combining two or three appetizers rather than getting an entrée—or ask the waiter for a simple grilled fish plus veggies. Every chef knows how to do that!

Make It Your Cheat Meal If you've decided you can handle the occasional "cheat," plan it for your night out, suggests Brooking. You can get right back on your keto regimen the next morning.

ANNOTATED MENU FOR OPTIMUM KETO

STARTERS

CLAM CHOWDER

Soups are iffy—you don't know what's in there. Many "cream" soups use pureed rice or starches to thicken them up.

HUMMUS & PITA
Olives, paprika, pita

Hummus is made from chickpeas; like other legumes, they're outlawed on keto because of their high carb count.

CHICKEN WINGS
Your choice of: Buffalo, brown sugar, chipotle BBQ or sweet chili sauce

Wings can be great—if they're simply grilled or fried, not battered. Also, many BBQ sauces have hidden sugars.

BEEF CARPACCIO
Paper-thin sliced beef on a bed of arugula, shaved Parmesan

Great choice! You could even combine it with one or two other keto-friendly appetizers to make a full meal.

PUMPKIN RISOTTO
Baby arugula, sage, carrots, green peas, Parmesan cheese

Nope. Risotto = rice.

ARTISAN CHEESE PLANK
Selection of cheeses, pecans, melba toast, charcuterie

If you can resist the bread that comes with this (ask the waiter to leave it off the plate), cheese, salami and nuts can be a great choice.

ENTRÉES

CAESAR SALAD
Romaine, Parmesan, croutons, soft boiled egg, Caesar dressing

Caesar is a no—unless you can either resist the croutons or the chef will agree to leave them out.

CRISPY CHICKEN SALAD
Lettuce, tomato, red onions, mushrooms, feta cheese, vinaigrette

"Crispy" is code for "breaded and fried," so opt for something else.

STEAK SALAD
Hanger steak, romaine, red onion, red peppers, Irish cheddar, buttermilk dressing

A good choice, though dressings can have hidden sugars. Ask for olive oil and vinegar instead.

SALMON BURGER
Chopped salmon, red onion, peppers, ginger aioli, Parker House bun

This can be keto, if you order it without the bun (ask for lettuce leaves to use in its place).

VEGETABLE BURGER
House-made wild rice–black bean burger, spiced hummus, seeded brioche bun

Ah, veggie burgers sound so healthy...but on keto they don't work. The rice, beans, hummus and bun are all loaded with carbs.

BRICK-ROASTED HALF CHICKEN
Farro, fingerling potatoes, green beans

All good—except for the potatoes and farro, an ancient wheat. Ask to sub in extra green beans or a side salad.

FISH & CHIPS
Ale-battered cod fillet, tartar sauce, garlic-lemon aioli, house fries

Fish is great, but a "battered" fillet plus fries puts this off the keto menu.

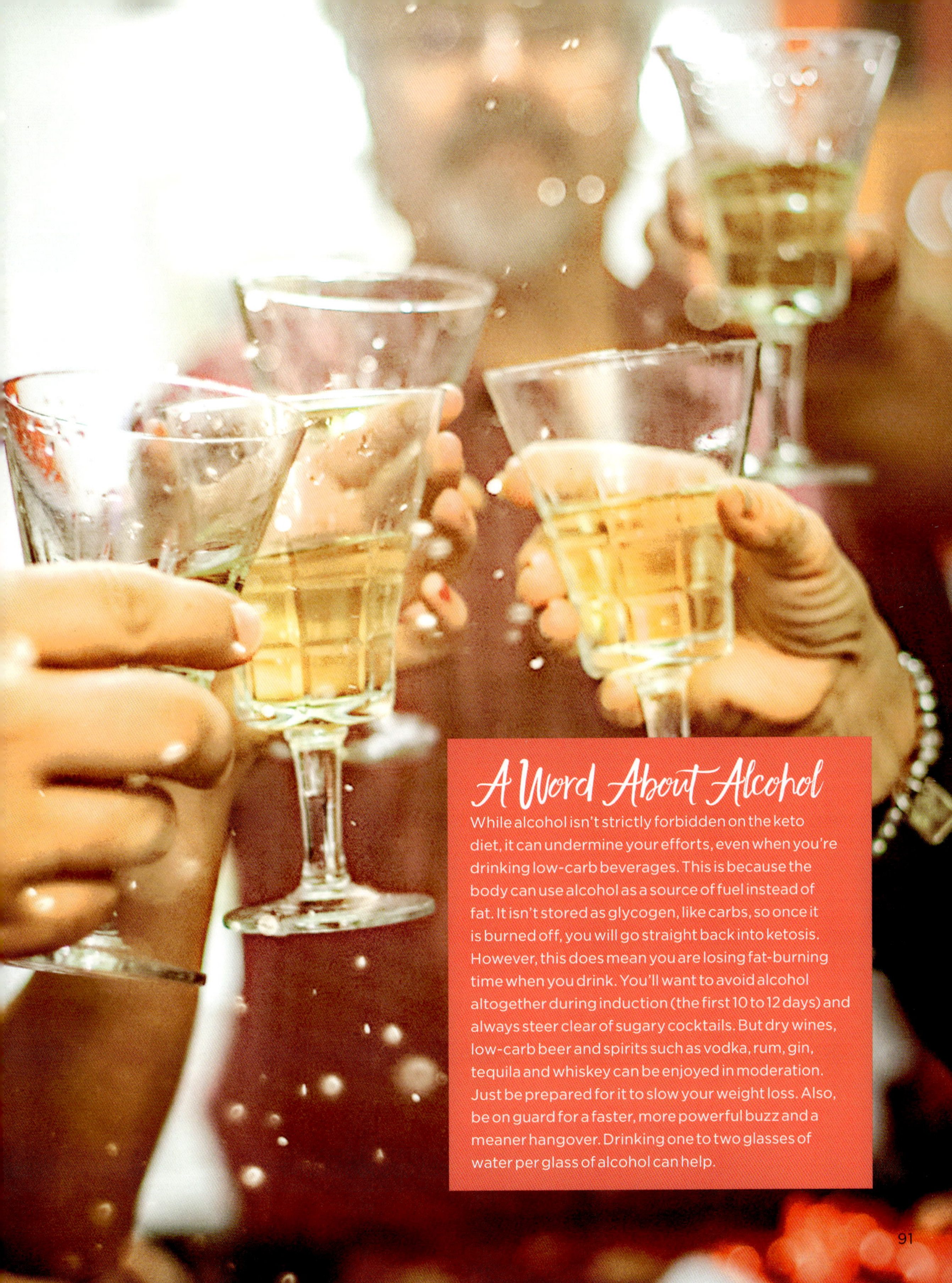

A Word About Alcohol

While alcohol isn't strictly forbidden on the keto diet, it can undermine your efforts, even when you're drinking low-carb beverages. This is because the body can use alcohol as a source of fuel instead of fat. It isn't stored as glycogen, like carbs, so once it is burned off, you will go straight back into ketosis. However, this does mean you are losing fat-burning time when you drink. You'll want to avoid alcohol altogether during induction (the first 10 to 12 days) and always steer clear of sugary cocktails. But dry wines, low-carb beer and spirits such as vodka, rum, gin, tequila and whiskey can be enjoyed in moderation. Just be prepared for it to slow your weight loss. Also, be on guard for a faster, more powerful buzz and a meaner hangover. Drinking one to two glasses of water per glass of alcohol can help.

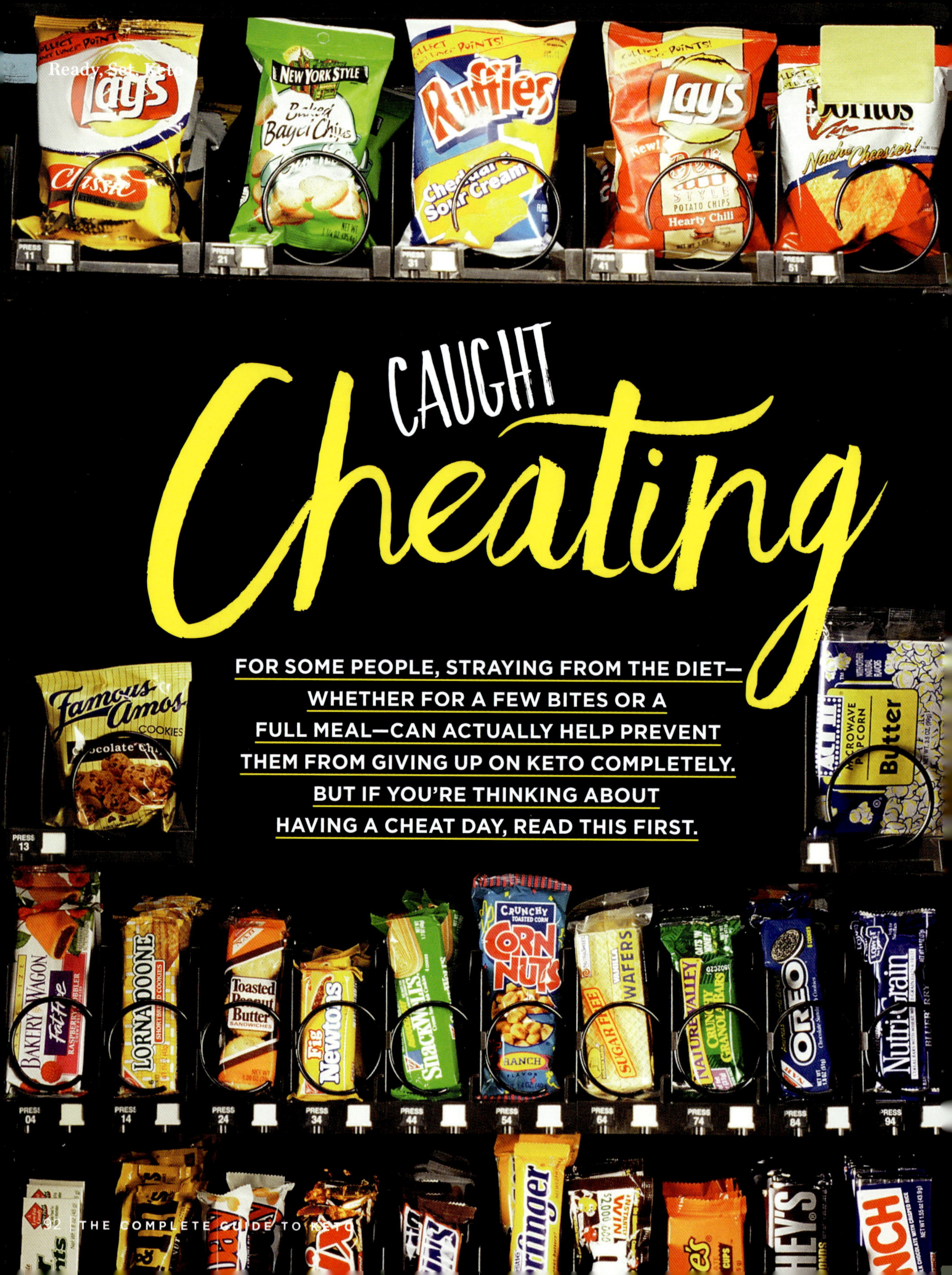

CAUGHT *Cheating*

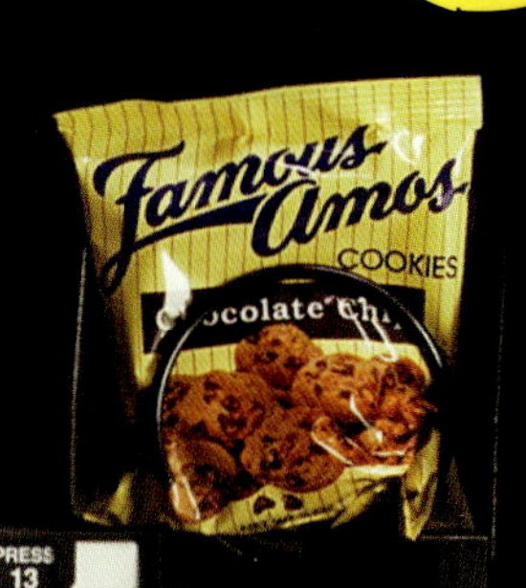

FOR SOME PEOPLE, STRAYING FROM THE DIET—WHETHER FOR A FEW BITES OR A FULL MEAL—CAN ACTUALLY HELP PREVENT THEM FROM GIVING UP ON KETO COMPLETELY. BUT IF YOU'RE THINKING ABOUT HAVING A CHEAT DAY, READ THIS FIRST.

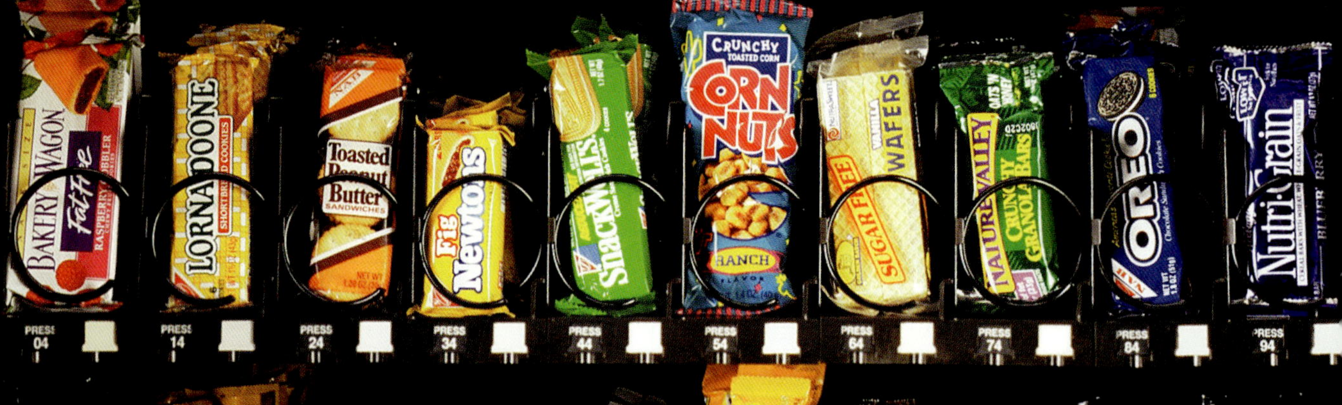

WE GET IT. When there's a gooey slice of pecan pie or a basket of freshly baked rolls staring you down, it can be difficult to remain faithful to a keto diet. And after days, weeks or even months of staying on plan, you may wonder: How bad is a cheat day, really?

In fact, many keto followers swear by cheat days and say that being able to indulge in carbs every now and then actually makes it easier to stick to the diet in the long run. But before you go breaking up with keto—even if it's only for a meal—read on to find out how adding in extra carbs could impact your weight loss and even your health.

Just like with relationships, keto will work better if you don't cheat.

The Dirt on Cheating

There's no getting around it. If you stray too far from keto-friendly foods, you'll fall out of ketosis. "If you eat carbs, your body will use them for fuel," says Amanda A. Kostro Miller, RD, LDN, a registered dietician in Chicago. That means that whether you have one binge meal or even a small non-keto treat, if it pushes you over your net carb goal, you'll fall out of ketosis. And getting back on the bandwagon isn't always easy.

"You may have to work really hard the next several days to get back to ketosis," explains Kostro Miller. Everyone is different, and the exact amount of time it will take to get back to ketosis depends on your level of carb restriction and the amount of carbohydrates you ate during your cheat day. And here's a real bummer: Kostro Miller says you could even experience the keto flu again.

Still Tempted to Cheat?

Ideally, Kostro Miller says even your "cheat days" should be within ketogenic guidelines, otherwise you can quickly jump out of ketosis. Keto cookies and bars, nut butter and keto-friendly candy can be lifesavers. (In fact, four pieces of Life Savers hard candy can soothe a struggling sweet tooth without steering you off a keto diet.) Other snacks such as keto-friendly cheese puffs and crackers can feed the need to eat indulgently without kicking you out of ketosis.

Rolling your eyes? We get it—those keto snacks are far from a slice of pizza or mashed potatoes and gravy. And like others, you may find that having the occasional flexibility to go off-plan could help you stick with keto—and that's OK! "If you want to follow the keto diet long-term, yet still want some true cheat days with non-keto foods, make sure you are OK with choosing to go out of ketosis on cheat days," urges Kostro Miller. "This way if you do jump out of ketosis, you're doing so on your own terms."

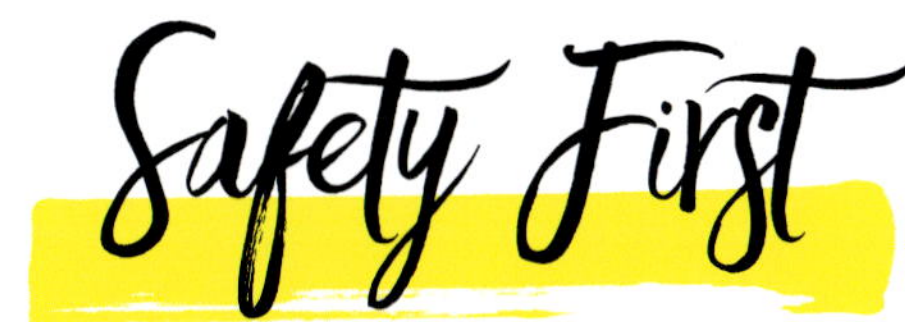

Falling out of ketosis isn't the only cheat-day concern. A new (albeit small) Canadian study shows that veering from a ketogenic diet may damage blood vessels. Blasting your body with sugar appears to undo some of the positive health benefits of living in ketosis. As a result, researchers advise against cheating—even just a little bit—when following a keto diet, especially if you're living a keto lifestyle for medical reasons.

While the data recommends against it, if you are tempted to take a break from keto, try to tread lightly. A small bite or sip (rather than an entire bowl or glass) of a non-keto food or drink may limit the negative health effects of cheating. "Sticking as close to your carb goal as possible is the best way to lessen the effects of cheating on a keto diet," says dietician Amanda Kostro Miller.

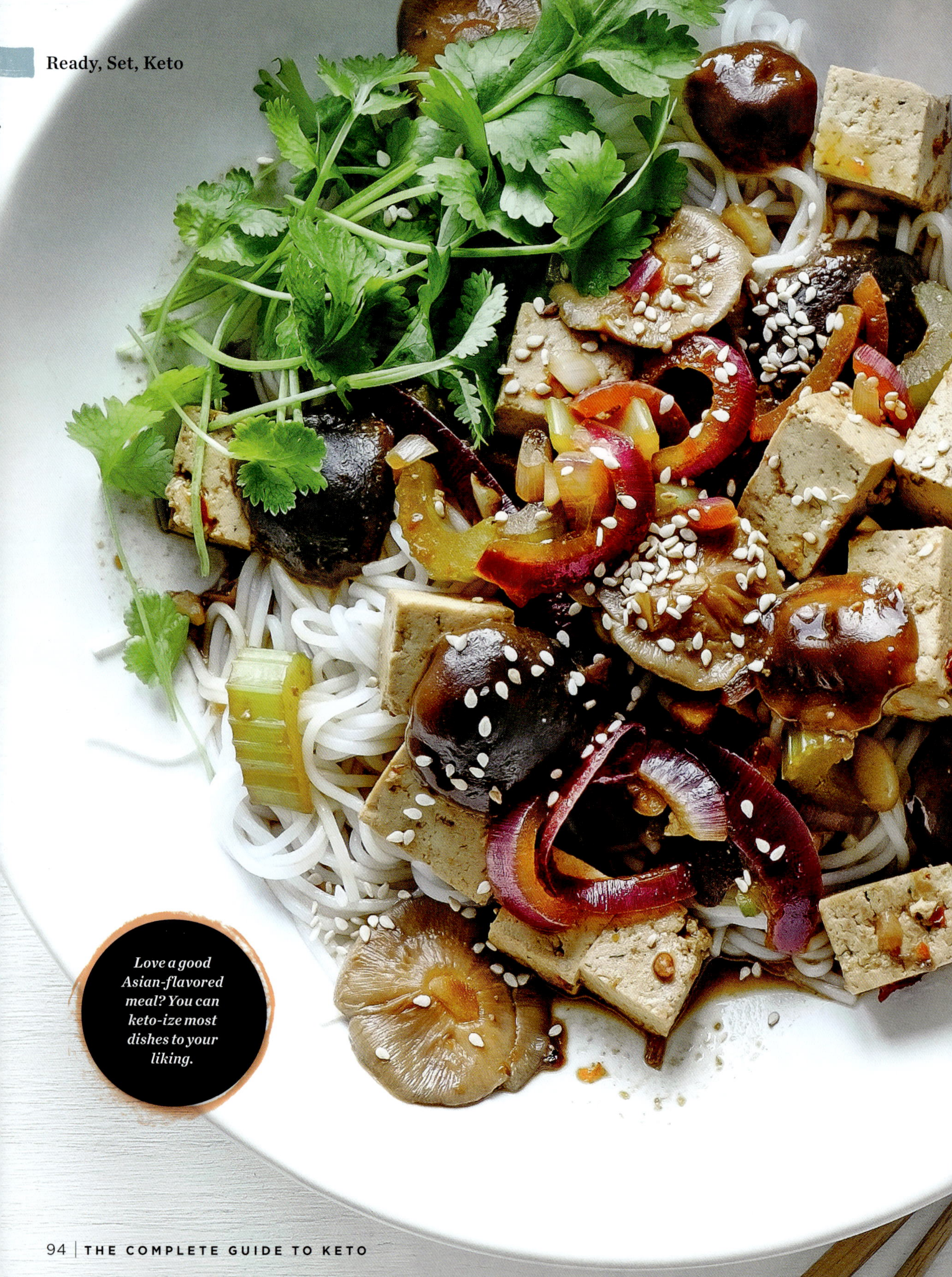

Love a good Asian-flavored meal? You can keto-ize most dishes to your liking.

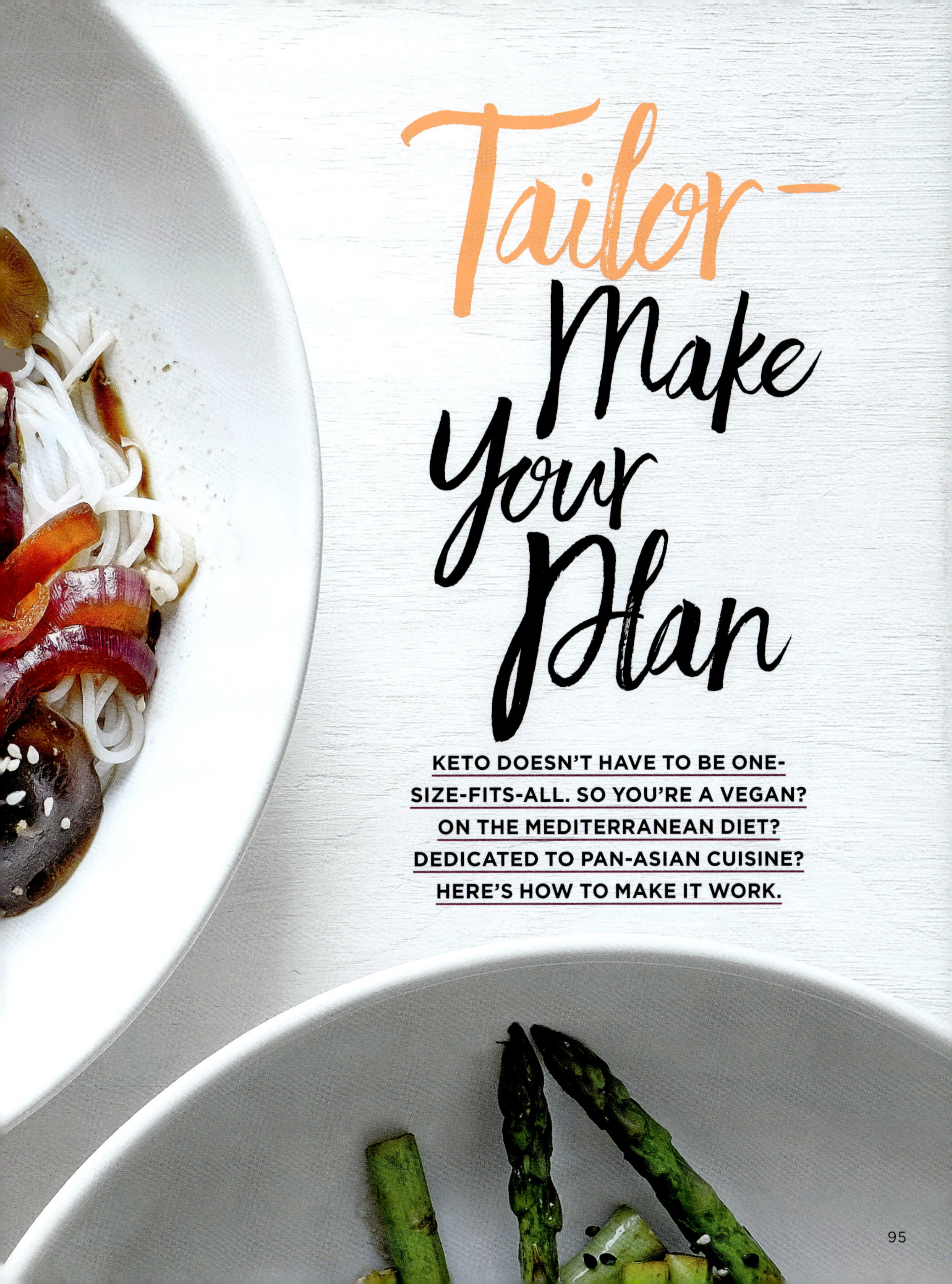

Tailor-Make Your Plan

KETO DOESN'T HAVE TO BE ONE-SIZE-FITS-ALL. SO YOU'RE A VEGAN? ON THE MEDITERRANEAN DIET? DEDICATED TO PAN-ASIAN CUISINE? HERE'S HOW TO MAKE IT WORK.

Vegan

Many people assume that "vegan" and "keto" just can't go together, because they picture a plate full of meat or fish. "It's not as hard as you think!" says Liz MacDowell, a certified holistic-nutrition consultant specializing in whole-food diets, food allergies/intolerances, special diets and nutritional support for digestive health who also runs the blog Meat Free Keto. "People ask, 'But where do you get your pro...' and I stop them right there. If you've been vegetarian or vegan for any amount of time, you've probably realized that there's protein in basically everything, even vegetables. If you do want to pump up your protein intake a little, you can add some nutritional yeast to your meals. It usually contains around 3 grams of protein per tablespoon and is very low-carb. There are also plenty of vegan protein powders on the market." Not to mention that the main point of keto is not protein but fat, partly because any excess protein is converted to glucose by your body. It may actually be harder to do Paleo or Atkins as a vegan than to do keto, because of those diets' emphasis on protein. For keto, fat—not protein—is where it's at.

"Oils are a vegan-keto freebie," says MacDowell, "because all oils are low in carbs, and are super fatty. You'll want to have a good-quality bottle of olive oil on hand, along with coconut oil. And oils contain vitamins, minerals and other phytochemicals when they're not overly processed—so they're not just 'empty calories.' I remind people of this, because when I was first getting into healthy eating years ago, it was drilled into my head that I should avoid using oil in my food, the reason being that there was no nutritional benefit and it was high in calories." While it's true that oils are high-calorie, that's not a concern on keto, which isn't a calorie-counting program. And most importantly, fats and oils form the basis of keto. In addition to using enough oil, MacDowell suggests looking to whole-food sources like coconut, avocados, olives, nuts and seeds.

If you want to ease into a vegan-keto program, try replacing high-carb foods over time. "If you eat a lot of pasta and rice-based dishes, for example, you could start by replacing all the pasta with zucchini noodles ["zoodles"] and the rice with cauliflower rice," says MacDowell. "Then start eliminating other high-carb foods, like bread and potatoes, and shift to eating lower-carb fruits, like berries. It's a fairly sustainable way of eating, and you end up developing new habits over time." Keto vegans can also choose fatty plant foods, advises Megha Barot, co-founder of KetoConnect: "Things like hemp hearts, chia seeds, avocados, coconut and low-carb nuts, like macadamias, walnuts or pecans. A great breakfast is to soak hemp hearts and chia seeds in coconut cream overnight—it's like a delicious keto 'oatmeal.'"

EXPERIMENT WITH PASTA SUBSTITUTES, LIKE SHIRATAKI NOODLES MADE FROM THE KONJAC YAM.

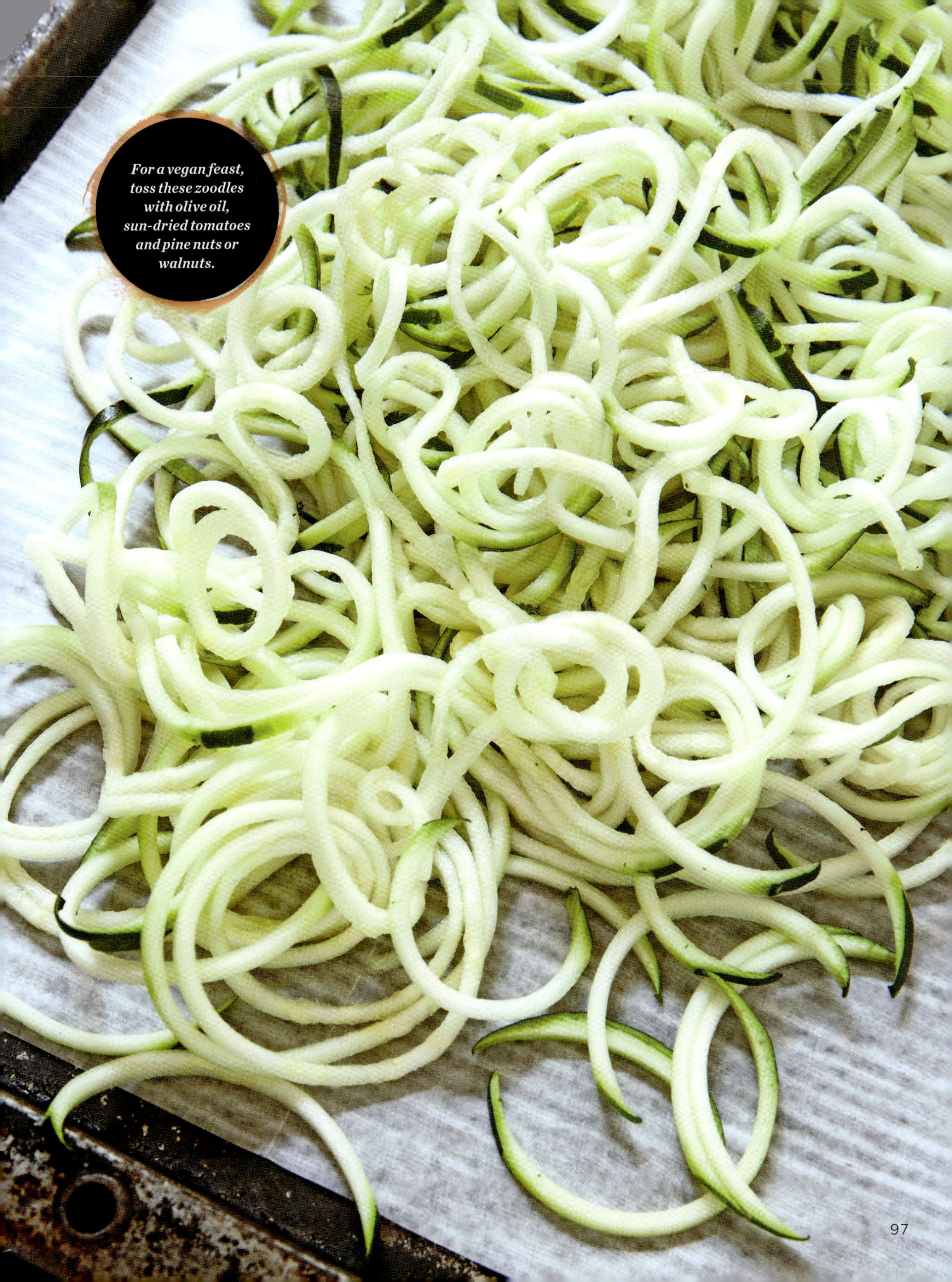
For a vegan feast, toss these zoodles with olive oil, sun-dried tomatoes and pine nuts or walnuts.

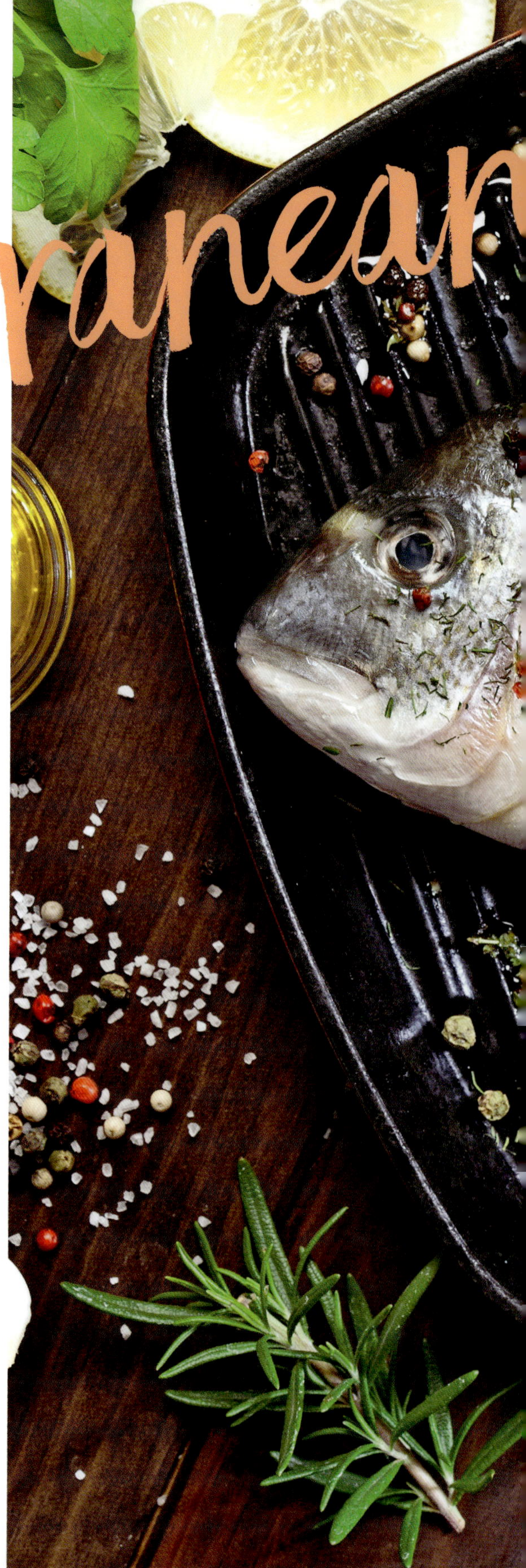

Mediterranean

The fish- and vegetable-rich Mediterranean diet can dovetail quite well with keto—it's mainly a matter of favoring fish over red meat and indulging in plenty of olive oil and leafy greens. A recent study of people following a combined keto and traditional Mediterranean plan found successful long-term weight loss and improvements in health risk factors like cholesterol, triglycerides and glucose levels. Perhaps most important, the study emphasized, compliance was very high. You could read that as saying, the diet was delicious and easy to follow—and when you see the list of foods on the diet, that's not surprising: poultry, fish, some beef and veal, raw and cooked green vegetables, eggs and cheeses like Parmesan.

"On Mediterranean, you go easier on things like butter and red meat," says Matt Gaedke, co-creator of KetoConnect. "But there's a nice crossover of the two with vegetable oils, such as olive, avocado and coconut, as well as seafood. Nuts and seeds are also a great way to up your fats and stay within the confines of both keto and Mediterranean."

Another thing the two diets share is an emphasis on whole foods and home cooking over processed foods, which are shunned on both regimens. The Mediterranean plan has certainly seemed to work for people who live in the Greek Islands, one of the so-called Blue Zones where people enjoy extraordinarily long and healthy lives. Picture a plate of grilled fish finished with olive oil, a salad of spinach, tomatoes, cucumbers and feta cheese, with a side of cured olives.

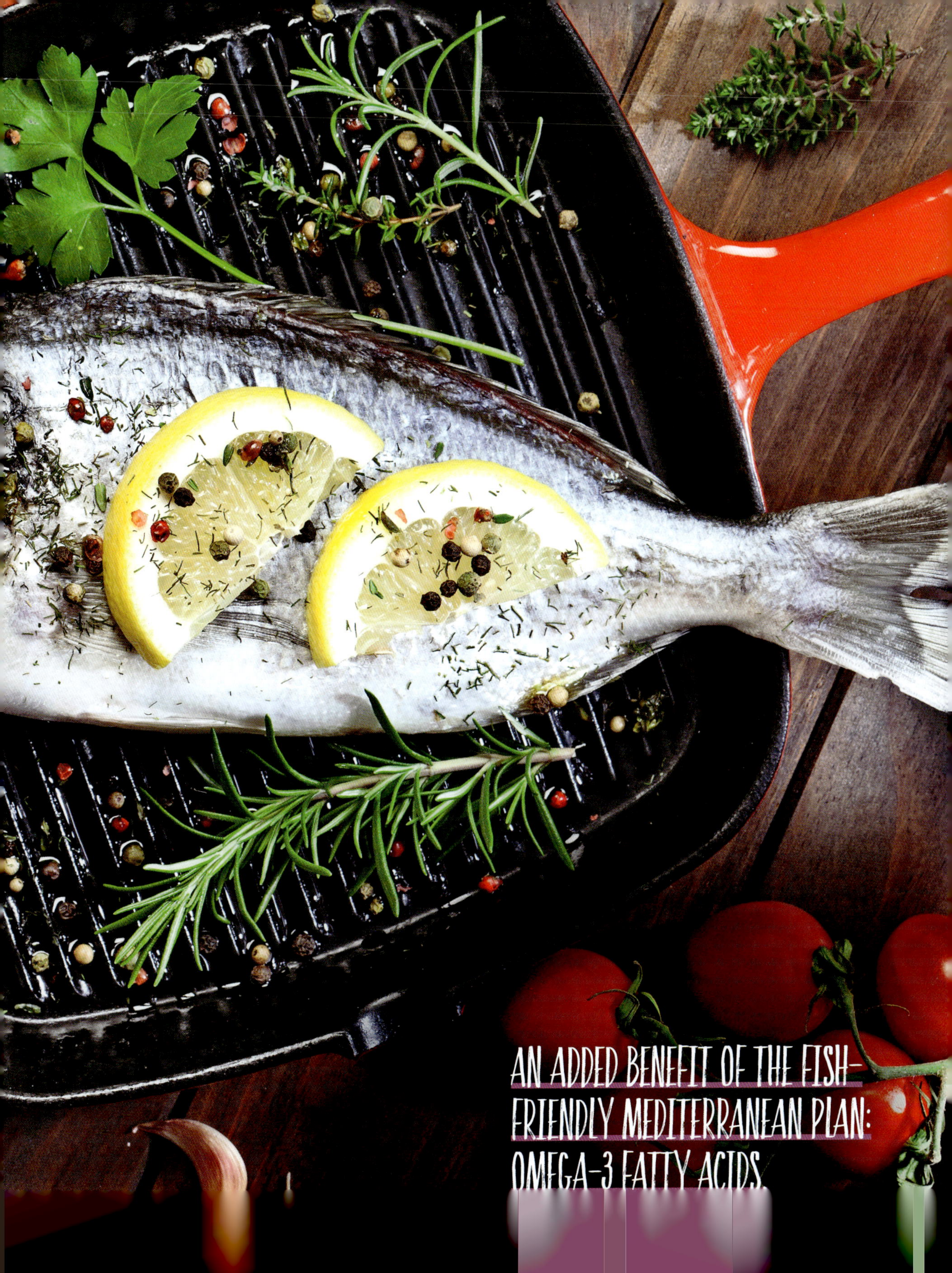
AN ADDED BENEFIT OF THE FISH-
FRIENDLY MEDITERRANEAN PLAN:
OMEGA-3 FATTY ACIDS.

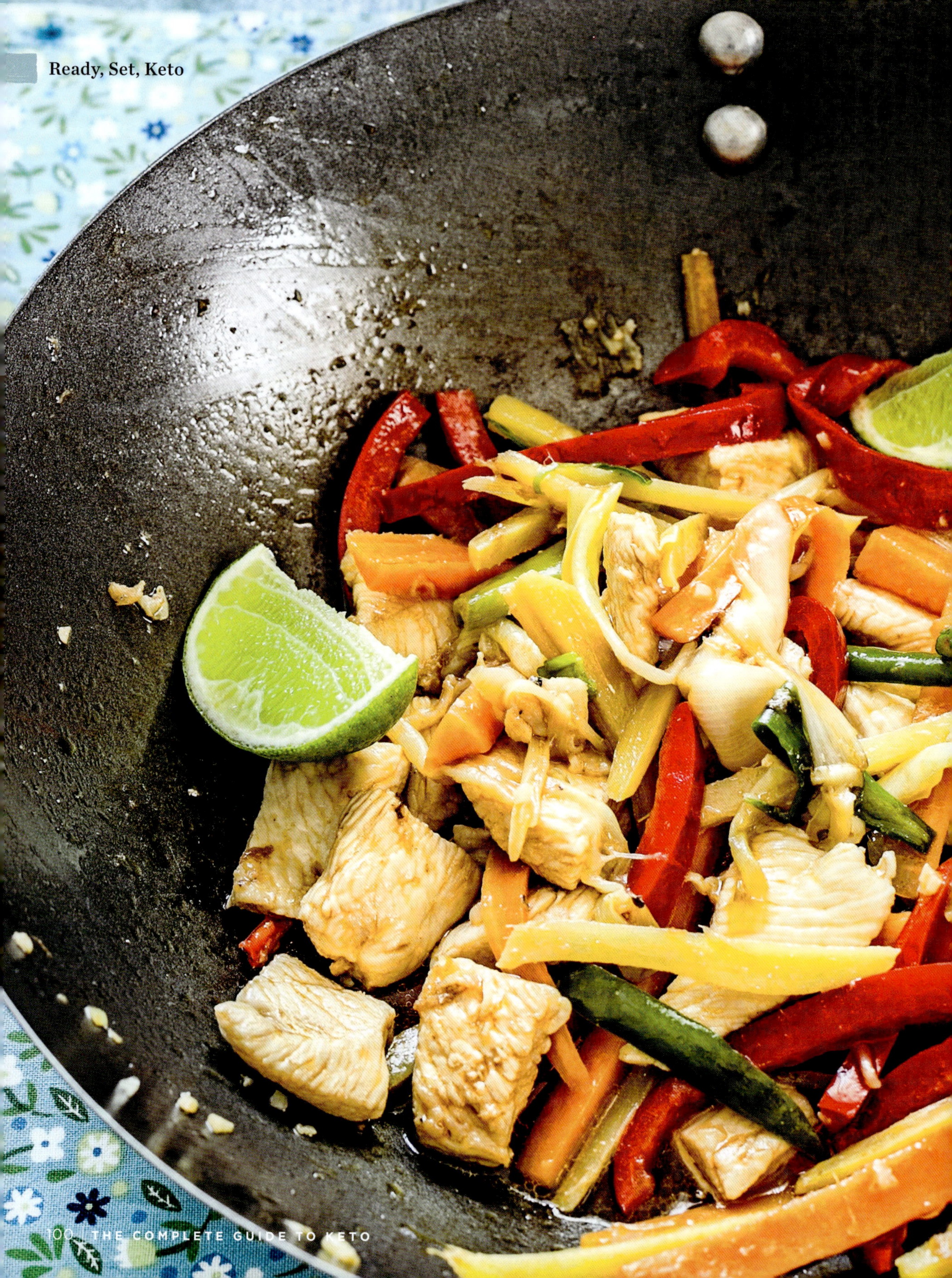

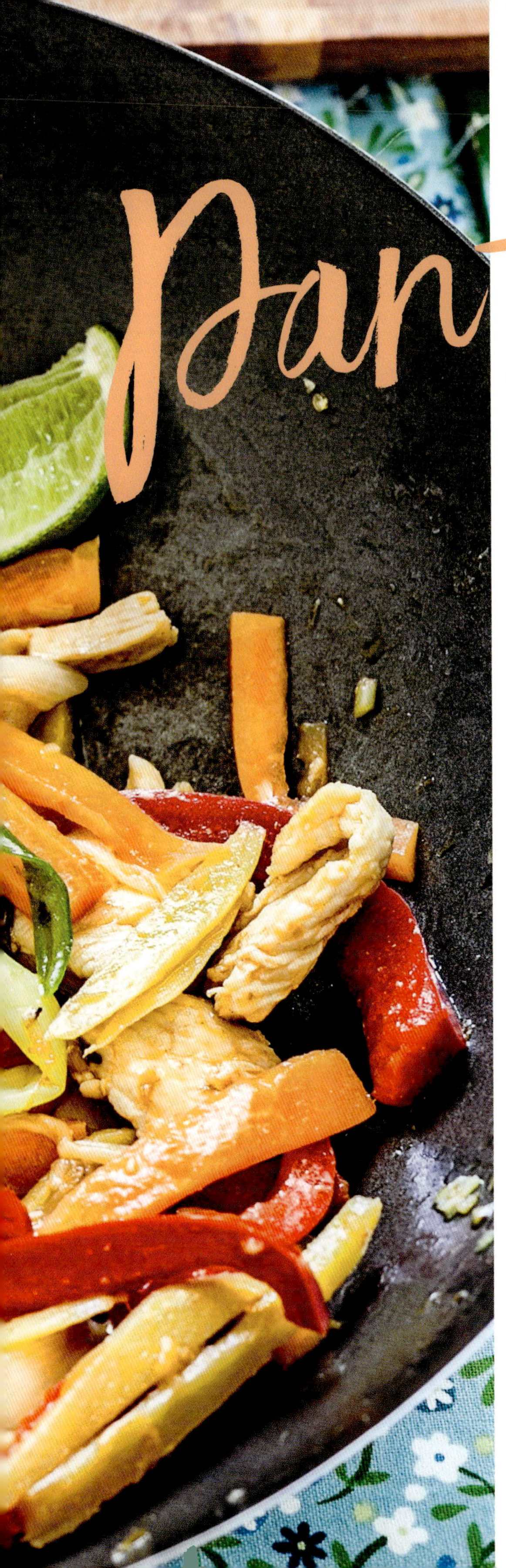

Pan-Asian

Asian on keto can be tough sometimes, because there's so much great food, whether it's Thai or Indian or Chinese, that's available and tempting in restaurants," says Gaedke. "But a lot of restaurants add sugar or use cornstarch or breading without listing those ingredients on the menu, so you might not realize it." You can deal with that by asking the waiter what's in the dish, requesting sauces or gravies on the side, and getting extra steamed vegetables to add volume and texture, Gaedke says. But Asian keto is also easily accomplished at home.

Think stir-fries and/or curried chicken, served over cauliflower rice. Or use your cauliflower rice to make a delicious fried "rice" with eggs or shredded pork. You do need to keep an eye out for any added sugars in teriyaki sauce or coconut milk, though. "Make sure to use unsweetened canned coconut milk or heavy cream to make a gravy or curry," says Gaedke. "Stick with lower-carb veggies, like broccoli, asparagus and green beans, and amp up the flavor with garlic and shallots." Fresh ginger and sesame oil are also flavor boosters. And remember: Any kind of delicious Asian filling can be served in butter lettuce as wraps, so you can still have your moo shoo pork, just minus the pancakes.

THOUGH BELL PEPPERS ARE ALLOWED ON KETO, THEY CONTAIN MORE CARBS THAN LEAFY GREEN VEGGIES, SO DON'T GO OVERBOARD.

Working Out on Keto

JUST SWITCHED TO A LOW-CARB LIFESTYLE? HERE'S HOW TO KEEP FIT.

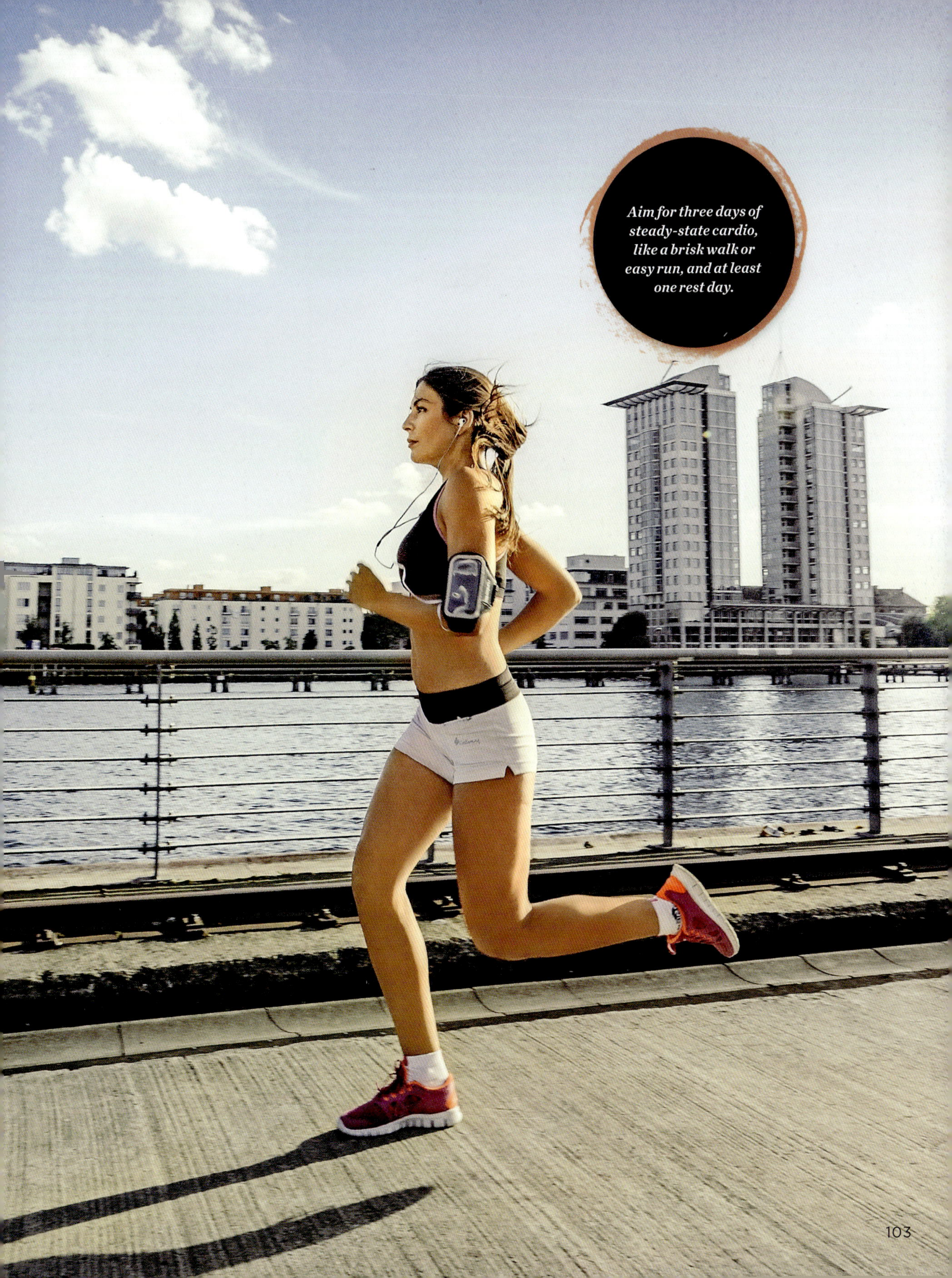
Aim for three days of steady-state cardio, like a brisk walk or easy run, and at least one rest day.

IF YOU'RE NEW TO THE KETO DIET, you might ask yourself: How will my diet affect my regular fitness routine? Do I need to do anything differently? While you should always consult your doctor before making drastic changes to your diet and workout plan, these are the basic rules to follow when it comes to exercising as a ketoer.

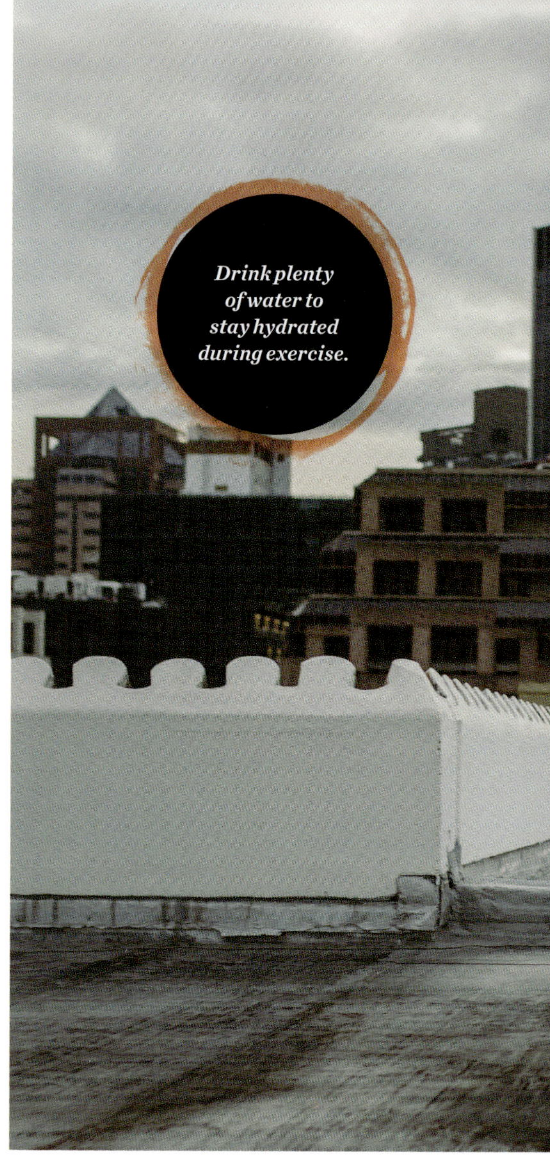

Drink plenty of water to stay hydrated during exercise.

Don't Try Anything New

When you first make the switch over to the keto diet, it's likely that you'll experience "keto flu," symptoms, says Jim White, CPT, RD. You may feel mentally foggy and low in energy while your body transitions to burning more fat as fuel. "Don't perform exercises that may require a quick reaction," he says. This could be anything from road cycling (where being alert is critical) to a long, challenging hike. "Avoid trying new exercises for the first few weeks. The body is still trying to adjust, and [you don't want to] overwhelm it."

In General, Avoid High-Intensity Exercises

"High intensity [interval training] or HIIT can have negative effects when used in combination with the keto diet," says White. When you have an extremely low intake of carbohydrates and your body is put into a starved state, "muscle cells become deprived of the sugar that's needed to have enough energy for these types of exercises." This means that any type of activity that requires a significant burst of energy within the first two minutes—like sprinting or powerlifting—may not be safe or beneficial.

Ironman and keto athlete Ramsey Bergeron, CPT, recommends focusing on resistance training and lower-intensity cardio. "You need resistance training to maintain and build muscle to keep your metabolism up."

Fuel Your Body the Right Way

When you're starting and maintaining this plan, it's critical to fuel your body, depending on the type of exercise you're doing. "Gauge your food choices and macronutrient ratios based on the exercise that you want to perform," says White. If you do want to incorporate higher-intensity training into your regimen, you can slightly adjust your carbohydrate intake for a "targeted keto diet."

Although everyone's body is different, the general guidelines dictate that you should consume 15 to 30 grams of carbohydrates about 30 minutes before high-intensity or anaerobic exercise, and roughly 30 grams of carbohydrates 30 minutes after exercise, to allow your body to properly recover. This will give you the energy you need to perform higher-intensity workouts;

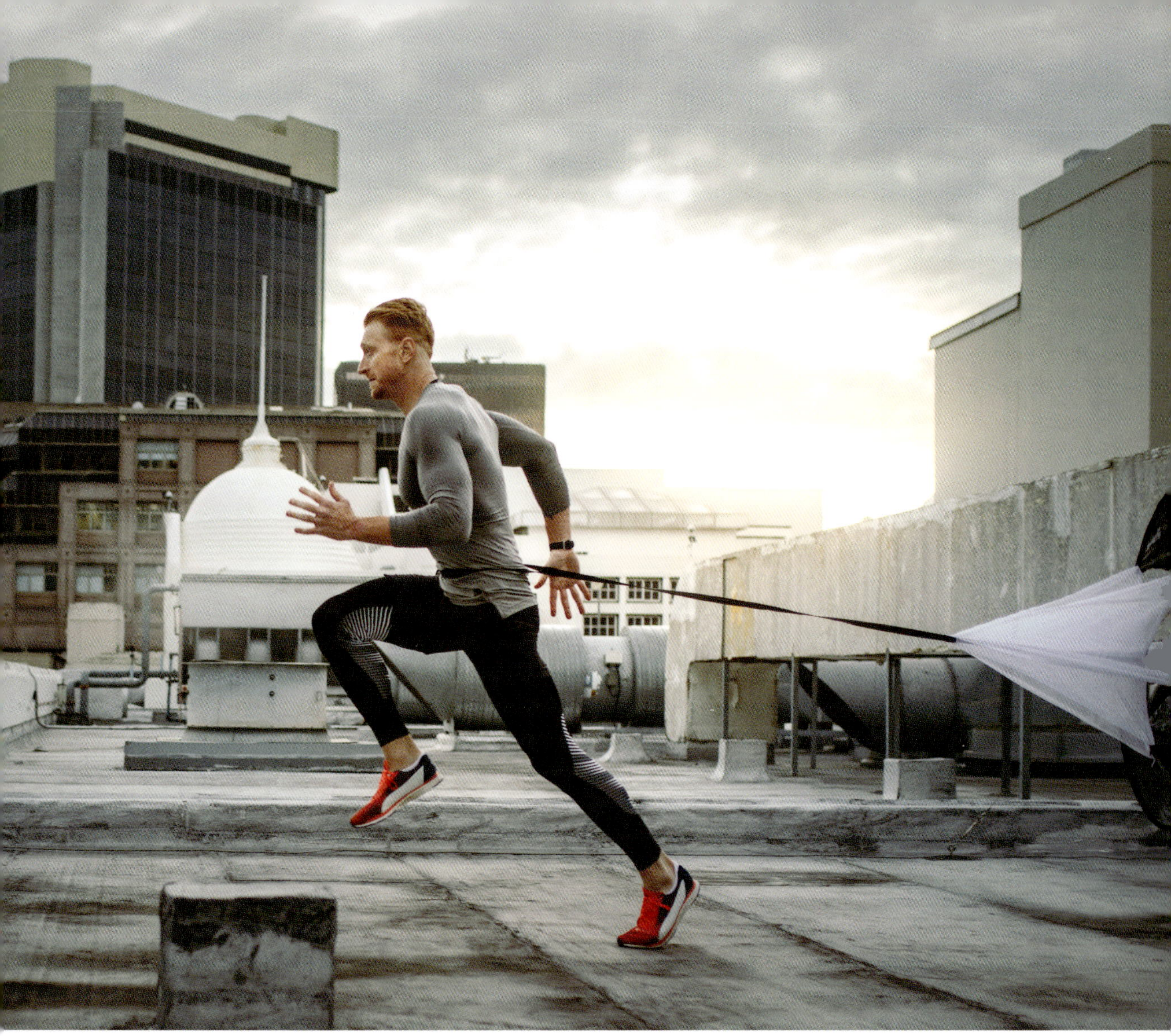

on days when you are not performing high-intensity exercise, stick to your regular keto diet. Experiment with your carb intake around exercise to learn what keeps you in ketosis.

While training for and competing in Ironman competitions, Bergeron fuels his body according to his heart rate. Although he spends most of the race in fat-burning mode, during a high-intensity portion (like swimming), his body may shift to burning sugar—so he takes gels to avoid crashing later. "Doing an Ironman is an incredibly challenging event, and having an expert nutrition coach to help you is crucial."

ONCE YOUR BODY IS FULLY KETO-ADAPTED, YOU MAY WANT TO TAKE ON MORE INTENSE, ENDURANCE-BASED WORKOUTS THAT WILL USE MORE FAT AS FUEL.

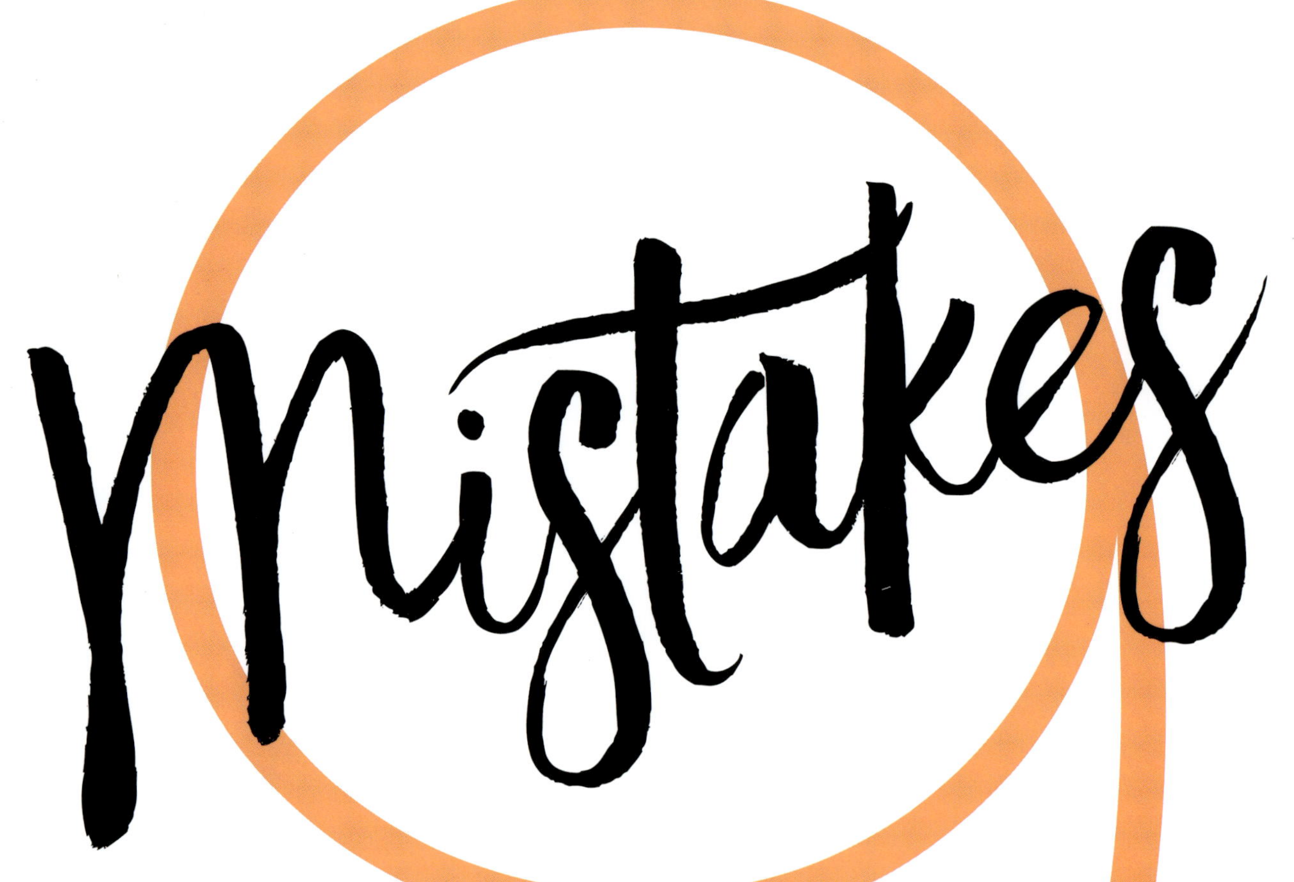

YOU MAY BE MAKING

SIMPLE STRATEGIES CAN HELP YOU GET THE MOST OUT OF THE DIET.

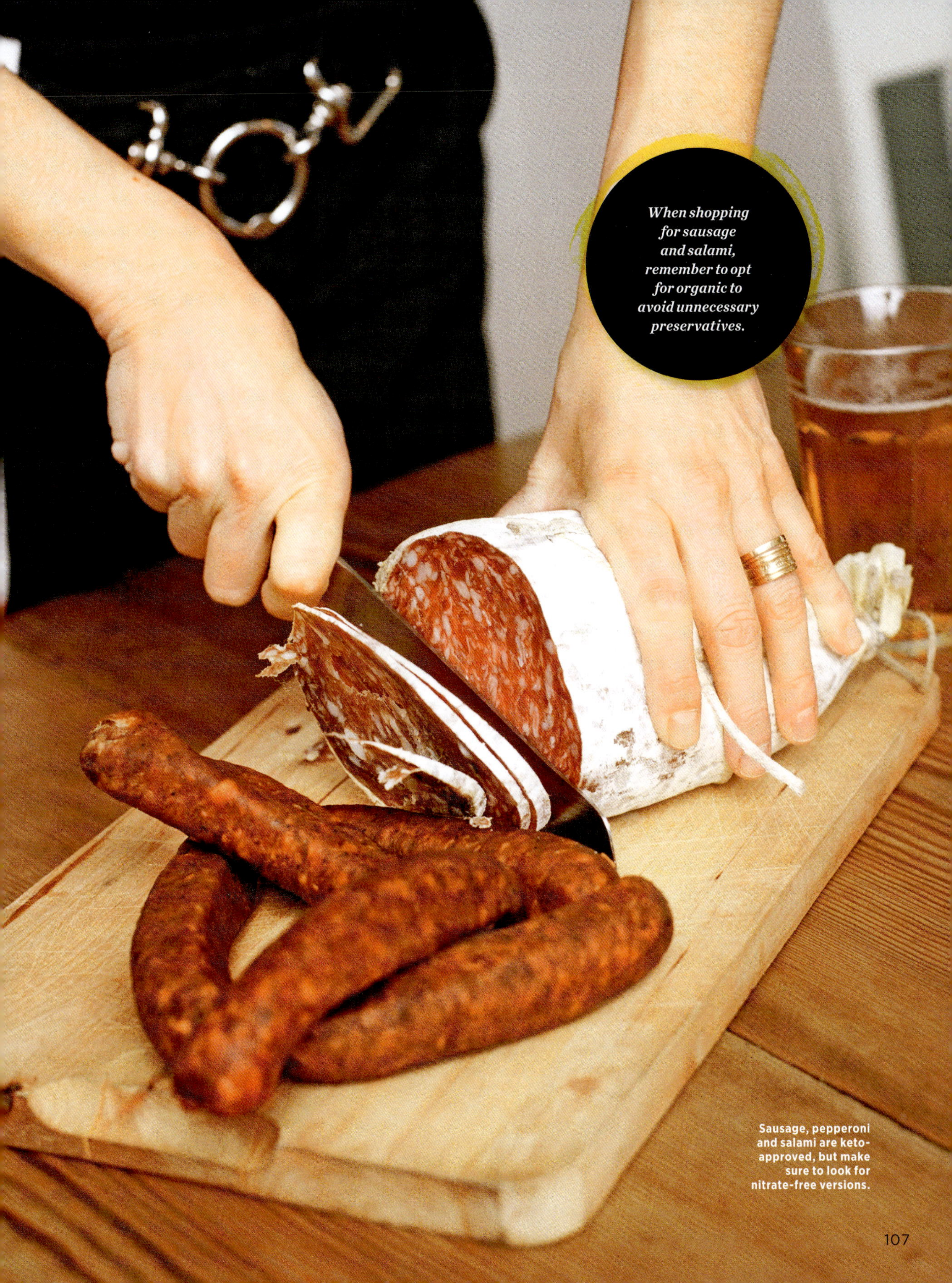

When shopping for sausage and salami, remember to opt for organic to avoid unnecessary preservatives.

Sausage, pepperoni and salami are keto-approved, but make sure to look for nitrate-free versions.

DESPITE ITS RECENT SURGE IN popularity, the keto diet is widely misunderstood. For starters, there is the complicated physiological process the body has to go through to get into ketosis. Since it's low-carb, many people associate it with Atkins or Paleo. But not all low-carb diets will put your body into ketosis, says Brit Inez, body-goals specialist and transformation coach. Keto comes with its own set of rules that are worth following. Here, the most common missteps dieters make when going keto, and how to fix them.

1 Jumping Straight Into a Keto Plan

If you regularly consume a Western diet of red and processed meats, prepackaged carb-heavy foods and convenience foods, you might think that a ketogenic diet won't be too hard—you'll simply cut carbs, right? Not so fast: Switching straight from a diet high in processed foods into a strict ketogenic diet is a disaster waiting to happen, says holistic nutritionist Jennifer Hanway. "A ketogenic diet can be tricky for even the healthiest eater to navigate, so making gradual changes is a more realistic option for success," Hanway says. She recommends transitioning through a Whole30- or Paleo-style diet first, where you'll begin by following a lower-carb plan, and then eventually switch over to a full ketogenic diet. This allows you to become familiar with a whole-foods approach (including healthy proteins and low-carb veggies), ensuring consistency and balance within your nutrition plan. "Once these approaches are adopted, sticking to a keto diet will be much easier—and symptoms of the 'keto flu' [nausea, tiredness, brain fog] should be nonexistent," says Hanway.

2 Thinking You'll Eat Unlimited Amounts of Cheese and Bacon

While the ketogenic diet calls for an unusually high recommended daily dose of fat, it's worth noting that not all fat is created equal. Before you start chowing down on bunless bacon cheeseburgers daily, know that this could cause issues with inflammation and blood sugar levels. "One of the benefits of a ketogenic diet is its ability to lower systemic inflammation, but processed meats and dairy can cause inflammation to rise—not to mention being high in sodium and nitrates," explains Hanway. "Additionally, consuming dairy products can cause a spike in our insulin levels, raising blood glucose...which is the opposite of what a ketogenic diet is intended to do." Keep processed meats to a minimum and choose nitrate-free options whenever possible, says Hanway. Eat full-fat cheese and make sure to count your macros in an app or program to stay within daily goals.

3 Overdoing It on Protein

Many individuals eat too much protein on the keto plan, mistaking it for an Atkins-style diet, explains nutritionist Ann Louise Gittleman, PhD, CNS, author of *Radical Metabolism*. "Since fat is the primary source of fuel, less protein may actually be required for maintaining lean muscle mass," says Gittleman. "Heavy-duty protein is hard on the kidneys." Instead of piling your plate with protein, she recommends limiting your intake to about 60 to 100 grams daily, spread throughout the day.

4 Guesstimating Your Carbohydrate Intake

It's important to track your carb intake so that you can ensure your body reaches ketosis. The recommendation of 20 to 50 grams of carbs a day varies from person to person, depending on their size, activity level, body composition and insulin sensitivity. "It can be very easy to 'spill over' and switch the body back to glucose-burning mode if you eat too many carbs," says Hanway. "That's why it's so important to limit carbohydrate-containing keto staples such as nuts, seeds and avocados and ensure that the majority of carbohydrates comes from leafy and nonstarchy vegetables." She recommends using a tracking app, such as MyFitnessPal, especially during the first few weeks of adopting the diet.

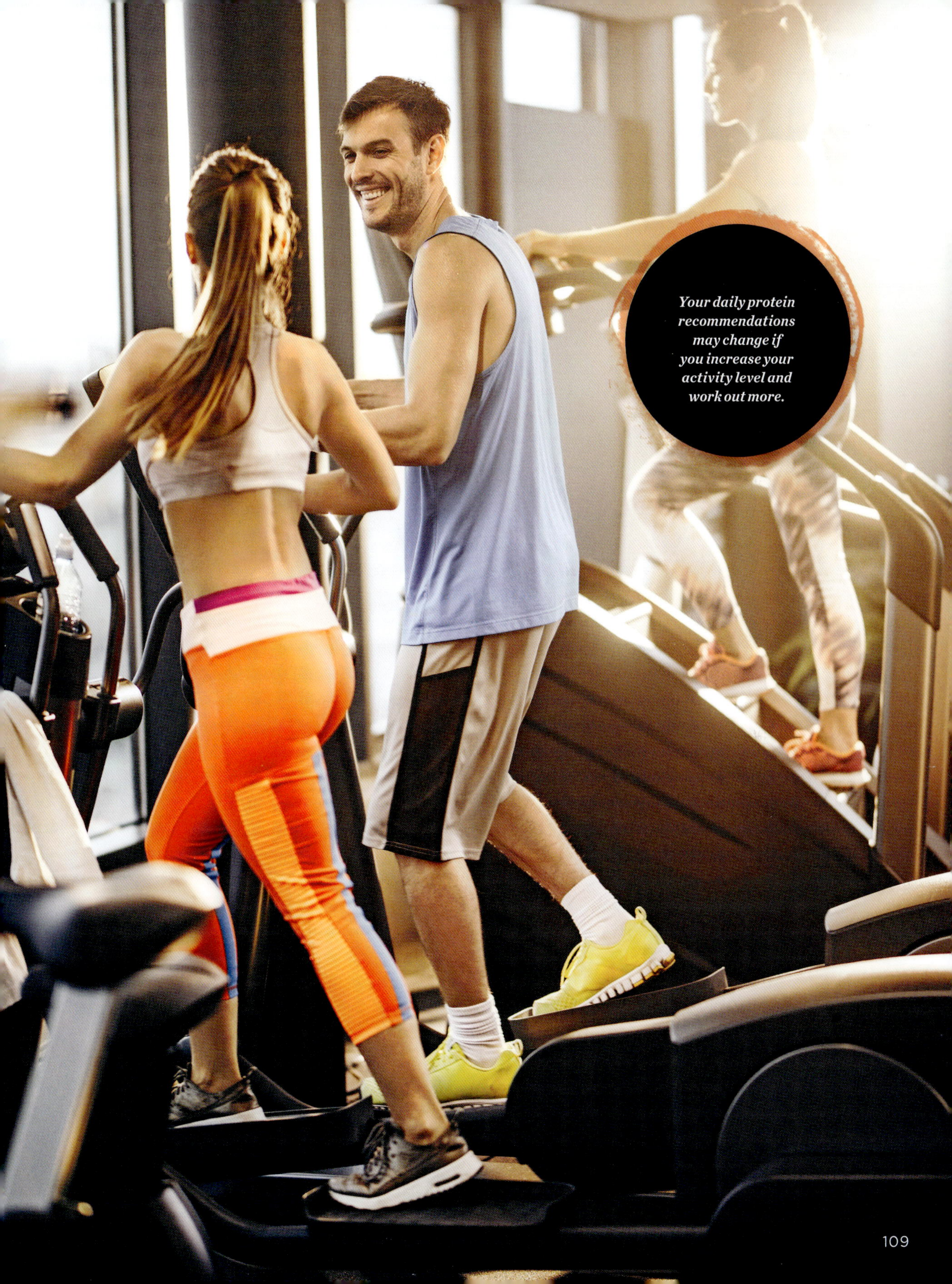

Your daily protein recommendations may change if you increase your activity level and work out more.

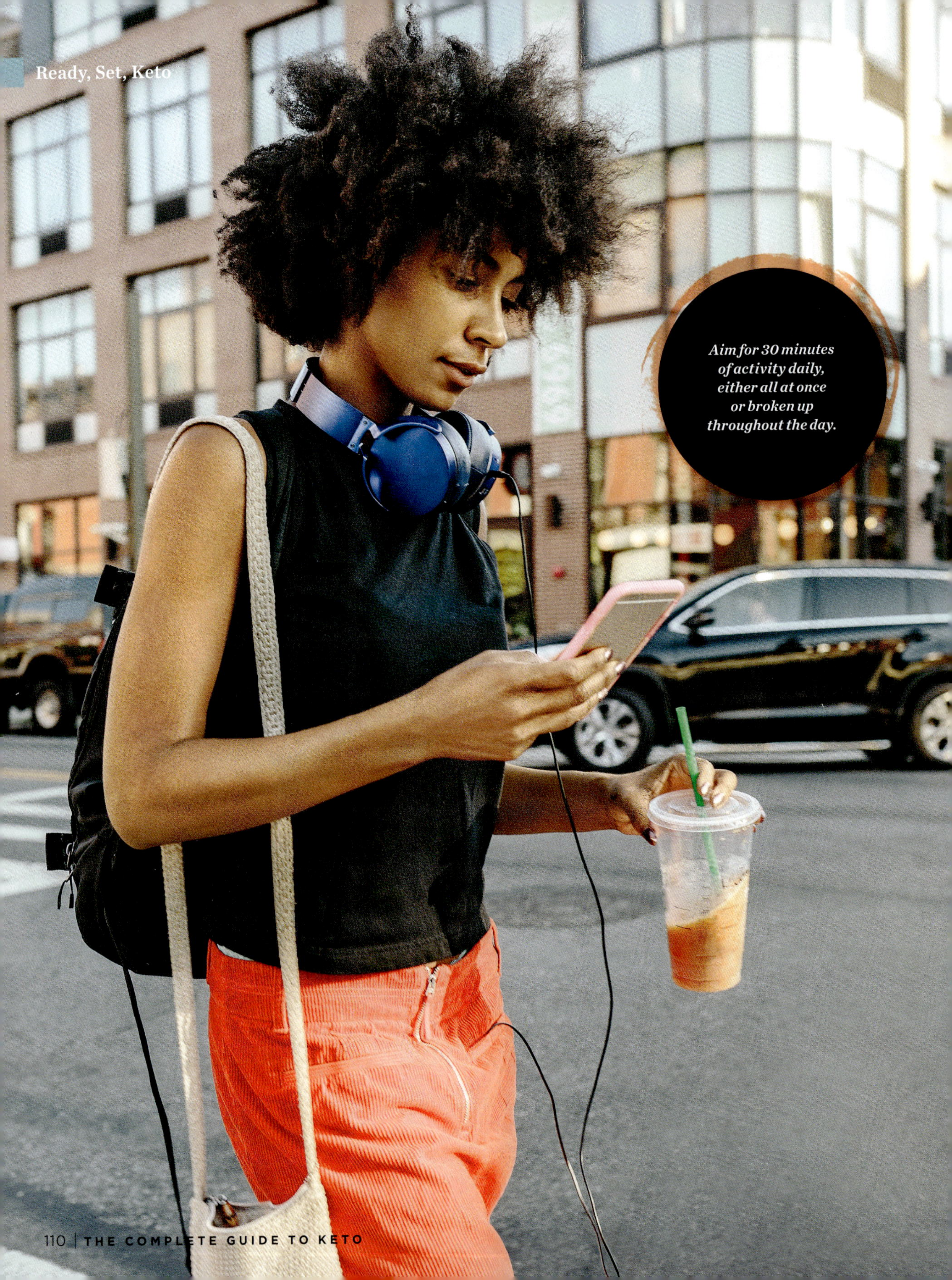

Aim for 30 minutes of activity daily, either all at once or broken up throughout the day.

5 Not Measuring Ketones

The only tangible way to confirm that your body has really reached a state of ketosis is to measure ketones. You can do this by testing your urine, breath or blood. "The Precision Xtra Blood Glucose and Ketone Monitor is considered to be one of the easiest to use, with accurate ketone monitors. A finger-prick test done once daily at the same time is the best way to ensure you're still in fat-burning mode," says Hanway.

6 Limiting the Amount of Exercise That You Do

Many people make the mistake of restricting exercise while they're on a keto diet, especially as their body adjusts. While it's true that exercising on strict carbohydrate deprivation is difficult, and strenuous exercise is discouraged as you get to ketosis, some movement is beneficial, explains Kelly Boyer, executive chef, wellness expert and founder of Paleta meal-delivery service. "You don't need to train for a marathon, but a 30-minute walk daily will do wonders for weight loss and brain fog and can greatly reduce stress and improve sleep!"

7 Eating Too Many Processed Low-Carb and Sugar-Free Foods

Not all low-carb and sugar-free sources are what they appear to be. Many packaged foods with these claims have hidden carbs in them or contain sugar alcohols that can impact blood sugar, says Inez. "Spiking blood sugar can take you out of ketosis. Try to steer clear of low-carb and sugar-free foods or stick with those that have a very low impact on glycemic levels." Foods made with sugar alcohols can also wreak havoc on some people's digestive systems. The sweeteners ketoers favor tend to be the sugar alcohol erythritol and Stevia.

8 Going Off a Keto Diet Too Quickly

Try as you might, most experts don't suggest you stay on keto forever. "The body eventually needs a break from such a low-carb lifestyle," says Inez. "Many make the mistake of following keto for a long time, becoming tired of it, and then going right back to the high-carb foods they were eating before." This can be detrimental because it doesn't give your body the time it needs to properly readjust to carbs, which can cause massive weight gain—usually from water weight—and slow down your metabolism. Instead, Inez recommends you gradually and slowly reintroduce carbs into your diet. "A good rule of thumb to follow is to add in 10 to 20 grams of carbs while taking out 5 to 10 grams of fat per week, until you reach a point where at least 35 percent of your macronutrients are coming from carb sources."

9 Throwing in the Towel if You Overeat Carbs

Whether you indulge in a few cookies or fall prey to carb-heavy appetizers at a party, chances are you might make a keto misstep.

But that doesn't mean you should give up and go on a carb binge. Start by expecting that you might knock your body out of ketosis; you'll likely see that reflected in urine strips, blood-prick tests or your ketone breath analyzer. Begin eating your regular keto meals right away and you should be able to get back into ketosis within 24 to 48 hours. Your body needs to process that glucose for energy after running on fat for so long, so you won't be back in fat-burning mode for a few days. Your weight might fluctuate by a few pounds quickly and you might experience bloating, gas or a number of other uncomfortable GI issues. Just give your body time to adjust. You might want to try "keto cycling" as part of your routine. Learn more about it on page 48.

"EXERCISE IS VITAL ON A KETO DIET—IT STIMULATES FAT LOSS AND BUILDS MUSCLE THAT HELPS BURN CALORIES ALL DAY LONG," SAYS WELLNESS EXPERT KELLY BOYER.

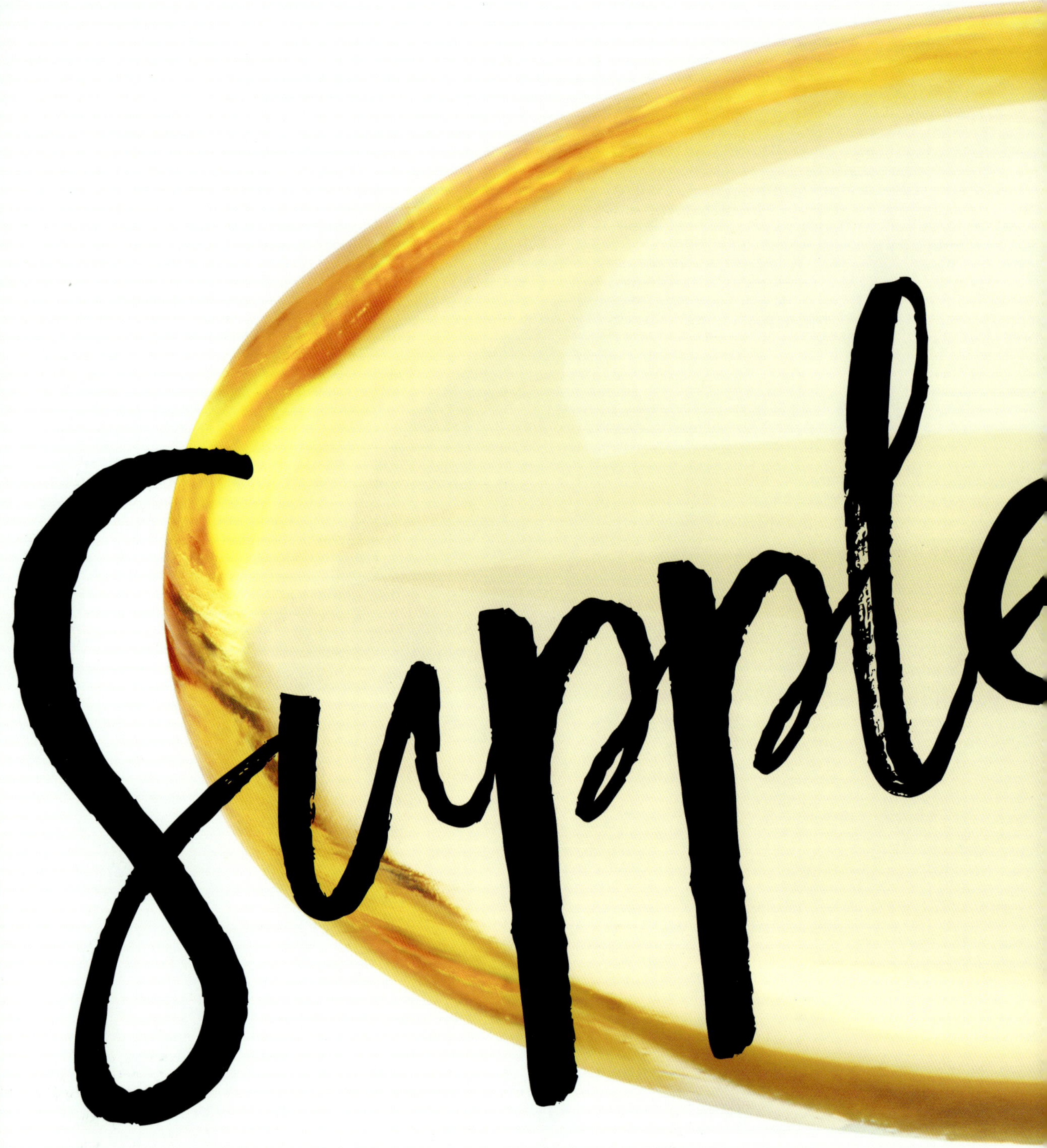
Supple

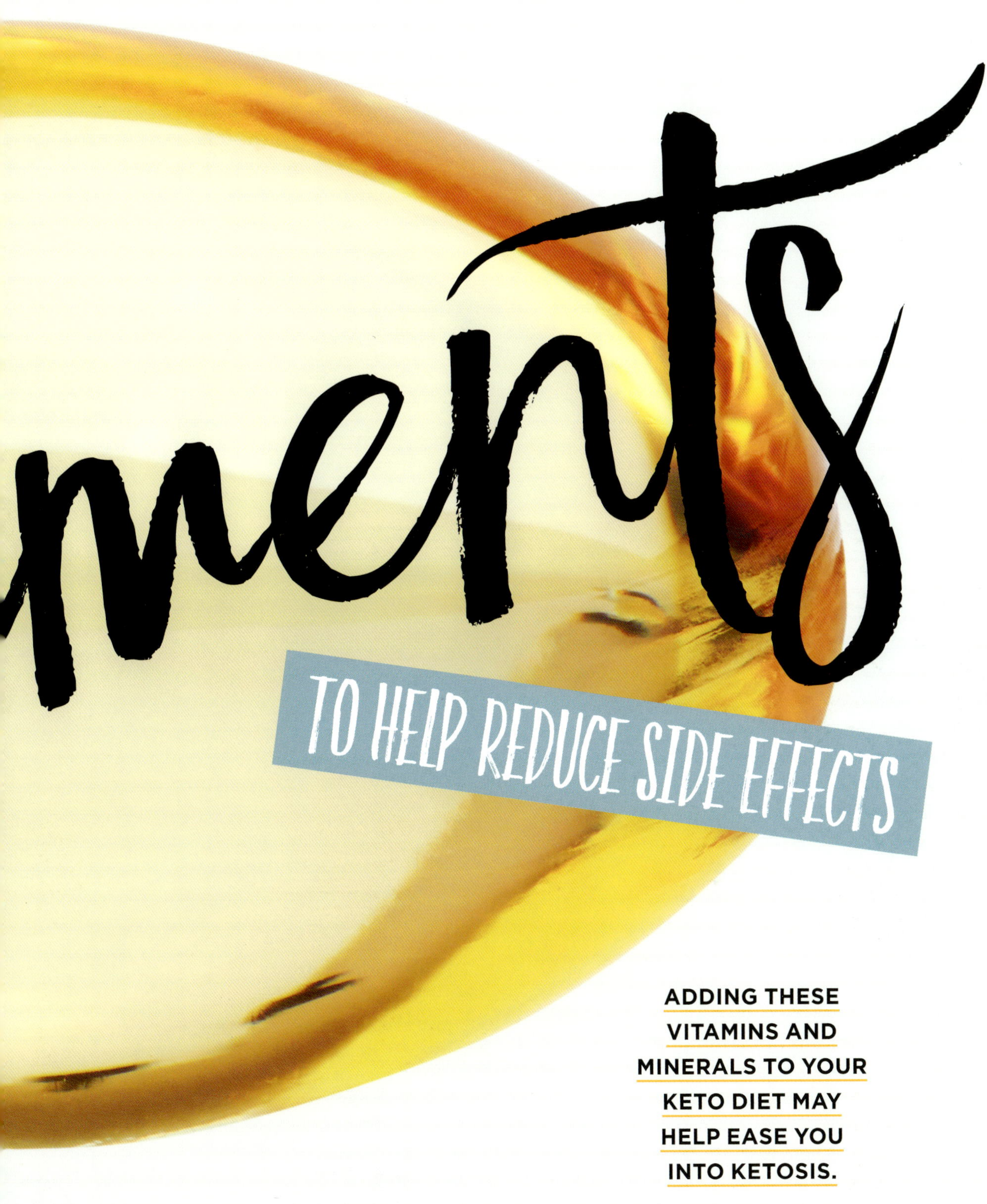

ments

TO HELP REDUCE SIDE EFFECTS

ADDING THESE VITAMINS AND MINERALS TO YOUR KETO DIET MAY HELP EASE YOU INTO KETOSIS.

SO YOU'VE BOARDED THE KETO TRAIN and have started shedding weight, and now you're looking to further your health goals with proper supplementation. That's not a bad idea, because supplements can help give you the energy and the edge you need to stick with keto over the long haul.

Since limiting or excluding food groups may cause your body to become deficient in key nutrients, it's wise to familiarize yourself with the supplements ketoers need—and why they're important.

Some supplements can help reduce undesirable side effects during early stages of ketosis and help bridge the gap of missed nutrients as you continue to find the right balance of macros while creating keto meals.

Taking supplements may also help you feel better during ketosis, provide needed nutrients and even help deliver a boost for workouts by picking up the slack that carbohydrates normally deliver. To know exactly what your body may need, it's always recommended that you meet with a licensed professional, like a registered dietitian.

Here, Ryan Gebo, RD, walks us through the top supplements recommended for keto followers. Always consult with your doctor before starting any supplement program, since they may interfere with current medications.

FISH OIL

Ketogenic dieters occasionally experience taste-bud fatigue from eating fatty fish, since it can be a daily staple on the plan. **But these fish contain the very important omega-3 fatty acids EPA and DHA, which are essential fatty acids,** Gebo explains. They have a number of benefits—namely, the reduction of high triglyceride levels in the body. Fish-oil supplements are convenient but they can taste "fishy"; if you can't stomach that flavor, know there are fish-oil pills with a lemon base that have a refreshing citrusy tang. Taking 2 to 6 grams of fish oil daily can ensure that you get the benefits of EPA and DHA without having to eat another bite of seafood.

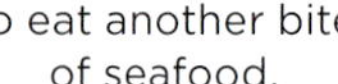

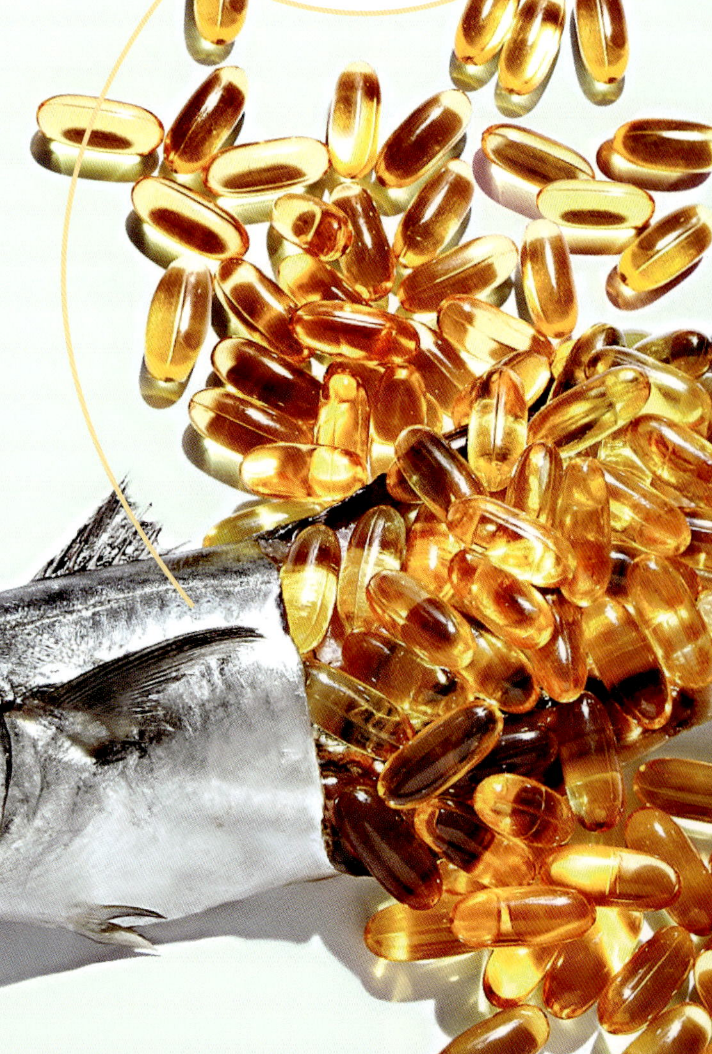

POTASSIUM AND MAGNESIUM

During the first one to three weeks of ketosis, there is a rapid flux of fluids in your body that can lead to an imbalance of electrolytes such as sodium, potassium and magnesium. **Daily intakes of potassium should reach 3.5 to 5 grams; get 400mg of magnesium for optimal health.** With that said, Gebo explains that sodium repletion can easily be accomplished with regular table salt, ensuring your nutritional requirement of 3 to 6 grams of sodium daily. Individuals with kidney dysfunction, heart disease or high blood pressure, or those who are on regular medication, should consult with their physician before supplementing with additional electrolytes.

A GOOD-QUALITY MULTIVITAMIN

Most dieters would benefit from a daily multivitamin, especially since many of us aren't always eating balanced meals that deliver optimal energy. With carbohydrates eliminated on a ketogenic diet, certain micronutrients that are abundantly found in those foods can be lacking in your diet. **A multivitamin will ensure that any micronutrient gaps are filled.** Look for an organic, non-GMO, whole-foods-based vitamin.

MCT OIL

Medium chain triglycerides (MCTs) are unique fatty acids with benefits that include improved blood sugar control, improved weight control and reduced appetite. MCTs convert to ketones quickly, due to their ability to bypass certain areas of digestion, unlike most other naturally occurring fats. Incorporate one to three tablespoons of high-quality **MCT oil into your diet daily.** Organic, extra-virgin, cold-pressed coconut oil is a great source of MCTs.

LIPASE

Lipase is a naturally occurring enzyme that helps break down the fat in foods into components, making it easier to digest, says Gebo. Ketoers often experience symptoms of inadequate fat breakdown, like GI distress such as bloating and diarrhea, due to the shift toward a fat-dominant diet. To help ease these symptoms, Gebo recommends 4,500 to 6,500 FIP of lipase taken with meals. (FIP is a term used to describe a high-quality enzyme; most supplements use this unit of measurement.) **Lipase helps your body better tolerate the additional fat intake and utilize it for energy.**

FISH OIL SUPPLEMENTS ARE A GOOD WAY TO MEET YOUR OMEGA-3 NEEDS.

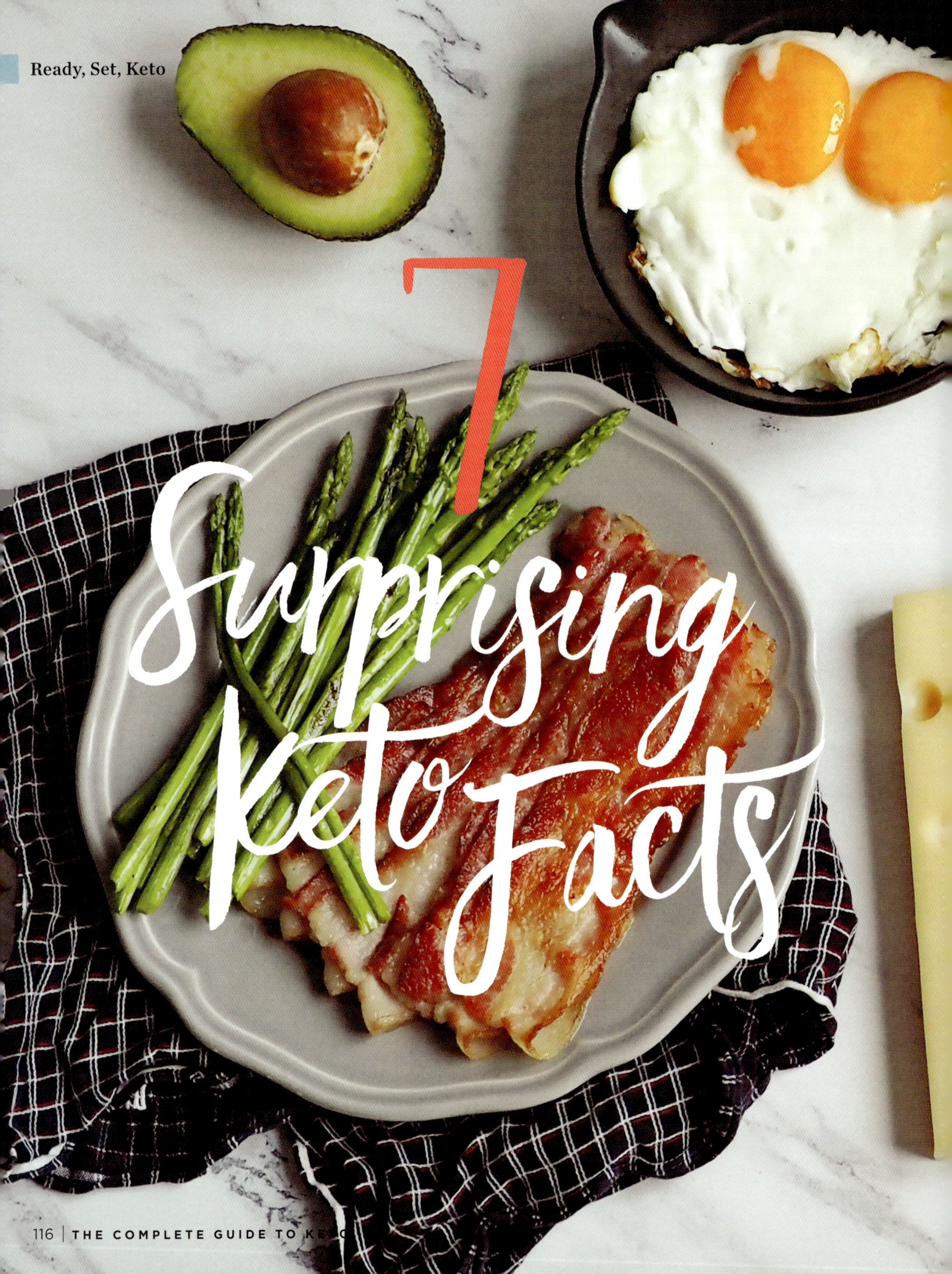

7 Surprising Keto Facts

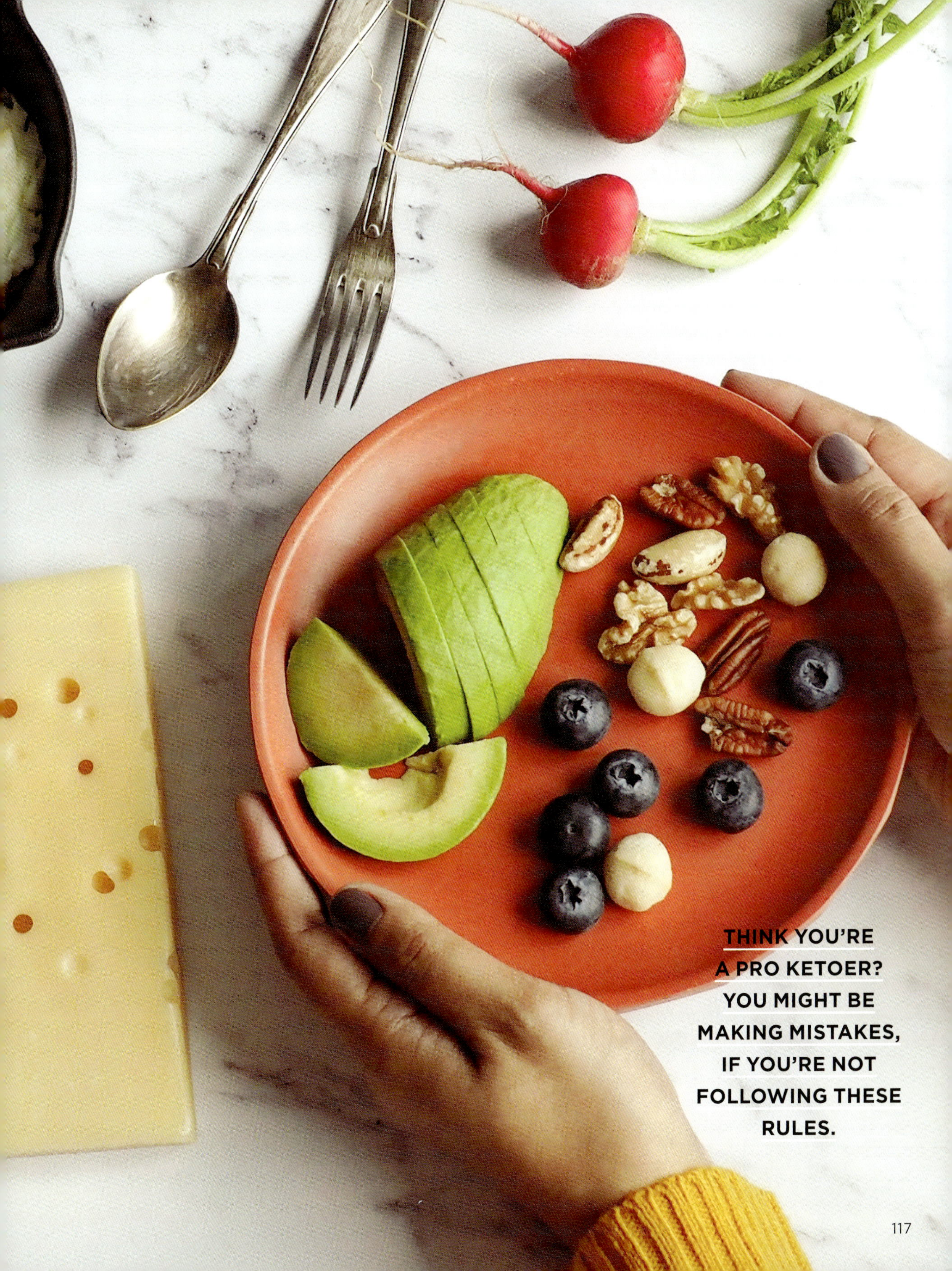

THINK YOU'RE A PRO KETOER? YOU MIGHT BE MAKING MISTAKES, IF YOU'RE NOT FOLLOWING THESE RULES.

IF YOU PUT FIVE KETO ENTHUSIASTS IN a room, you'll probably find they each practice their own individual version of the diet. That's because while all proponents of the plan know ketosis (when you're burning fat for fuel) can lead to many health benefits, including fat loss, increased energy and enhanced physical and mental performance, there are still many variations of the keto diet, ranging from casual to extreme.

The only essential rule for following keto is that you must keep your carb intake very low—and even that isn't incredibly specific, according to Mark Sisson, an early adopter of the keto diet and author of *The Primal Kitchen Cookbook*. "To some people, myself included, 'very low carb intake' means keeping it below 50 grams total per day, as this is the recommendation of ketogenic research pioneers—registered dietitian Jeff Volek [PhD] and Stephen Phinney [MD]," he explains. "Others argue that carbohydrates must be restricted to 20 to 30 grams per day, but this is mostly the case for people following a therapeutic ketogenic diet for conditions like epilepsy or perhaps as part of a treatment protocol for certain cancers, type 2 diabetes and the like." Beyond that, different keto approaches vary in terms of what foods they do and do not "allow" and how many fat and protein grams per day are recommended. Naturally, this can be confusing for beginners who are just starting out on the keto diet, because most of us prefer a specific set of guidelines to follow.

"In general, I recommend 75 percent of your dietary calories come from fat, 5 percent from carbs (25 net grams) and 15 percent from protein," says John Limansky, MD. This is based on original epilepsy studies. "This rough guide can be liberated somewhat, once people have improved their metabolic health and reached their weight-loss goal and insulin is improved."

But not everyone is in line with those numbers. "Keto diets really turn conventional dietary advice on its head, and with keto's exploding popularity, it's not surprising that we're seeing a backlash from mainstream nutrition circles," says Sisson. "There's a lot of fearmongering and misinformation swirling about on the internet and in the popular media." Still, ketosis is a normal and natural metabolic state, he says. "Not only is it safe, but throughout human history, our ancestors have followed a diet very similar to keto with the hunter-gatherer lifestyle."

If you're looking to follow the keto diet to a T—or, at least, get as close to the real thing as possible—here are some important facts you might not have known.

1 Most Cooking Oils Are Restricted on the Keto Diet

The majority of high-heat cooking oil—including vegetable, canola, sunflower-seed and grapeseed oils—aren't allowed on the ketogenic diet; however, alternative oils, such as coconut oil, avocado oil and ghee, are permitted, since they have higher smoke points (the point at which the oil begins to smoke and break down), explains Dana Murrell, executive research and development chef for Green Chef, which offers keto plans and other specialty diets.

2 Many Fruits Are Off-Limits

That's because plenty of fruits are high in carbs, including apples, bananas, pineapples and mangoes, to name a few. When following keto, the only fruits allowed are berries, avocados, olives and certain citrus fruits, explains Murrell. "Other fruits may be allowed, depending on individual carbohydrate goals, but should still be consumed in moderation." Berries should be viewed as a treat rather than heavily incorporated into meal planning.

3 Stress Management Is an Important Part of the Keto Diet

When most people think of following a diet, they focus all their efforts on what they eat. And while what you're putting into your body

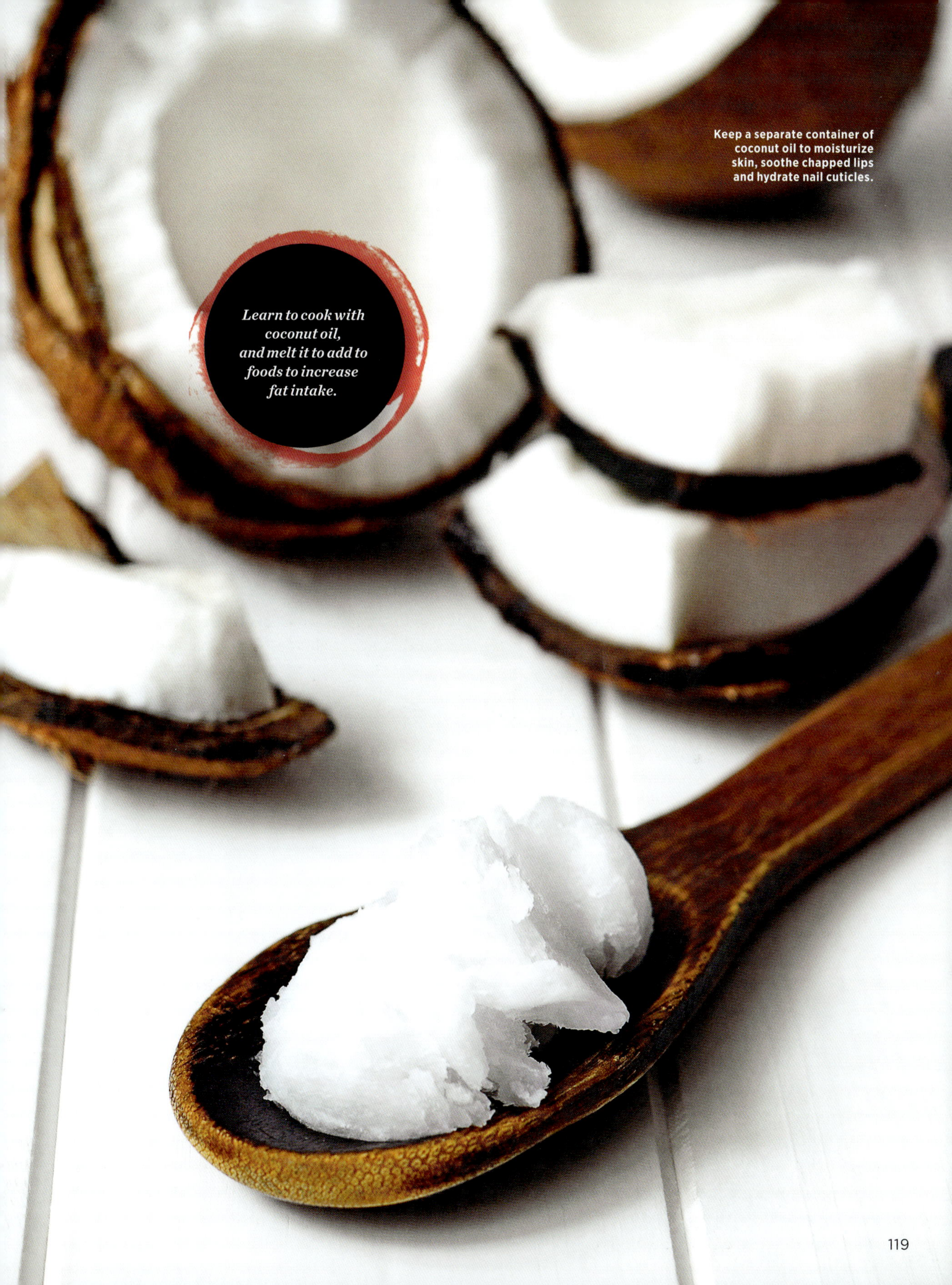
Keep a separate container of
coconut oil to moisturize
skin, soothe chapped lips
and hydrate nail cuticles.
Learn to cook with
coconut oil,
and melt it to add to
foods to increase
fat intake.

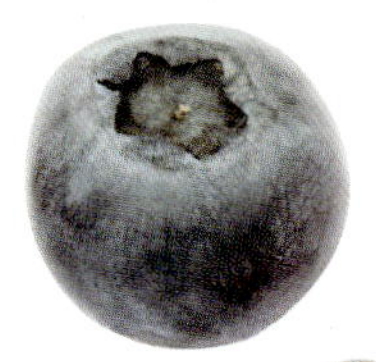

is incredibly important when it comes to following a weight-loss plan, stress also plays a major role, especially in keto. High stress levels may ruin your body's attempt at reaching a state of ketosis, says Sisson. "When you're operating from a place of high stress—whether it's due to your job, lack of proper sleep, overexercising or anything else—it triggers your sympathetic nervous system [SNS], or fight-or-flight response. The hormones involved in SNS activation are the opposite of what you want if you're trying to minimize sugar burning and maximize fat burning." He recommends reinforcing your keto efforts with effective stress management, plenty of sleep and daily movement.

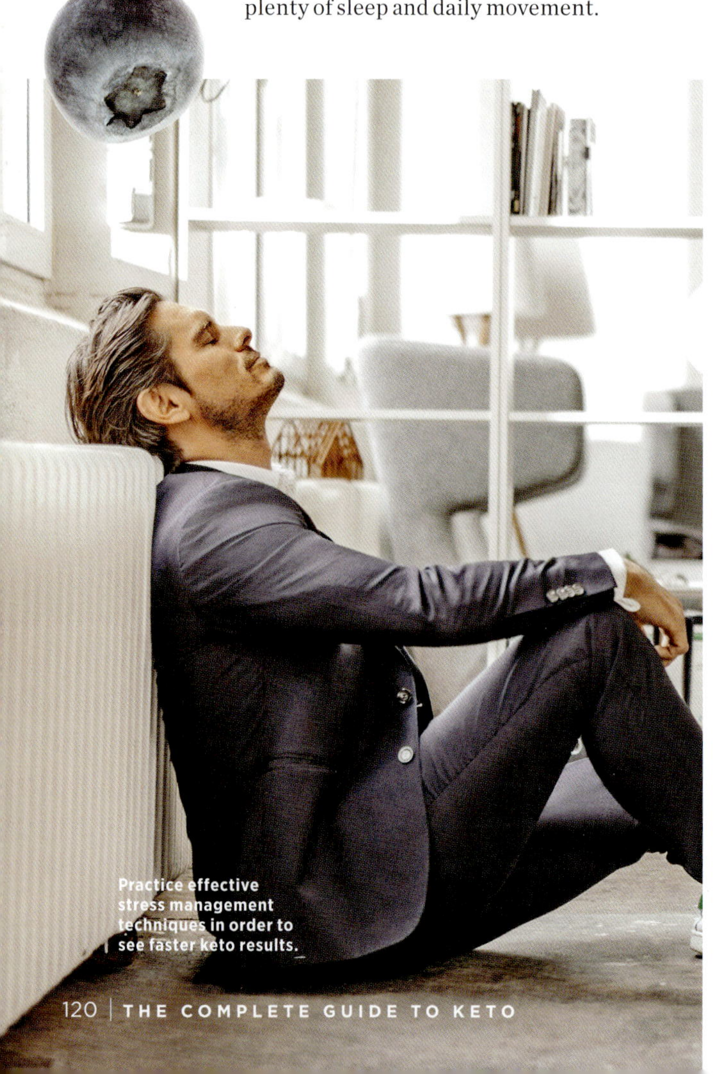

Practice effective stress management techniques in order to see faster keto results.

4 Nutrient Density Is of Utmost Importance on Keto

While it is possible to achieve a state of ketosis by eating artificially sweetened foods and replacing meals with butter coffee, it's not recommended, according to experts. Sisson believes this strategy is missing the point of keto entirely. "A ketogenic diet is meant to put you in an optimal metabolic state, help balance hormones and provide a variety of cognitive benefits," he says. "The best way to do that is by focusing on nutrient-dense foods —meat, poultry, seafood, eggs, nuts and seeds, plenty of vegetables and, if you tolerate it, some full-fat dairy."

5 Not All Fats Are Created Equal on the Diet

Choosing your fats wisely still reigns supreme. "Highly processed vegetable and seed oils and trans fats are incredibly inflammatory and damaging," warns Sisson. "While they might not interfere with ketosis, they will undermine health goals." Instead, he recommends opting for fats from animals raised on natural diets and in healthy conditions (pastured/organic lard, tallow, poultry fat, butter, ghee), as well as avocado, coconut and olive oils.

6 Higher Ketone Readings Are Not the Ultimate Goal

Measuring the amount of ketones that your body is creating can be reassuring for people following the keto diet. They might consider it tangible proof they're doing keto "right." However, Sisson has seen too many people get caught up in striving for higher and higher readings, even to the point of spending a lot of money on ketone supplements. "For the average keto dieter, there's no evidence that having higher ketone readings is better... anything over 0.5 mmol/L on a blood-ketone meter means you are in ketosis," he says.

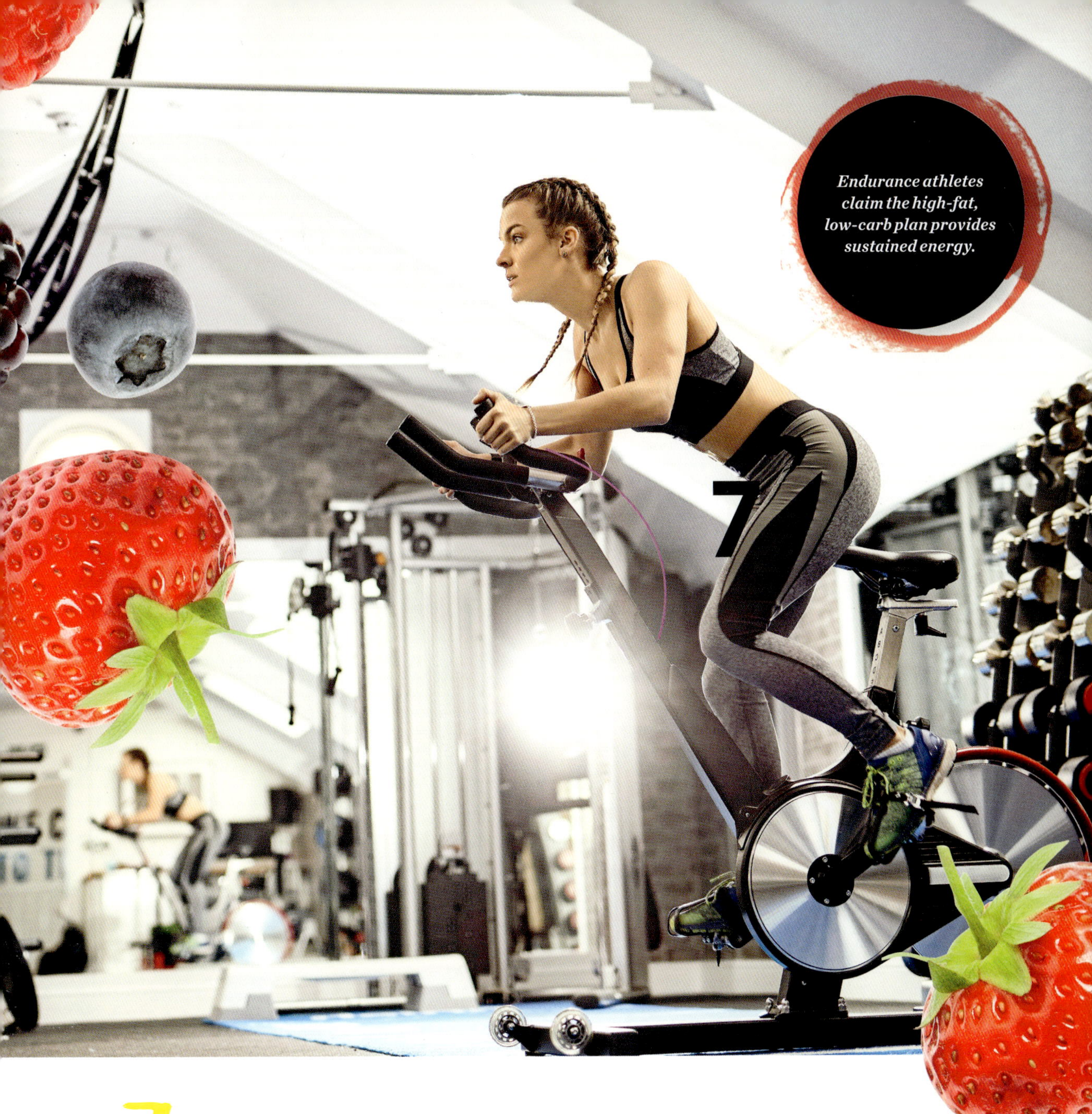

Endurance athletes claim the high-fat, low-carb plan provides sustained energy.

7 Gorging on Fats Is Not Recommended

While this diet calls for significantly higher amounts of fat than most nutrition plans, many people believe they need way more fat than actually required. "The reason keto followers need to eat plenty of healthy fats is to make up for the calories they aren't getting from carbs—not because eating fat is the goal in and of itself," says Sisson. "Yes, when you are brand-new to keto, it can be helpful to eat a lot of fat to ease the transition into being an efficient fat-burner. However, the ultimate goal is to burn fat." In other words, if you're already eating a diet high in fatty cuts of meat, eggs, avocados, coconut, nuts and seeds, plus some fat in the form of healthy condiments and marinades, you don't also need to slam down three fatty coffees and chase them with fat bombs—especially if you have a weight-loss goal in mind.

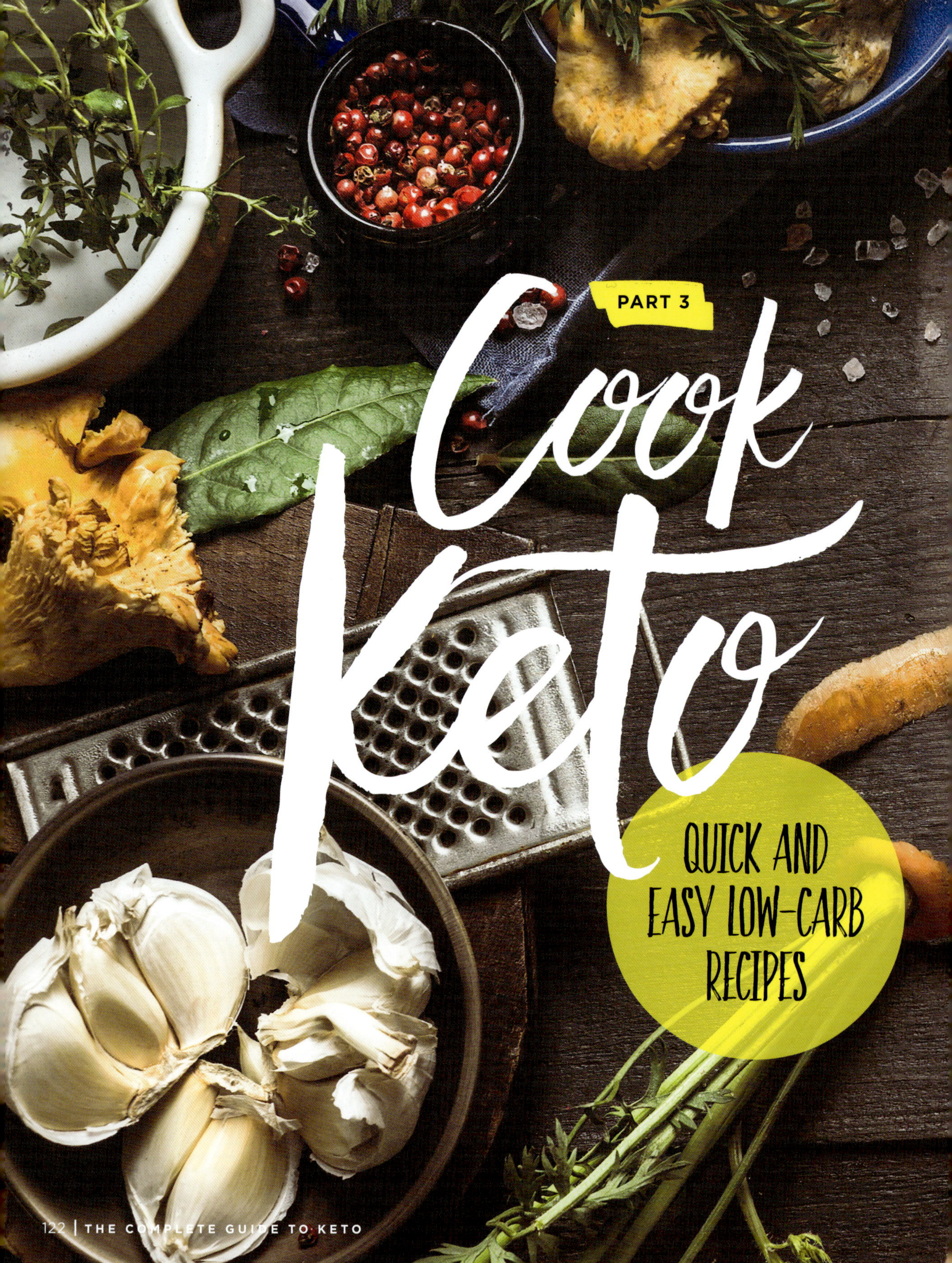
PART 3
Cook Keto
QUICK AND
EASY LOW-CARB
RECIPES

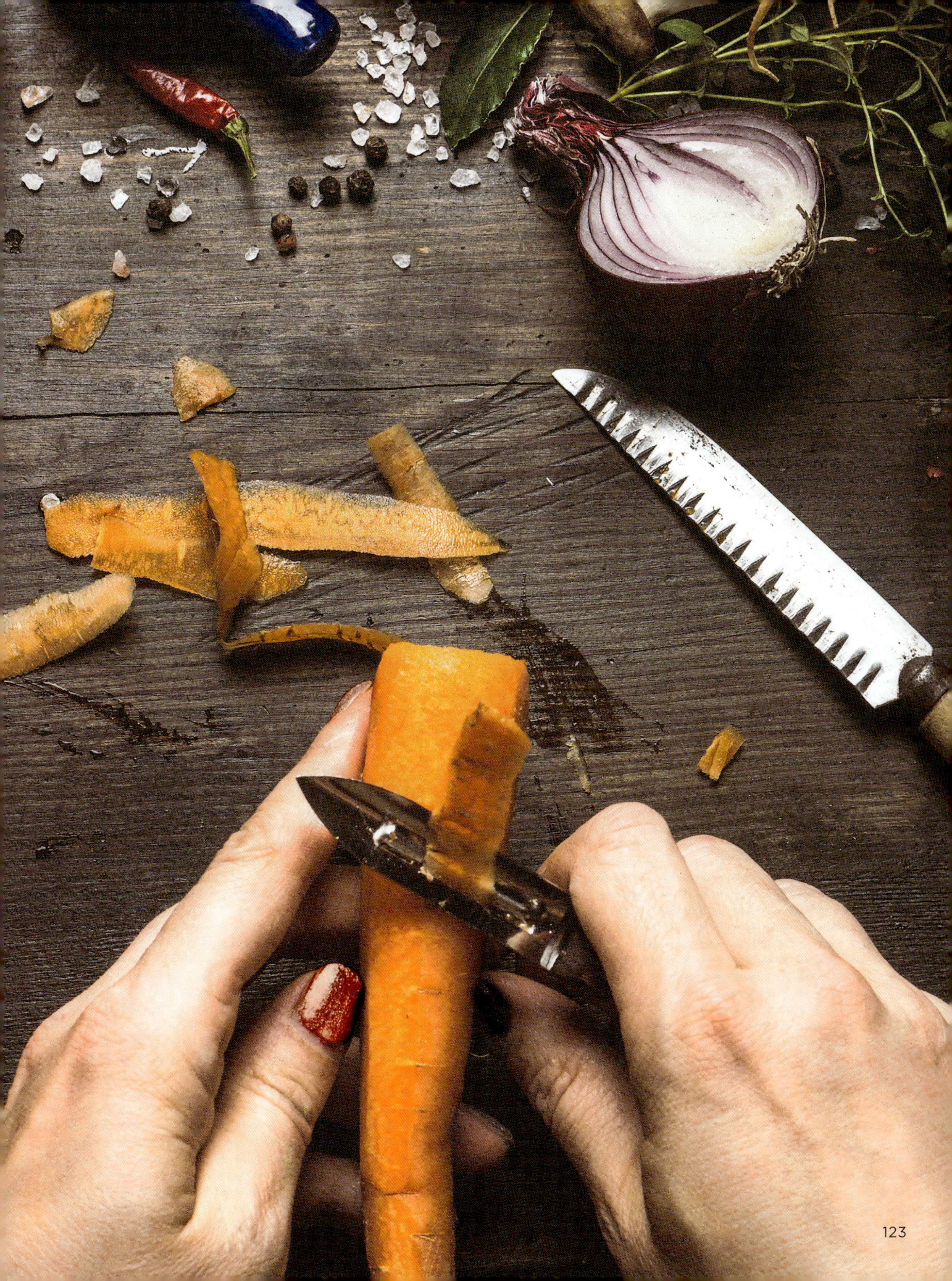

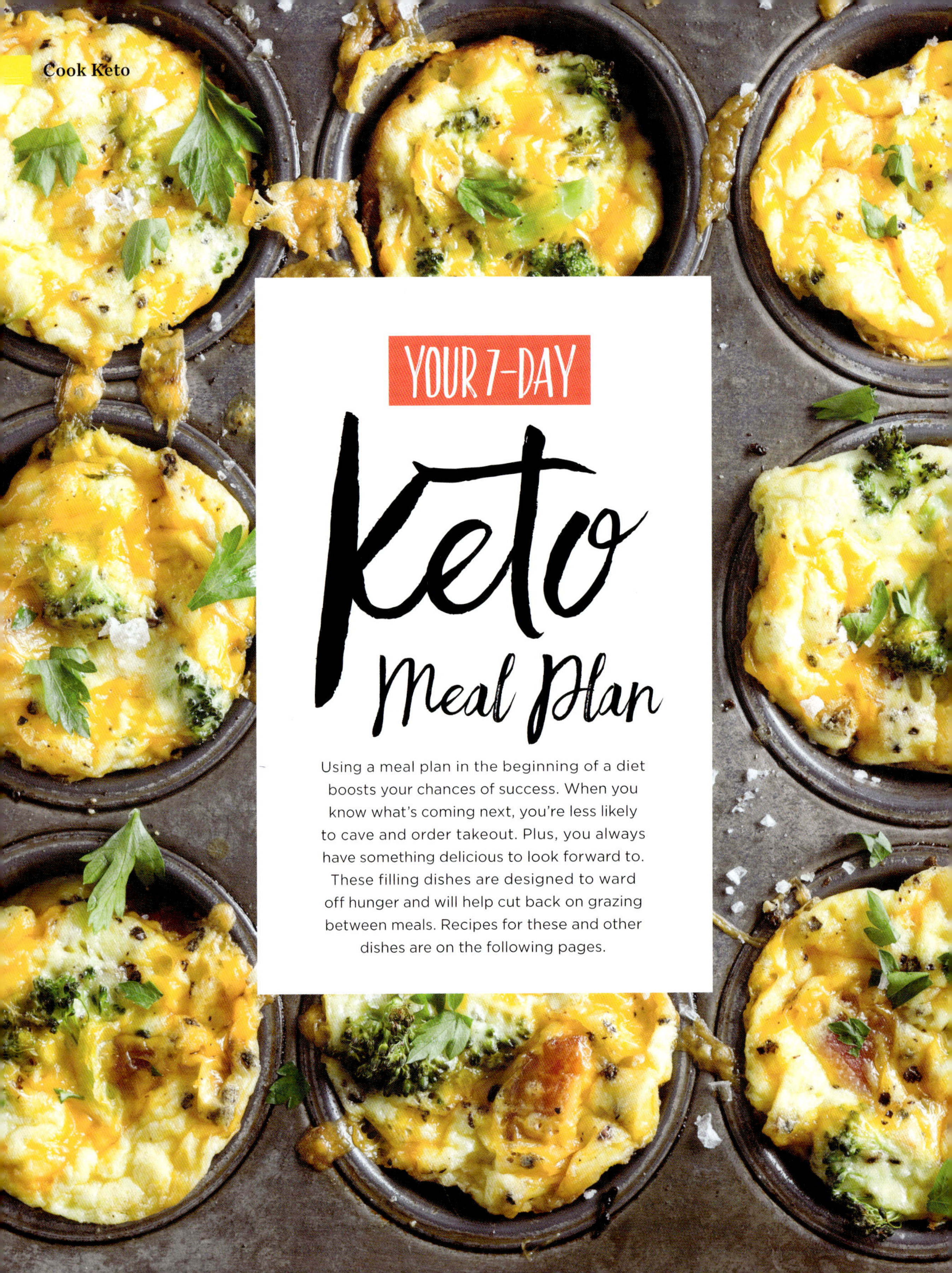

YOUR 7-DAY

Keto Meal Plan

Using a meal plan in the beginning of a diet boosts your chances of success. When you know what's coming next, you're less likely to cave and order takeout. Plus, you always have something delicious to look forward to. These filling dishes are designed to ward off hunger and will help cut back on grazing between meals. Recipes for these and other dishes are on the following pages.

	BREAKFAST	LUNCH	SNACK	DINNER	SNACK
MONDAY	Broccoli Cheddar Mini Frittata (pg. 130)	Chicken Cabbage Cups (pg. 140)	Ultimate Guacamole (pg. 174) With Celery Sticks	Oven BBQ Shrimp (pg. 150); Cheesy Broiled Tomatoes With Herbs (pg. 156)	Vanilla Pudding With Cream and Mixed Berries (pg. 182)
TUESDAY	Blueberry Basil Smoothie (pg. 132)	Tuna Niçoise Salad (pg. 138)	Loaded Deviled Eggs (pg. 172)	Skillet Garlic-Herb Pork Chops (pg. 148); Cauliflower Mash With Toppings (pg. 162)	Chocolate Lava Cake (pg. 181)
WEDNESDAY	Almond Pancakes With Raspberries and Cream (pg. 126)	Loaded "Potato" Soup (pg. 144)	1 to 2 Cups Bone Broth (homemade or purchased organic)	Lemon Baked Salmon Fillets (pg. 152); Parmesan Roasted Asparagus (pg. 160)	Chocolate-Peanut Butter Milkshake (pg. 184)
THURSDAY	Crustless Quiche Lorraine (pg. 134)	Grilled Salmon and Romaine Caesar Salad (pg. 142)	Mini BLT Bites (pg. 168)	Beef and Pork Meatballs Over Butternut Noodles (pg. 146)	Chocolate Chip Cookies (pg. 176)
FRIDAY	Blueberry Basil Smoothie (pg. 132)	Pad Thai Noodles (pg. 136)	Baked Cheese Crisps (pg. 73)	Oven BBQ Shrimp (pg. 150); Cheesy Broiled Tomatoes With Herbs (pg. 156)	Individual Strawberry Shortcake Trifles (pg. 178)
SATURDAY	Avocado Eggs Benedict With Hollandaise (pg. 128)	Loaded "Potato" Soup (pg. 144)	Baked Wings With Blue Cheese Dressing (pg. 170)	Whole Roasted Chicken With Brussels Sprouts (pg. 154)	Chocolate Lava Cake (pg. 180)
SUNDAY	Almond Pancakes With Raspberries and Cream (pg. 126)	Tuna Niçoise Salad (pg. 138)	Cauliflower Tot-chos (pg. 166)	Skillet Garlic-Herb Pork Chops (pg. 148); Steakhouse Creamed Spinach (pg. 158)	Vanilla Pudding With Cream and Mixed Berries (pg. 182)

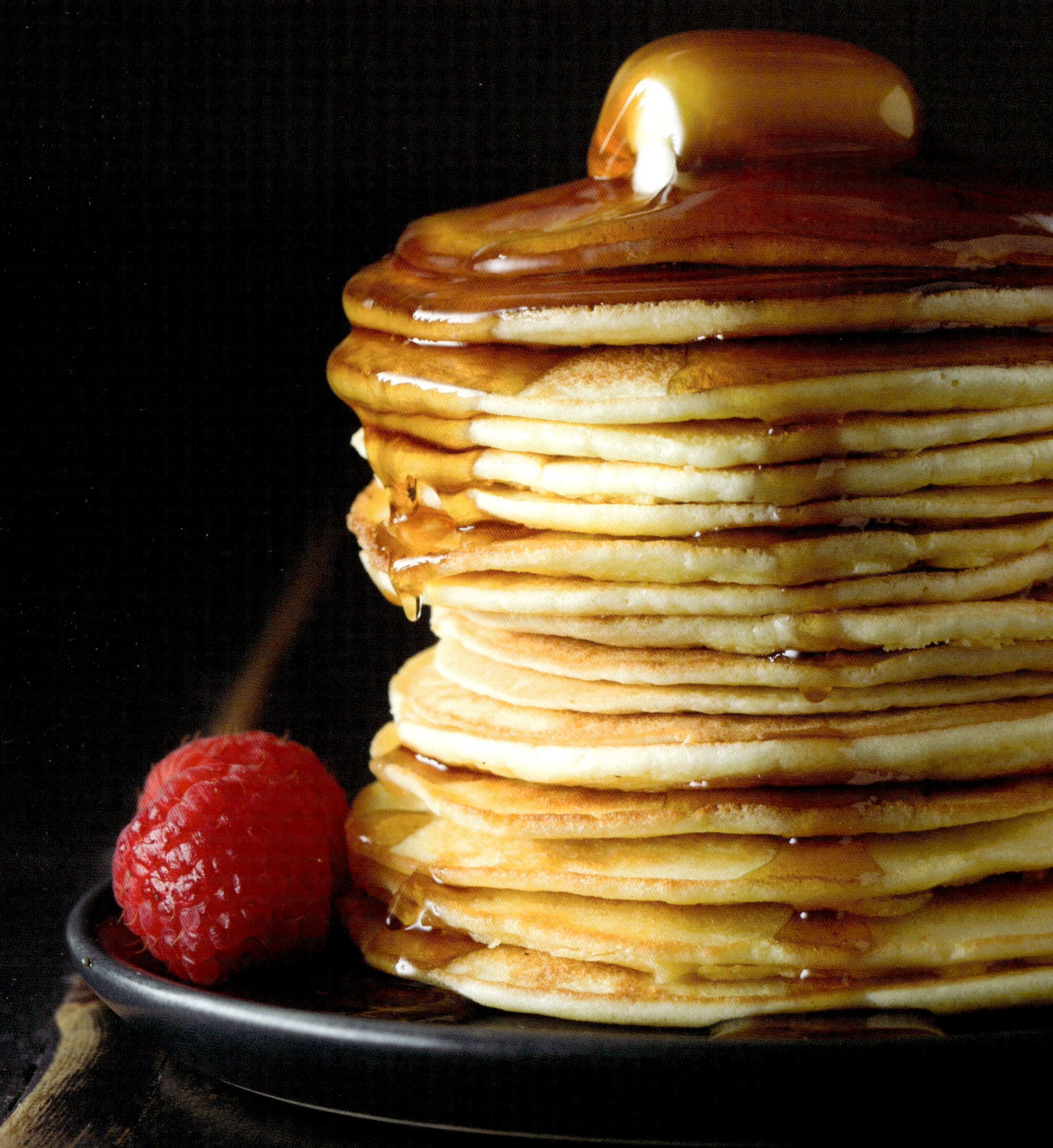

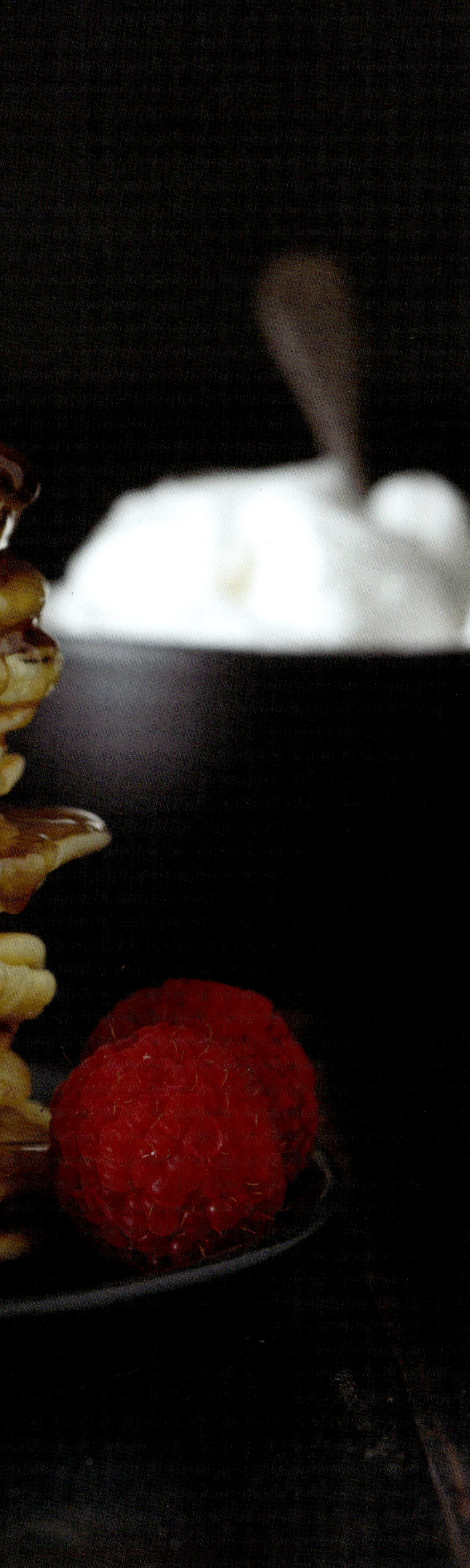

Breakfast

ALMOND PANCAKES WITH RASPBERRIES AND CREAM

START TO FINISH 20 minutes (5 minutes active)
SERVINGS 16 (1 pancake)

INGREDIENTS

- 1 cup almond flour
- 1 (8-ounce) package cream cheese, softened
- 8 eggs
- 2 teaspoons granulated sweetener
- 1 teaspoon baking powder
- ¼ cup butter

GARNISHES sugar-free syrup, butter, raspberries, whipped cream

DIRECTIONS

1 In a blender, mix almond flour, cream cheese, eggs, sweetener and baking powder.
2 In a large skillet or griddle, melt butter over medium-high heat. For each pancake, place 1/4 cup of batter in skillet; cook, 3 minutes per side, or until the edges are browned.
3 Serve with syrup, butter, raspberries and whipped cream on the side.

NUTRITION INFORMATION

CALORIES 80; **PROTEIN** 3.5g; **FAT** 7g; **CARBS** 2g; **FIBER** 6g; **NET CARBS** 0g

AVOCADO EGGS BENEDICT WITH HOLLANDAISE

START TO FINISH 15 minutes (10 minutes active)
SERVINGS 2

INGREDIENTS

- 4 egg yolks
- 1 tablespoon mayonnaise
- 1 teaspoon lemon juice
- ¼ teaspoon pepper
- ½ teaspoon salt
- ½ cup melted butter
- 2 slices bacon, cooked
- 1 avocado, sliced
- 1 tomato, sliced
- 2 eggs, poached

GARNISHES cracked pepper, snipped chives

DIRECTIONS

1 In a medium glass bowl, whisk together egg yolks and next 4 ingredients until smooth.
2 Slowly pour in melted butter, whisking constantly until mixture is no longer lumpy.
3 Heat the entire mixture in the microwave for 15 seconds and then stir. Return to microwave and heat for another 10 seconds and stir. Heat again for 15 seconds and stir until smooth. The hollandaise will thicken as it sits.
4 Arrange bacon, avocado and tomato slices on plates. Top with a poached egg and half the sauce. Garnish with cracked pepper and chives.

NUTRITION INFORMATION

CALORIES 604; **PROTEIN** 17g; **FAT** 39g; **CARBS** 15g; **FIBER** 8g; **NET CARBS** 7g

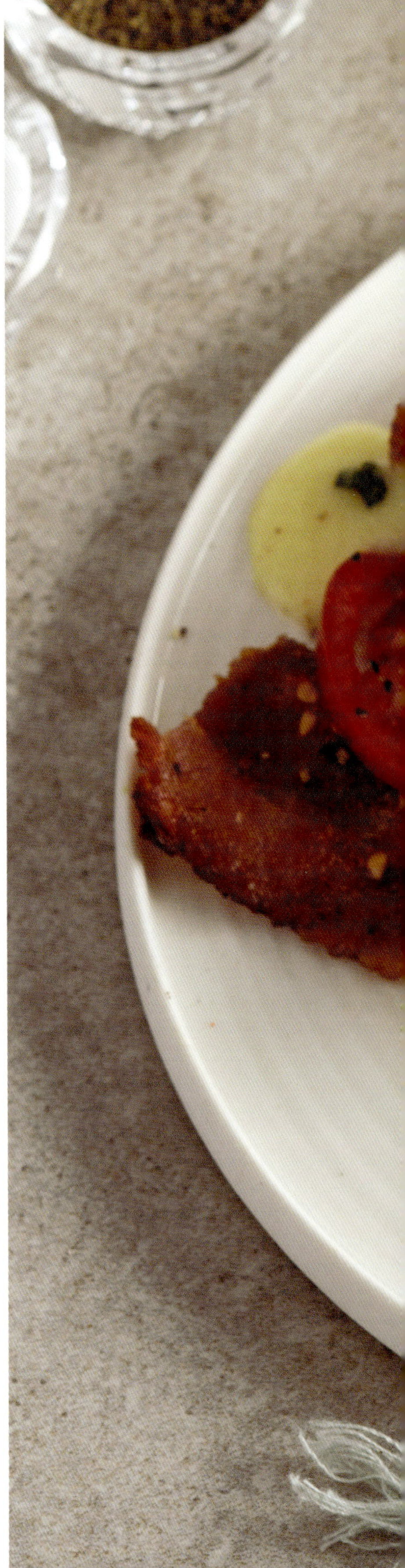

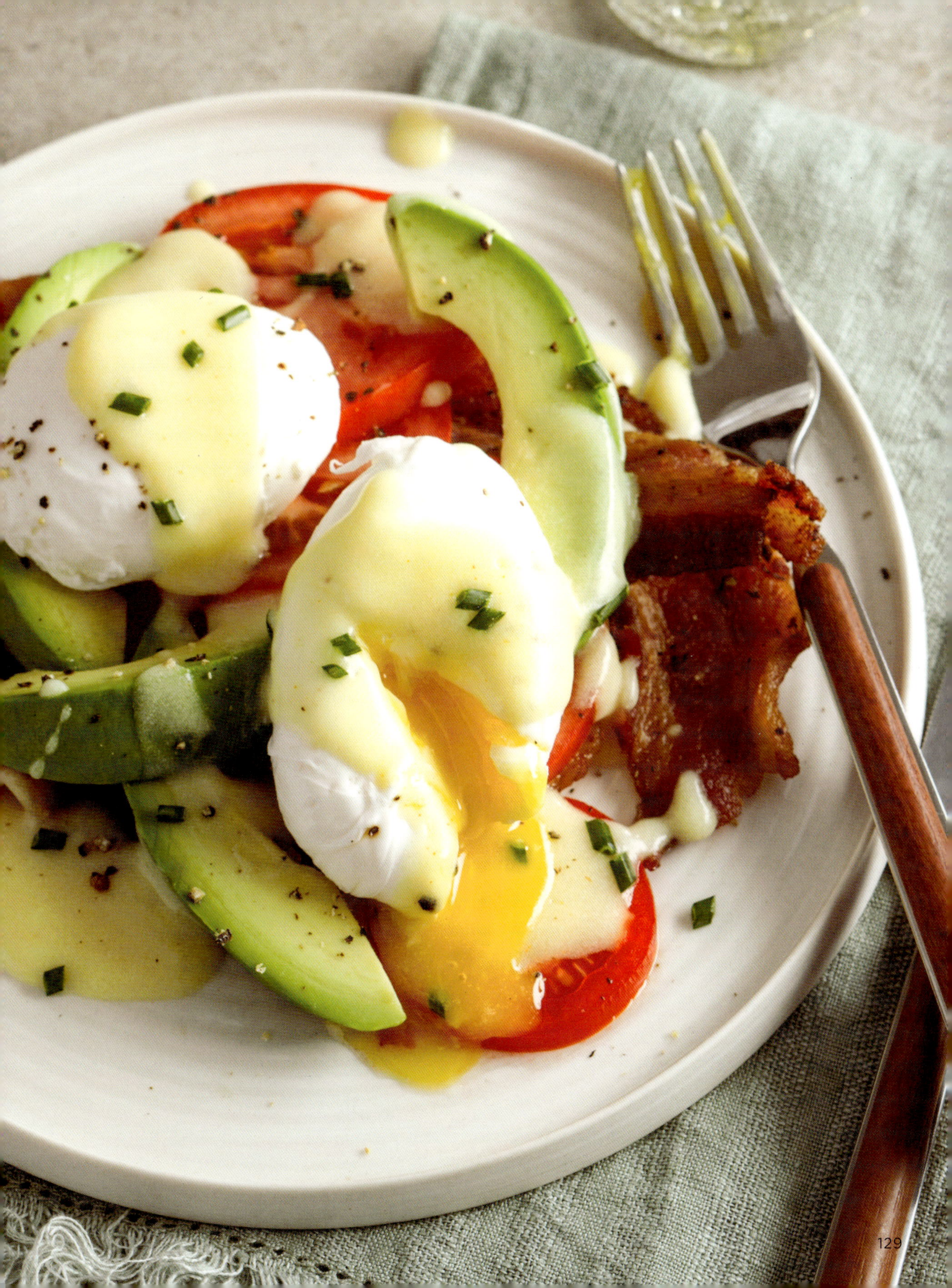

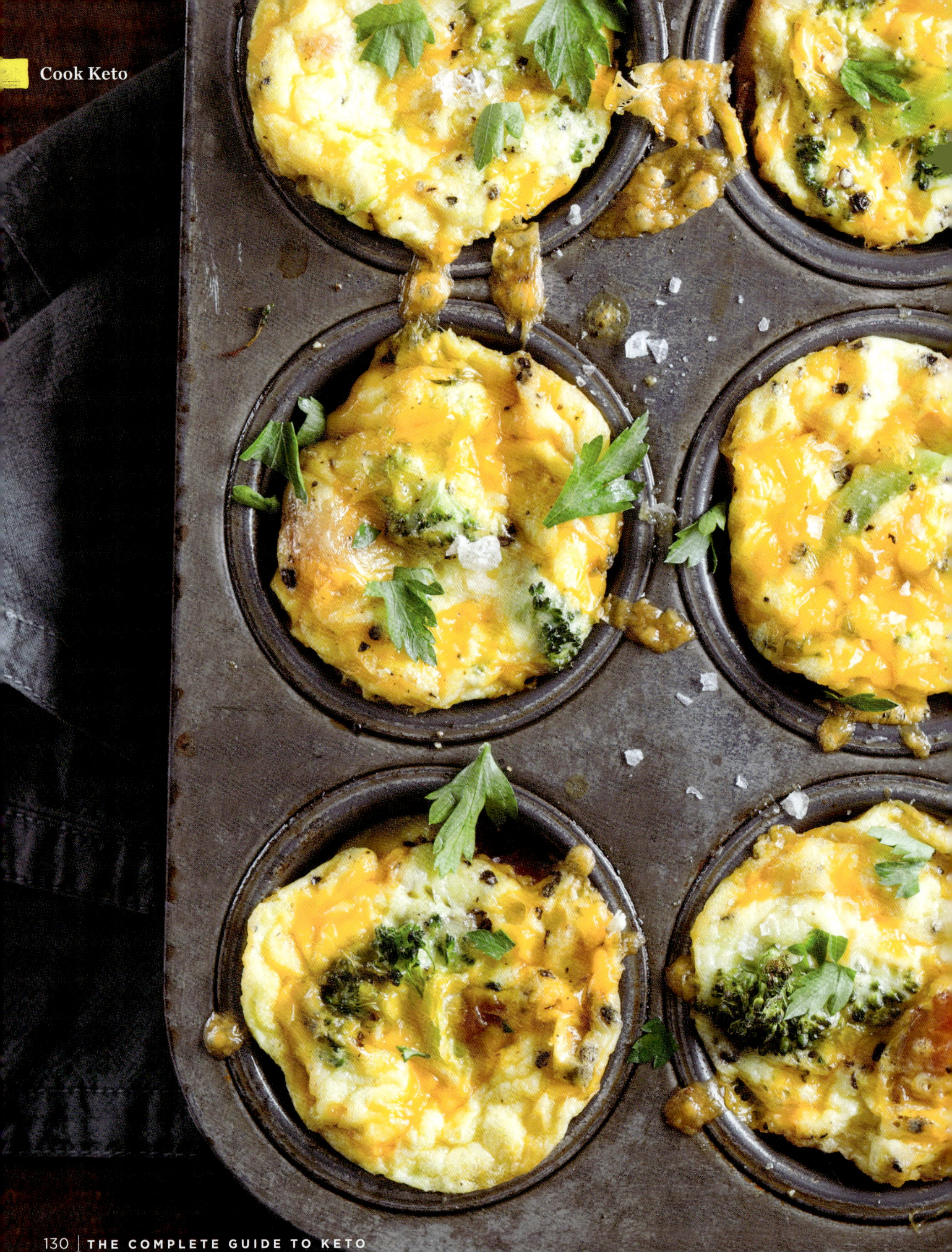

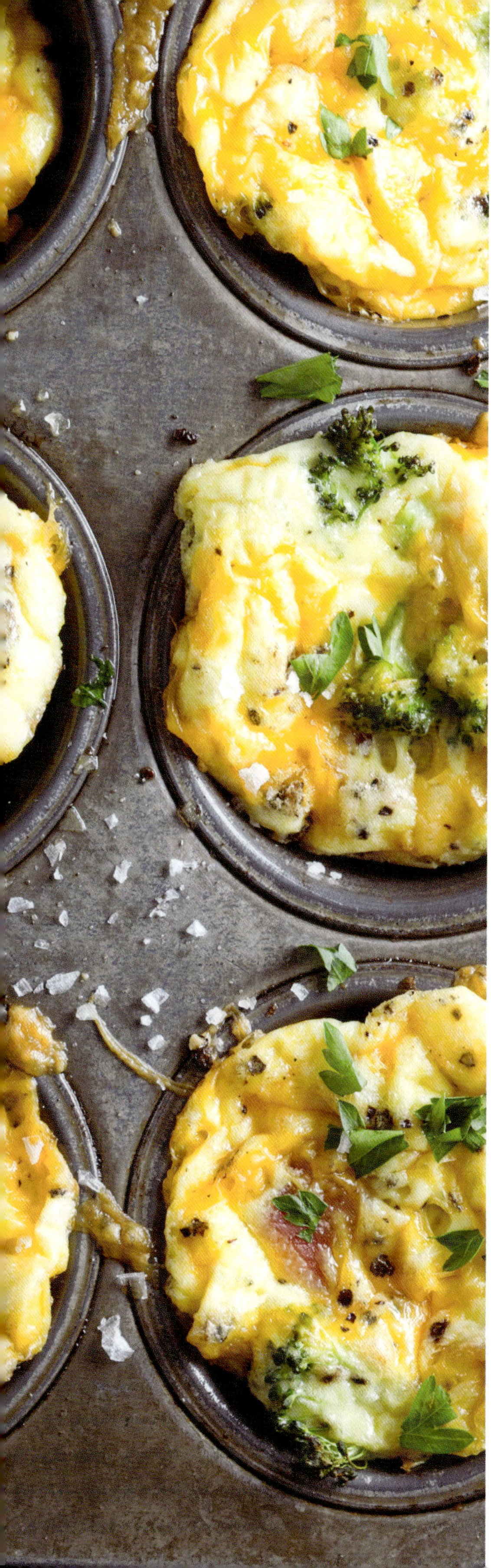

BROCCOLI AND CHEDDAR MINI FRITTATAS

START TO FINISH 35 minutes (10 minutes active)
SERVINGS 6 (2 frittatas)

INGREDIENTS

- 4 bacon slices, cooked and crumbled
- 2 cups cooked broccoli florets
- ⅓ cup shredded sharp cheddar
- 10 eggs, beaten
- ½ cup heavy cream
- ½ teaspoon salt
- ½ teaspoon pepper

GARNISH chopped parsley

DIRECTIONS

1 Preheat oven to 350°F.
2 Spray a 12-cup muffin tin with cooking spray; divide bacon, broccoli and cheese among the cups.
3 In a medium bowl, whisk together eggs, cream, salt and pepper until combined. Divide egg mixture among the cups.
4 Bake at 350°F for 16-18 minutes or until set. Cool on a wire rack for 5 minutes before serving. Garnish with chopped parsley.

NUTRITION INFORMATION

CALORIES 186; **PROTEIN** 14g; **FAT** 12g; **CARBS** 4g; **FIBER** 1g; **NET CARBS** 3g

BLUEBERRY BASIL SMOOTHIE

START TO FINISH 5 minutes (all active)
SERVINGS 1

INGREDIENTS

- ¼ cup almond or coconut milk
- ⅓ cup frozen blueberries
- 1 teaspoon vanilla
- 1 teaspoon coconut oil
- ¼ cup protein powder
- 1 tablespoon chopped fresh basil

GARNISH blueberries, coconut flakes, basil leaves

DIRECTIONS

1 Place all ingredients in a blender and process until smooth.
2 Serve and garnish with blueberries, coconut and basil leaves, if desired.

NUTRITION INFORMATION

CALORIES 109; **PROTEIN** 3g;
FAT 5g; **CARBS** 13g; **FIBER** 2g; **NET CARBS** 11g

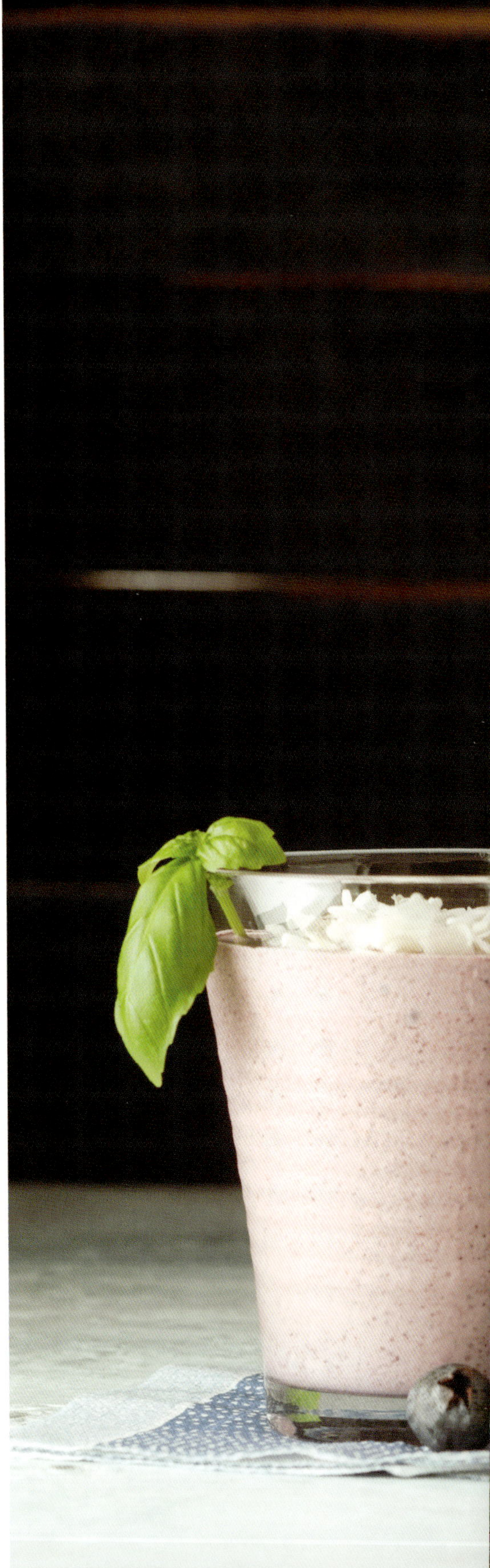

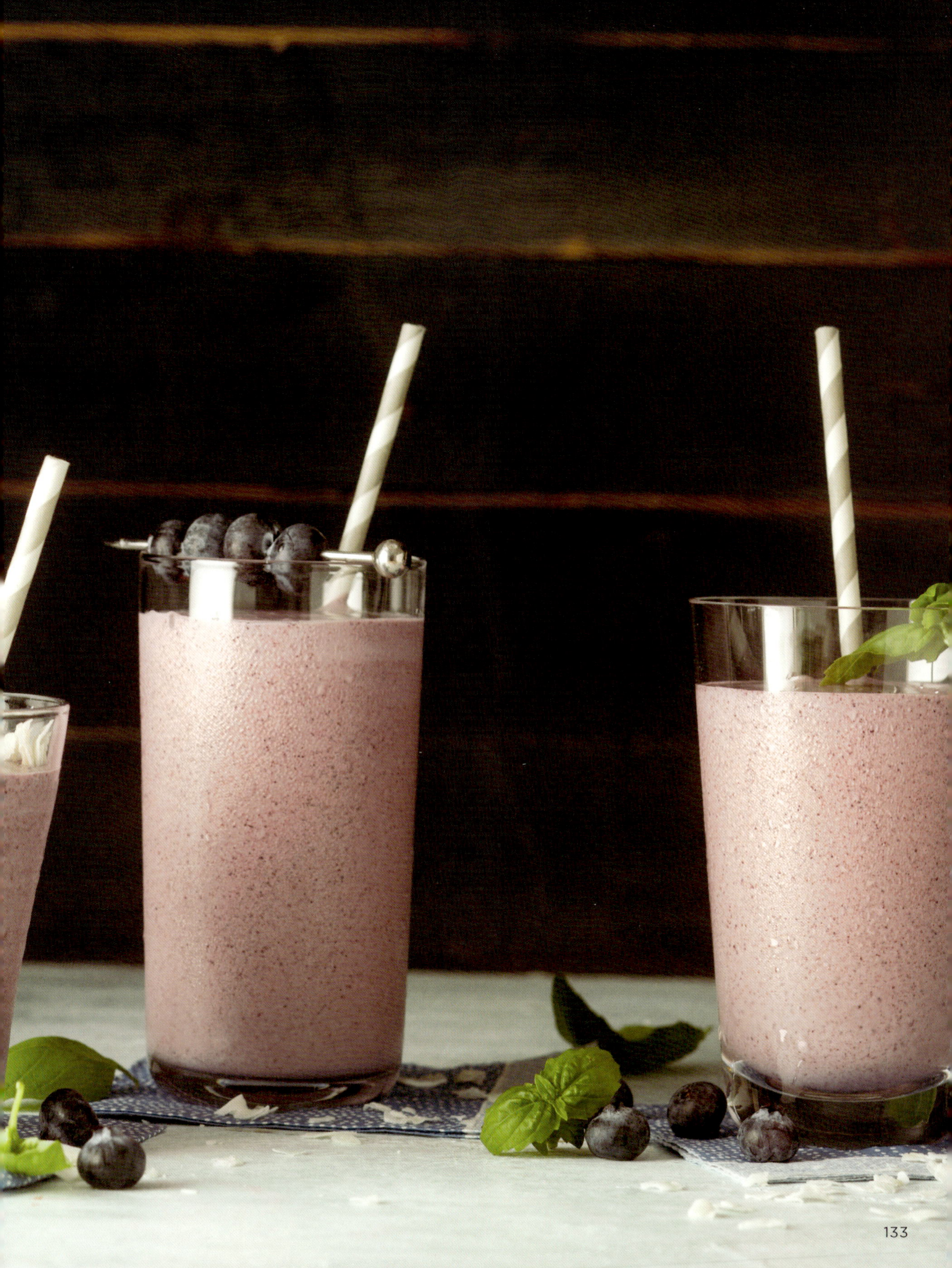

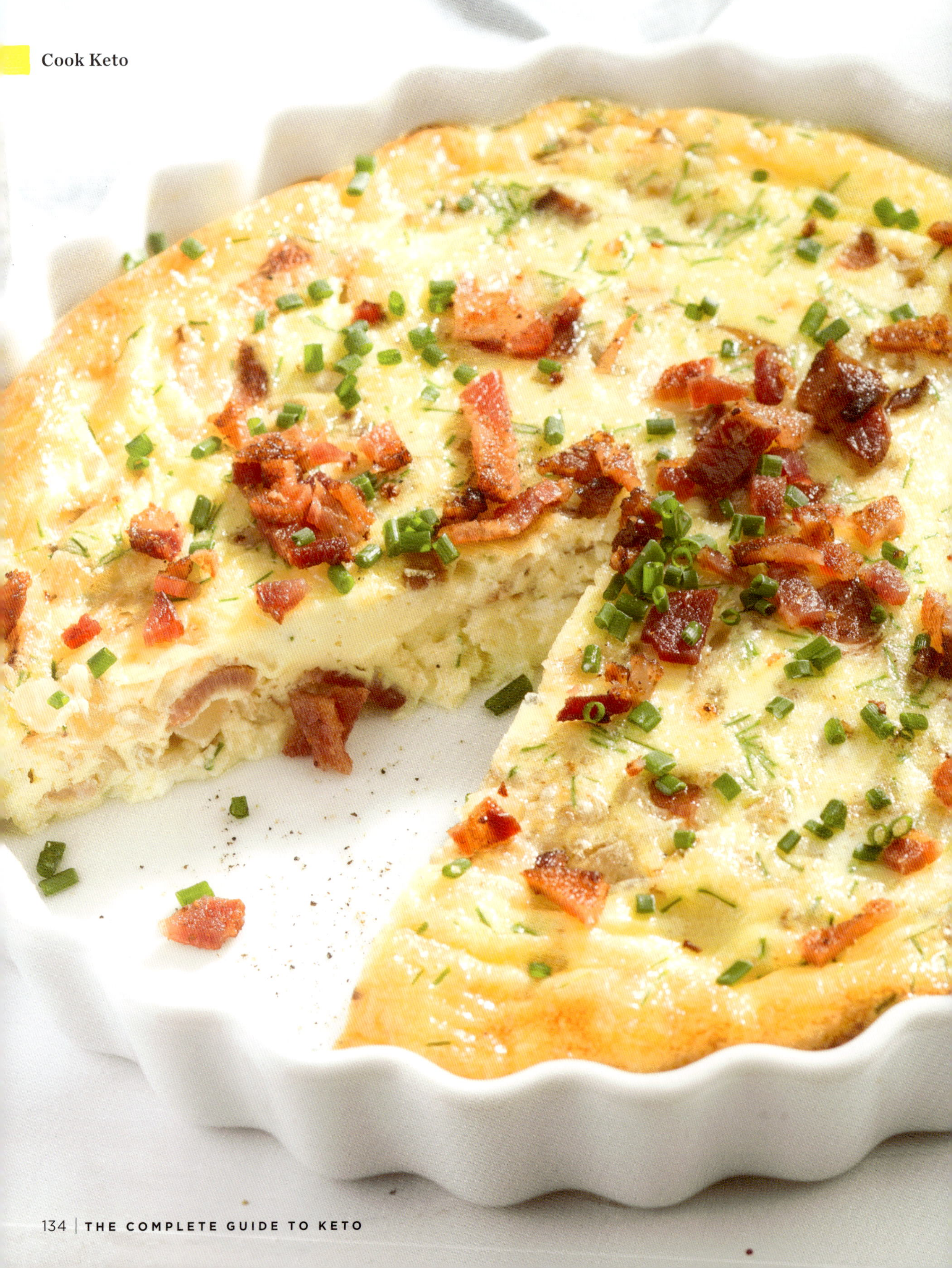

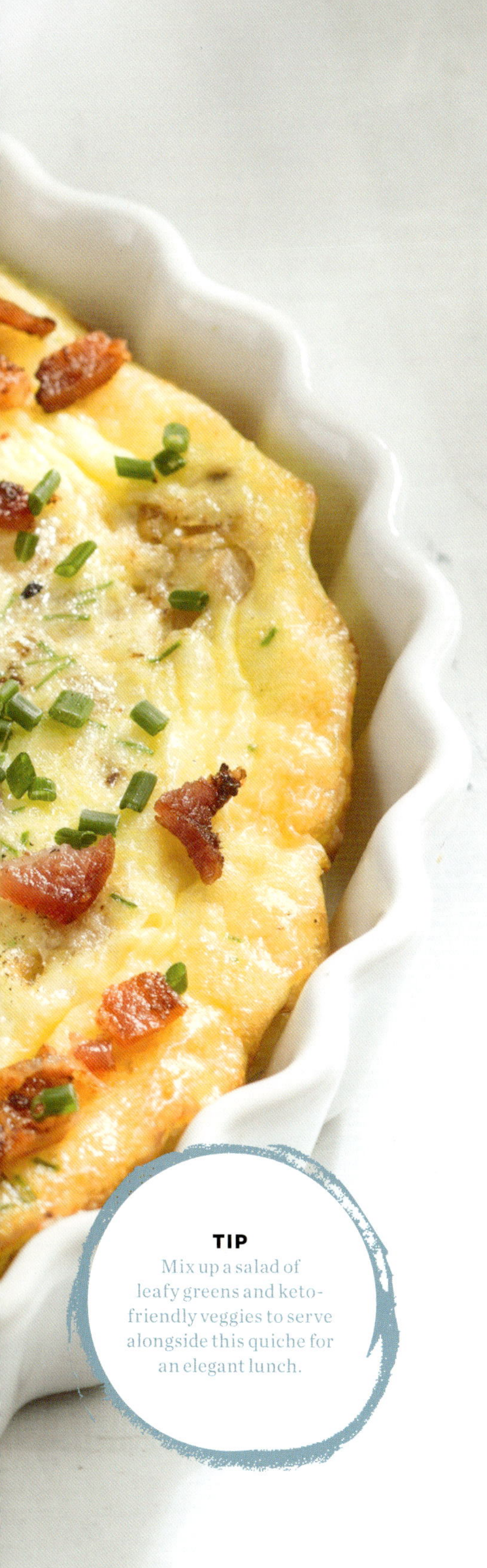

TIP
Mix up a salad of leafy greens and keto-friendly veggies to serve alongside this quiche for an elegant lunch.

CRUSTLESS QUICHE LORRAINE

START TO FINISH 1 hour 15 minutes (15 minutes active)
SERVINGS 6

INGREDIENTS

- 1 tablespoon olive or avocado oil
- ½ cup chopped onion
- ¾ cup cooked, crumbled bacon
- 6 eggs
- 3 egg whites
- 1 cup heavy cream
- ⅔ cup shredded Swiss cheese
- ½ teaspoon salt
- ½ teaspoon pepper
- 2 tablespoons snipped chives, divided

DIRECTIONS

1 Heat oil in a large nonstick skillet. Add onion and cook until tender; add bacon and heat through.
2 In a large mixing bowl, combine eggs, egg whites and cream and mix well. Stir in cheese, salt, pepper and half the chives. Add onion and bacon mixture and mix until combined.
3 Pour into a greased 9-inch tart pan or pie tin.
4 Bake at 350°F for 45-55 minutes or until puffed and browned.
5 Remove from oven and place on a cooling rack. Garnish with remaining chives. Cut into 6 equal slices to serve.

NUTRITION INFORMATION

CALORIES 344; **PROTEIN** 23g; **FAT** 24g; **CARBS** 3g; **FIBER** 0.2g; **NET CARBS** 2.8g

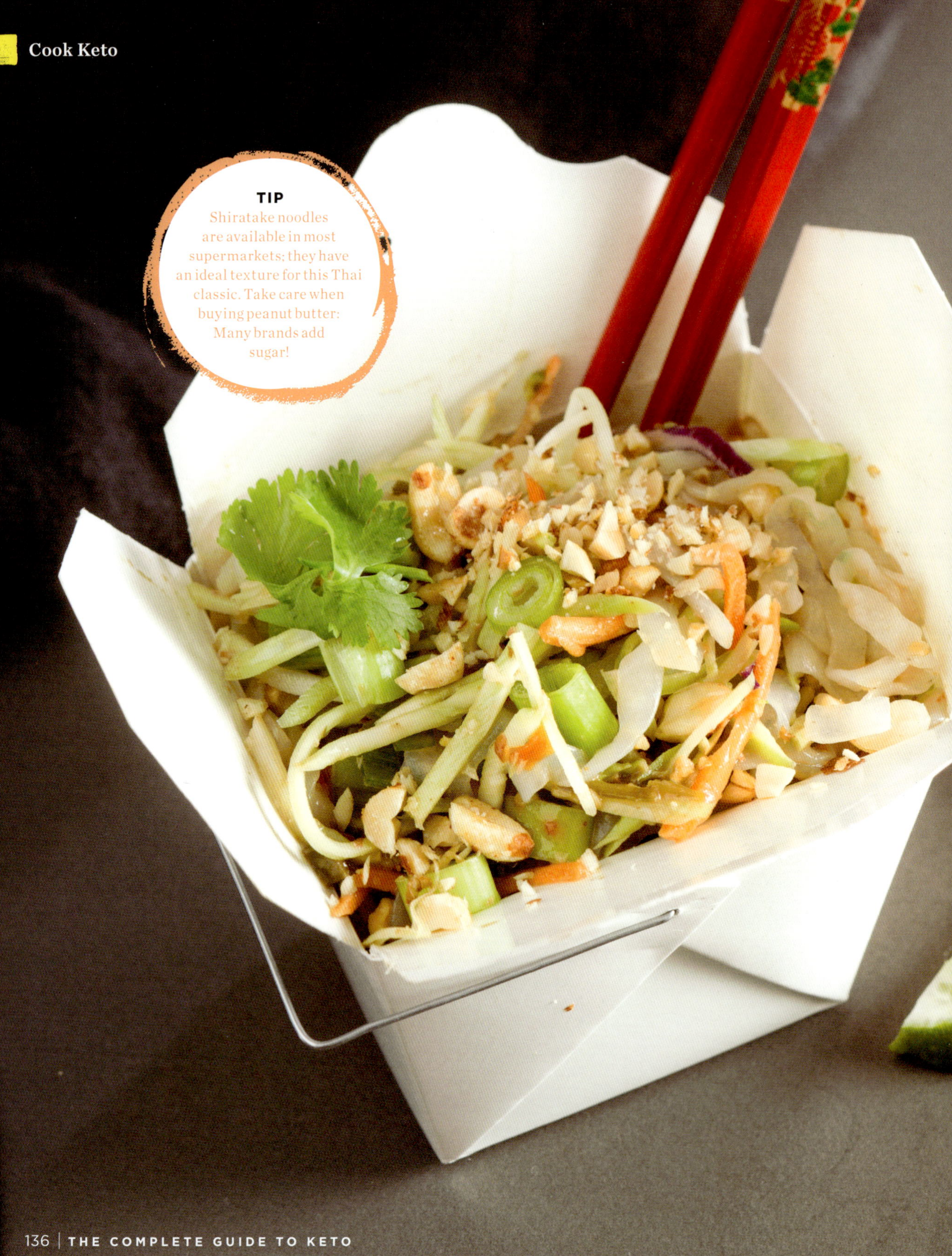

TIP

Shiratake noodles are available in most supermarkets; they have an ideal texture for this Thai classic. Take care when buying peanut butter: Many brands add sugar!

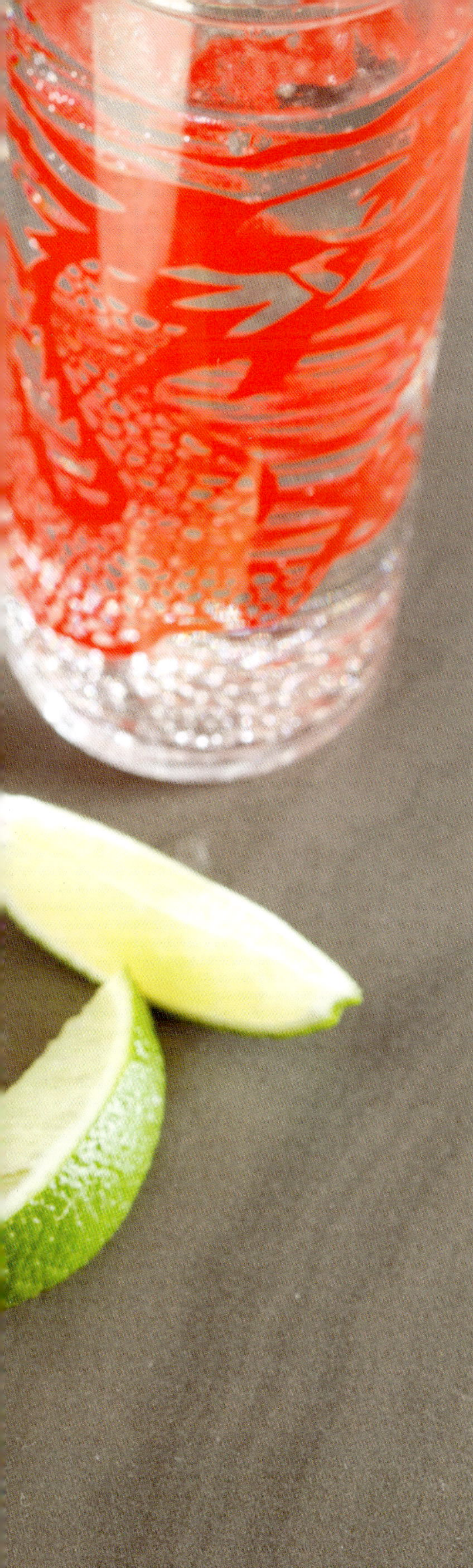

Lunch

PAD THAI NOODLES

START TO FINISH 10 minutes (all active)
SERVINGS 4

INGREDIENTS

1 (12-ounce) bag broccoli slaw mix
¼ cup sliced green onions
4 cups shiratake noodles, drained and rinsed (Skinny Pasta® konjac fettuccine)
¼ cup chopped dry-roasted peanuts
½ cup sugar-free peanut butter
2 tablespoons sesame oil
2 tablespoons lime juice
2 tablespoons water
1 teaspoon chopped ginger
1 teaspoon chopped garlic
½ teaspoon salt

GARNISH cilantro sprigs, lime wedges

DIRECTIONS

1 Combine slaw mix and next 3 ingredients in a large bowl.
2 Combine peanut butter and remaining ingredients in blender and mix until smooth.
3 Pour dressing over salad and serve.
4 Garnish with cilantro and limes, if desired.

NUTRITION INFORMATION

CALORIES 195; **PROTEIN** 6g; **FAT** 12g; **CARBS** 23g; **FIBER** 7g; **NET CARBS** 16g

TUNA NIÇOISE SALAD

START TO FINISH 15 minutes (10 minutes active)
SERVINGS 4

INGREDIENTS

- 1 tablespoon olive oil
- 8 ounces haricots verts, trimmed
- 1 teaspoon minced garlic
- 4 hard boiled eggs, quartered
- 4 Campari tomatoes, quartered
- ½ cup sliced red onion
- 1 small tin quality oil-packed tuna, drained
- 1 cup sliced cucumber
- 1 cup sliced radish
- ½ cup pitted kalamata olives
- No-Carb French Vinaigrette (such as Brianna's Real French Vinaigrette)

DIRECTIONS

1 In a large skillet, heat oil over medium-high heat and add green beans and garlic. Cook 4-5 minutes. Cool.

2 Divide ingredients among 4 individual plates or serve on a large platter as shown in the photo, so guests can assemble their own salads. Season with salt and pepper. Drizzle with dressing.

NUTRITION INFORMATION

CALORIES 193; **PROTEIN** 12g; **FAT** 10g; **CARBS** 11g; **FIBER** 3g; **NET CARBS** 8g

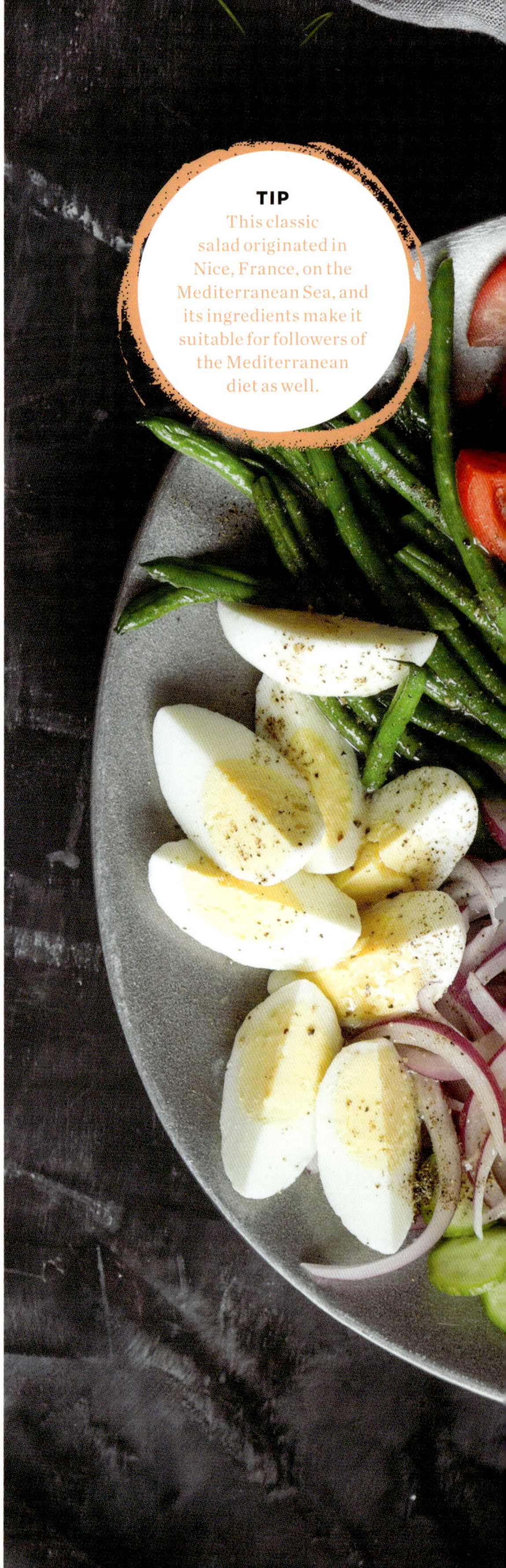

TIP
This classic salad originated in Nice, France, on the Mediterranean Sea, and its ingredients make it suitable for followers of the Mediterranean diet as well.

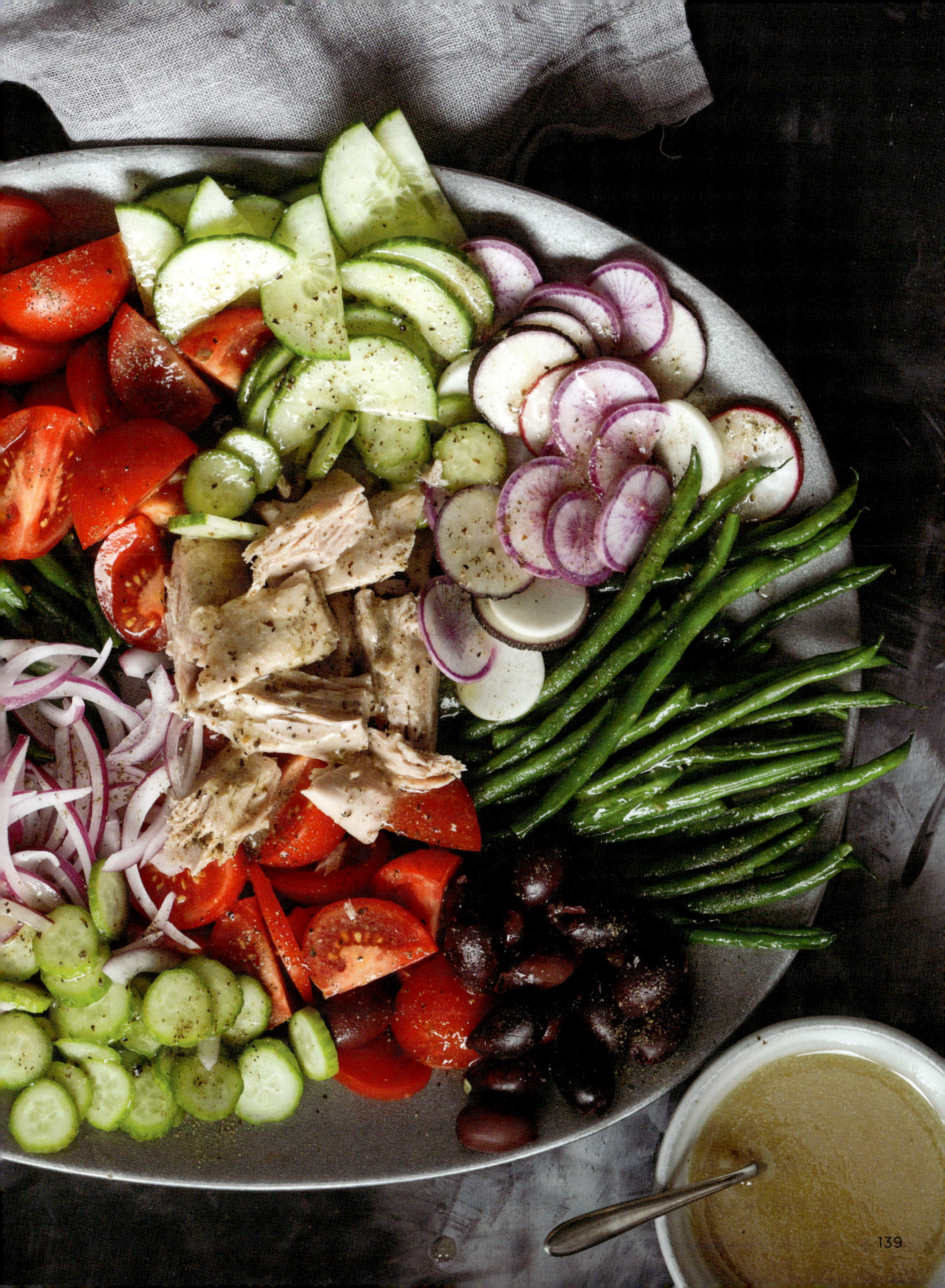

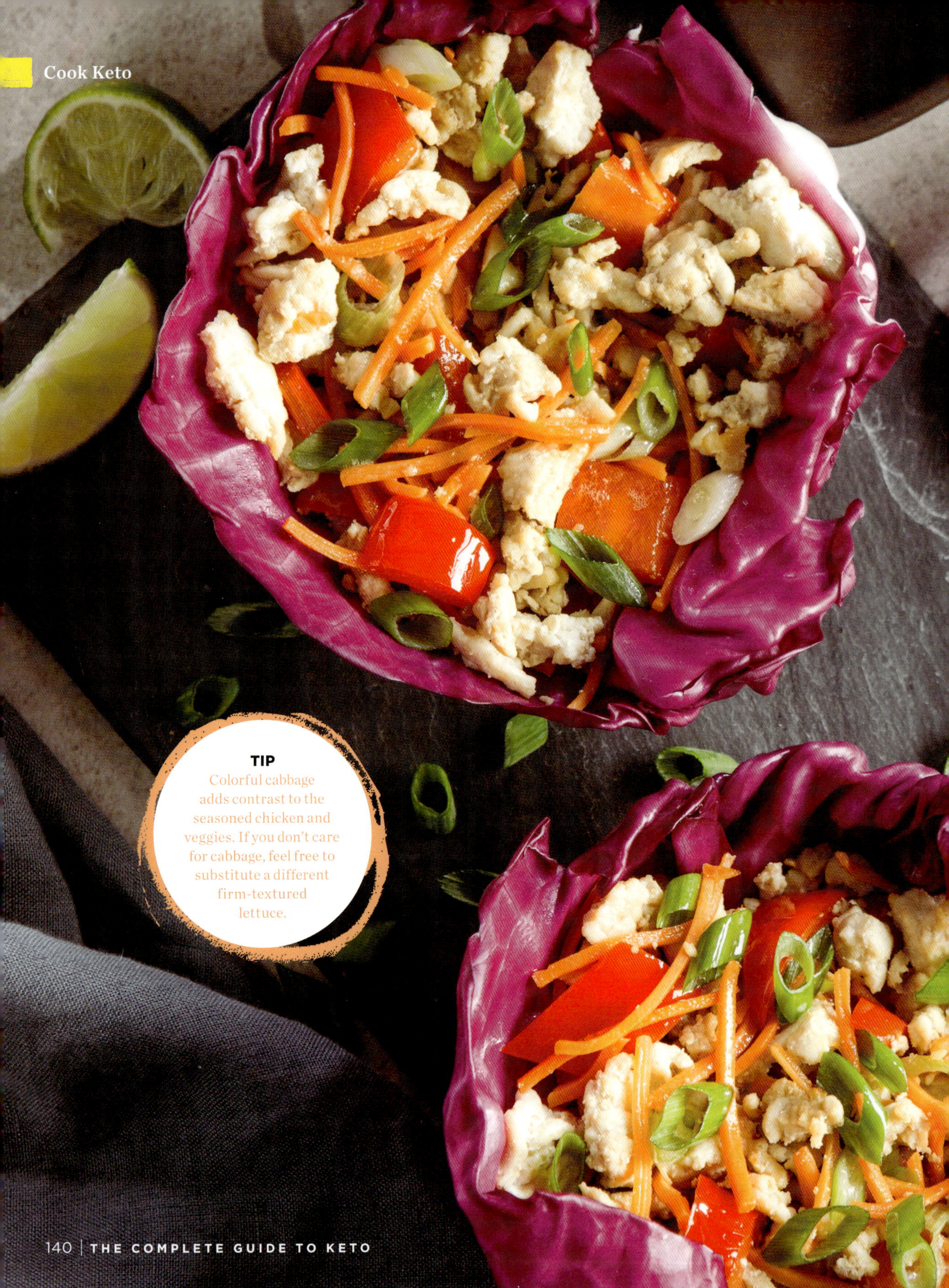

TIP

Colorful cabbage adds contrast to the seasoned chicken and veggies. If you don't care for cabbage, feel free to substitute a different firm-textured lettuce.

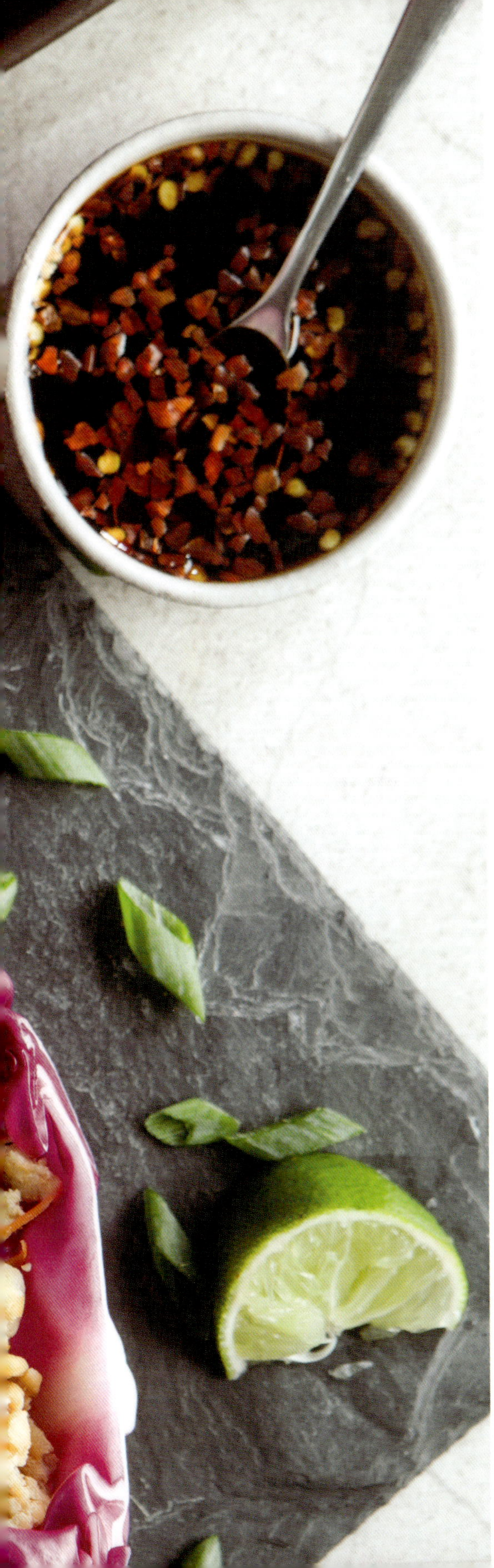

CHICKEN CABBAGE CUPS

START TO FINISH 25 minutes (10 minutes active)
SERVINGS 4

INGREDIENTS

- 1 tablespoon sesame oil
- 1 tablespoon olive or avocado oil
- 1 cup sliced green onion
- 1 cup shredded carrots
- ½ cup diced red bell pepper
- 1 tablespoon ginger
- 1 tablespoon garlic
- 1 pound ground chicken
- ¼ cup tamari
- 1 tablespoon rice wine vinegar
- ½ teaspoon red pepper flakes
- 4 cup-shaped purple cabbage leaves
- 1 tablespoon rice wine vinegar

GARNISHES green onion, red pepper flakes, sesame seeds, hot sauce

DIRECTIONS

1 In a large skillet, over medium heat, add oils and green onion, carrots, bell pepper, ginger and garlic.
Add ground chicken and cook for 8 minutes or until no longer pink.
2 In a small bowl combine tamari, vinegar and red pepper flakes. Add to skillet and cook 1 minute.
3 Spoon into cabbage cups and add desired toppings.

NUTRITION INFORMATION

CALORIES 390; **PROTEIN** 14g; **FAT** 23g; **CARBS** 38g; **FIBER** 11g; **NET CARBS** 27g

GRILLED SALMON AND ROMAINE CAESAR SALAD

START TO FINISH 25 minutes (15 minutes active) **SERVINGS** 2

INGREDIENTS

- 1 (8 ounce) salmon fillet
- ¼ teaspoon salt
- ¼ teaspoon pepper
- 2 romaine hearts, halved
- 2 eggs
- 2 tablespoon Dijon mustard
- 1 clove garlic
- 3 anchovies
- Salt and pepper to taste
- 2 cups olive oil
- ⅓ cup grated Parmesan cheese
- 1 tablespoon lemon juice
- 6 slices of bacon, cooked and crumbled
- 1 cup baby heirloom cherry tomatoes, halved
- ½ cup chopped pecans, toasted

DIRECTIONS

1 Preheat a grill skillet over medium-high heat.

2 Sprinkle salmon with salt and pepper. Grill for 4-5 minutes on each side. Flake with a fork. Set aside.

3 Grill romaine halves for 2 minutes. Chop.

4 To make dressing, in a food processor, blend eggs, mustard, garlic, anchovies, salt and pepper on high for 2 minutes.

5 While food processor is running, slowly add oil in a thin stream. Add cheese and lemon juice.

6 In a large bowl, add chopped romaine, then top with flaked salmon, bacon, tomatoes and pecans. Drizzle with dressing to serve.

NUTRITION INFORMATION

CALORIES 600; **PROTEIN** 42g; **FAT** 45g; **CARBS** 8g; **FIBER** 3g; **NET CARBS** 5g

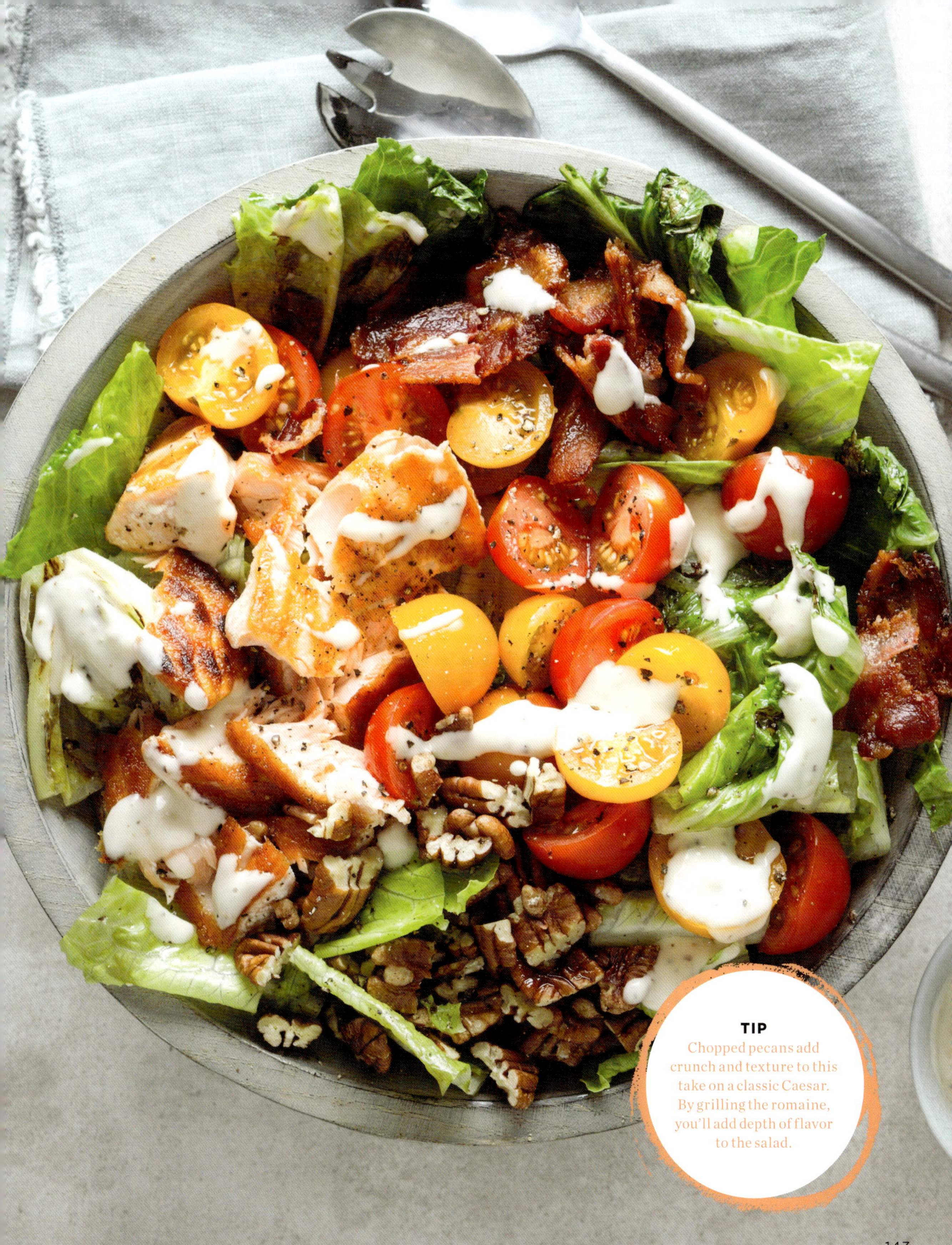

TIP

Chopped pecans add crunch and texture to this take on a classic Caesar. By grilling the romaine, you'll add depth of flavor to the salad.

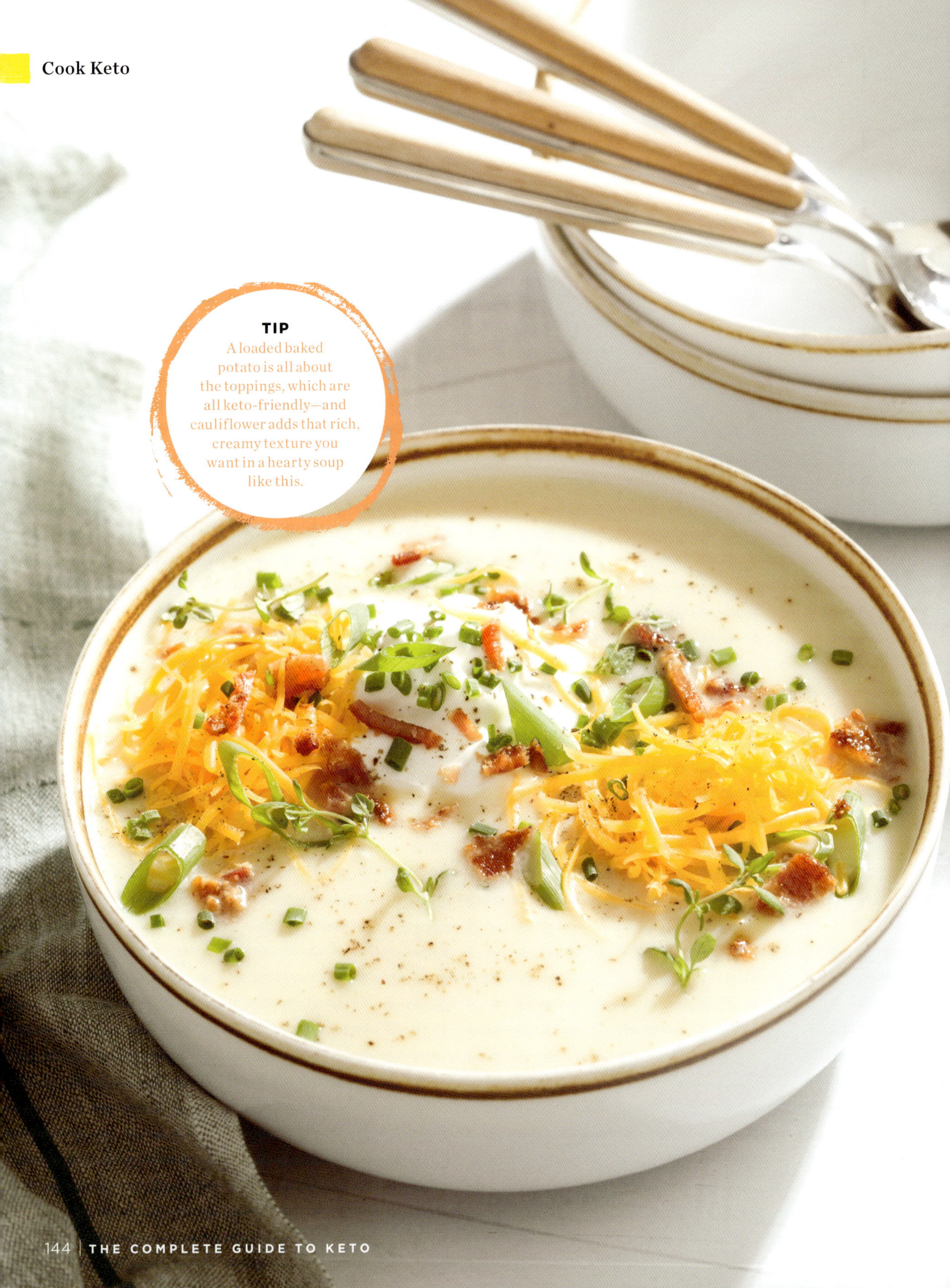

TIP
A loaded baked potato is all about the toppings, which are all keto-friendly—and cauliflower adds that rich, creamy texture you want in a hearty soup like this.

LOADED "POTATO" SOUP

START TO FINISH 1 hour (15 minutes active) **SERVINGS** 8

INGREDIENTS

- 1 (10 ounce) bag cauliflower florets
- 2 tablespoons olive oil
- Salt and pepper
- 6 thyme sprigs
- 4 slices uncooked bacon, chopped
- 1 small onion, chopped
- 2 teaspoons garlic, minced
- 6 cups chicken stock
- 1 bay leaf
- 1½ cups heavy cream

GARNISHES sour cream, shredded cheddar cheese, green onion, chives, thyme sprigs

DIRECTIONS

1 Preheat oven to 425°F. Divide the florets evenly between two large baking sheets. Drizzle with oil and season with salt and pepper. Scatter thyme sprigs on top.

2 Bake about 15-20 minutes or until golden.

3 In a large Dutch oven, over medium-high heat, cook bacon until brown and crispy, about 8-10 minutes. Drain bacon on a paper towel–lined plate.

4 Add onion to reserved bacon fat and cook until tender, about 5 minutes. Stir in garlic and cook an additional minute.

5 Add roasted cauliflower to the pot; add stock and bay leaf. Bring to a boil, reduce heat and simmer until the cauliflower is falling apart, about 15-20 minutes. Remove bay leaf.

6 Using an immersion blender, puree soup until smooth. Season with salt and pepper. Stir in heavy cream.

7 Garnish with sour cream, shredded cheddar cheese, green onion, chives and thyme sprigs.

NUTRITION INFORMATION

CALORIES 106; **PROTEIN** 6g; **FAT** 7g; **CARBS** 4g; **FIBER** 1g; **NET CARBS** 3g

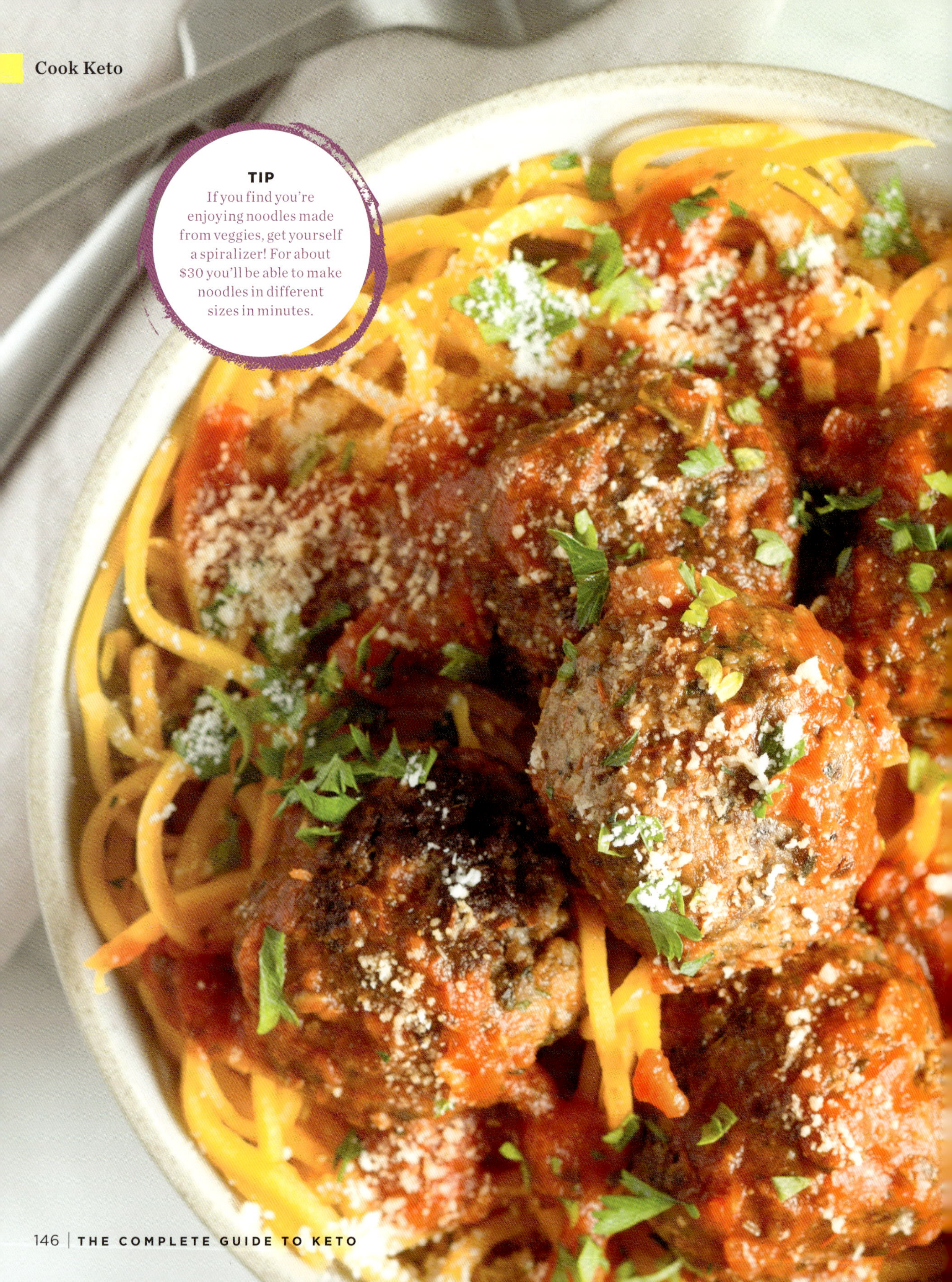

TIP
If you find you're enjoying noodles made from veggies, get yourself a spiralizer! For about $30 you'll be able to make noodles in different sizes in minutes.

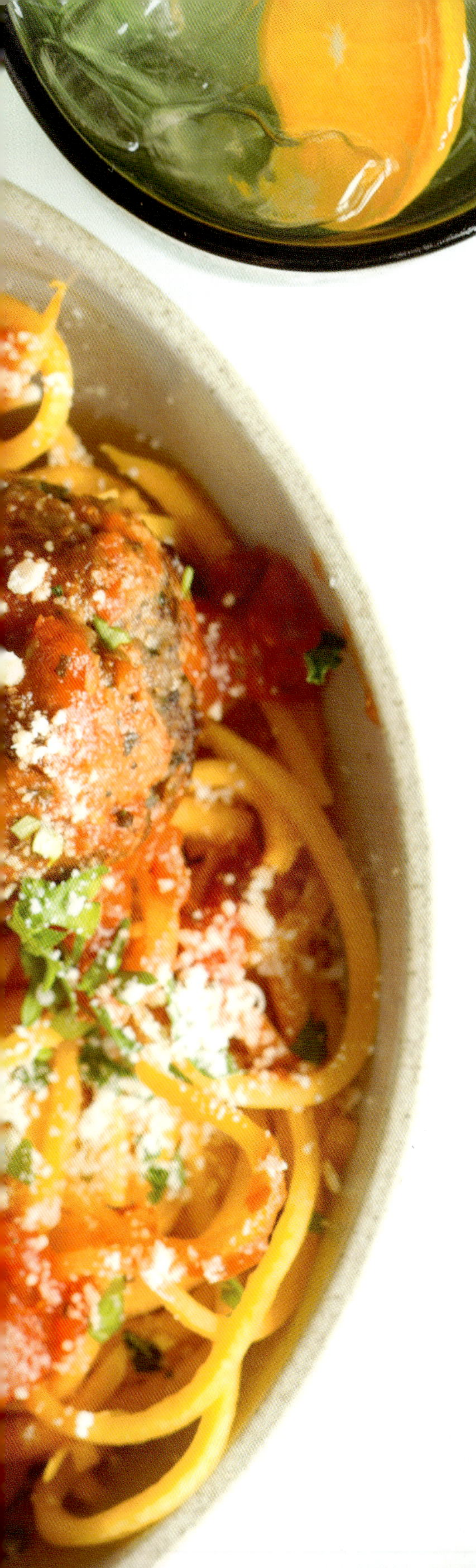

Dinner

BEEF AND PORK MEATBALLS OVER BUTTERNUT NOODLES

START TO FINISH 40 minutes (15 minutes active) **SERVINGS** 4

INGREDIENTS

- 1 pound ground beef
- 1 pound ground pork
- ¾ cup grated Parmesan cheese
- ½ cup almond flour
- 2 tablespoons minced parsley
- 1 teaspoon salt
- 1 teaspoon pepper
- 2 cups sugar-free marinara sauce
- 1 (10-ounce) container of butternut squash "noodles"

GARNISHES grated Parmesan, chopped parsley

DIRECTIONS

1 Preheat oven to 350°F.
2 In a medium bowl, combine beef, pork, cheese, almond flour, parsley, salt and pepper. Form into 16 meatballs. Place on greased baking sheet.
3 Bake for 20 minutes or until cooked through.
4 In a large skillet, heat up marinara and butternut squash noodles. Divide evenly between 4 plates. Top with meatballs and serve.
5 Garnish with grated Parmesan and chopped parsley, if desired.

NUTRITION INFORMATION

CALORIES 750; **PROTEIN** 55g; **FAT** 45g; **CARBS** 22g; **FIBER** 6g; **NET CARBS** 16g

SKILLET GARLIC-HERB PORK CHOPS

START TO FINISH 25 minutes (5 minutes active)
SERVINGS 2

INGREDIENTS

- 2 (12-ounce) bone-in pork chops
- 1 teaspoon salt
- 1 teaspoon pepper
- ¼ cup butter, melted
- 1 teaspoon thyme leaves
- 2 garlic cloves, minced
- 1 garlic bulb, halved
- 3 rosemary sprigs
- 2 tablespoons olive oil

GARNISHES thyme sprigs, sage leaves

DIRECTIONS

1 Preheat oven to 375°F.
2 Sprinkle salt and pepper over both sides of chops.
3 In a small bowl, combine butter, thyme and minced garlic. Set aside.
4 Heat oil in cast-iron skillet over medium high heat. Add chops, garlic halves and rosemary sprigs and cook 2 minutes per side. Remove garlic and rosemary. Set aside.
5 Pour butter mixture over chops. Place in oven and bake for 10-12 minutes or until internal temperature reaches 145°F. Let rest 10 minutes. Add herbs and garlic back to skillet.
6 Serve chops with the butter sauce and fresh herbs.

NUTRITION INFORMATION

CALORIES 369; **PROTEIN** 24g; **FAT** 28g; **CARBS** 5g; **FIBER** 0.5g; **NET CARBS** 4.5g

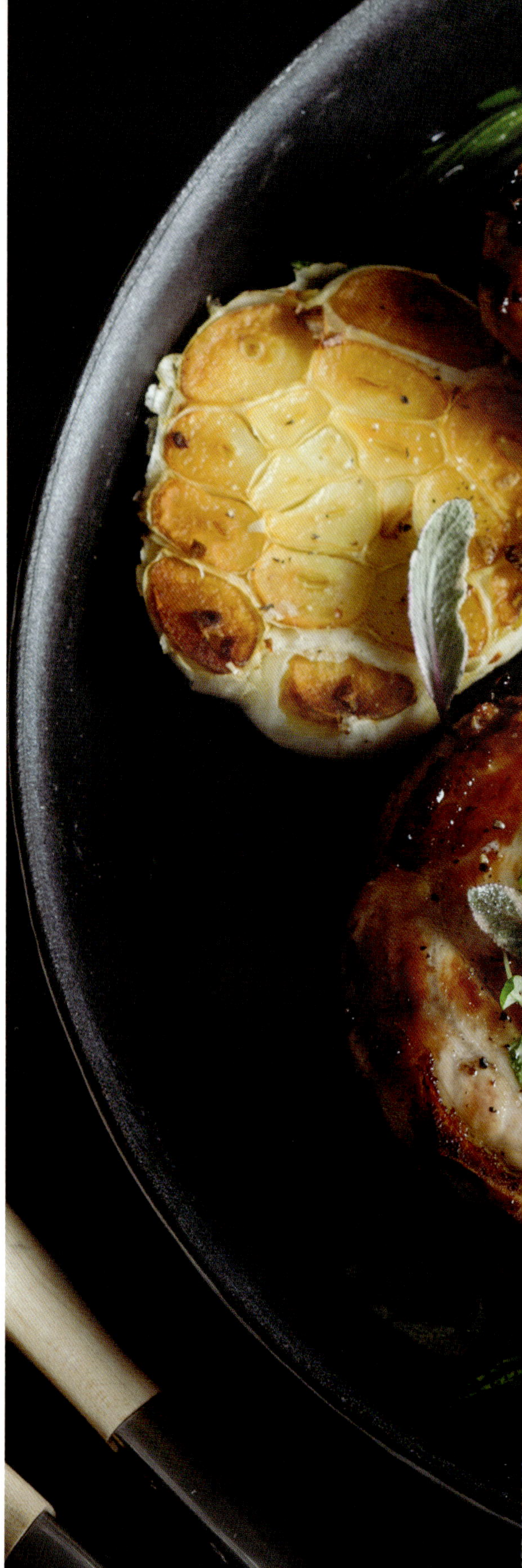

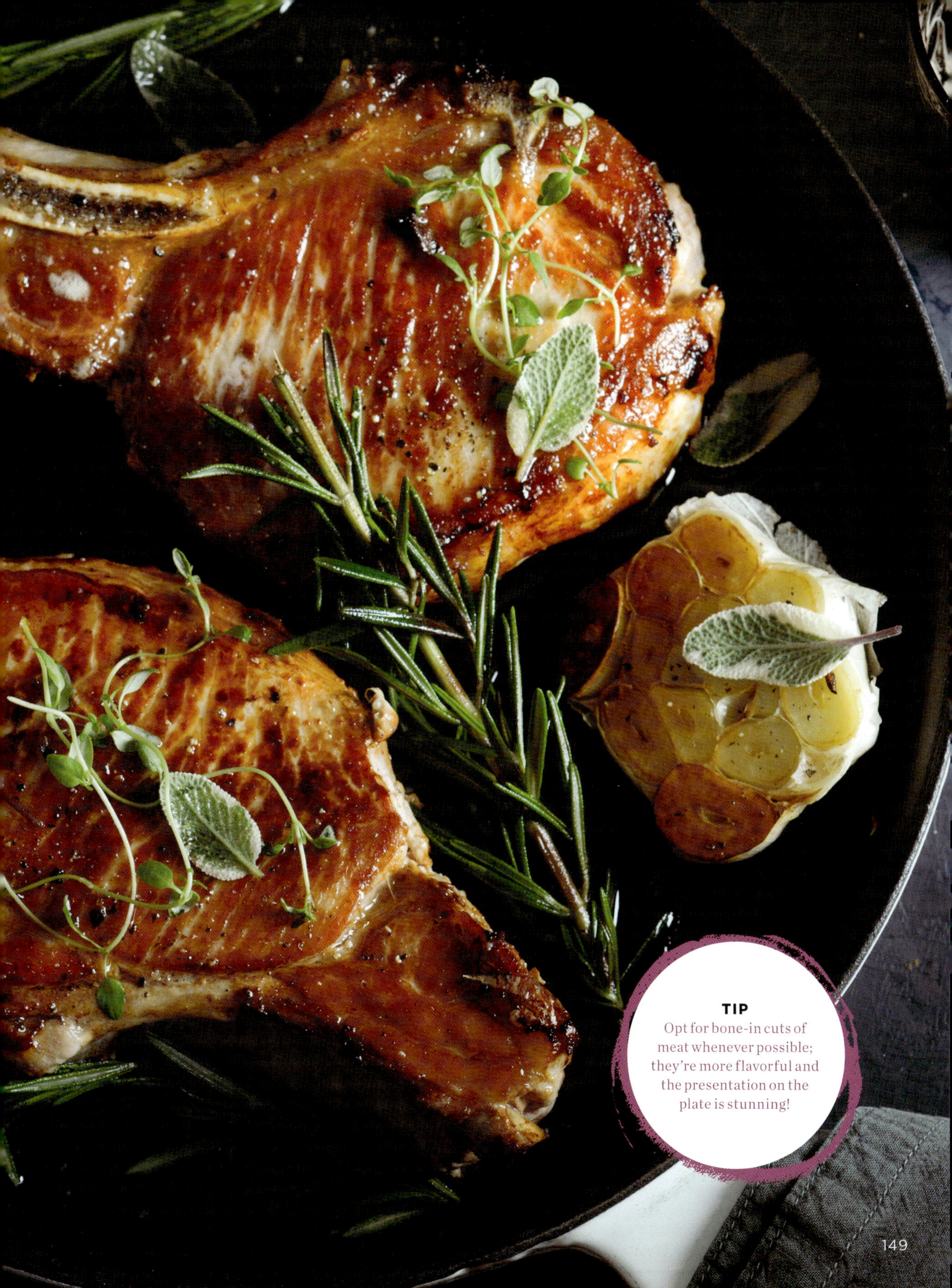

TIP
Opt for bone-in cuts of meat whenever possible; they're more flavorful and the presentation on the plate is stunning!

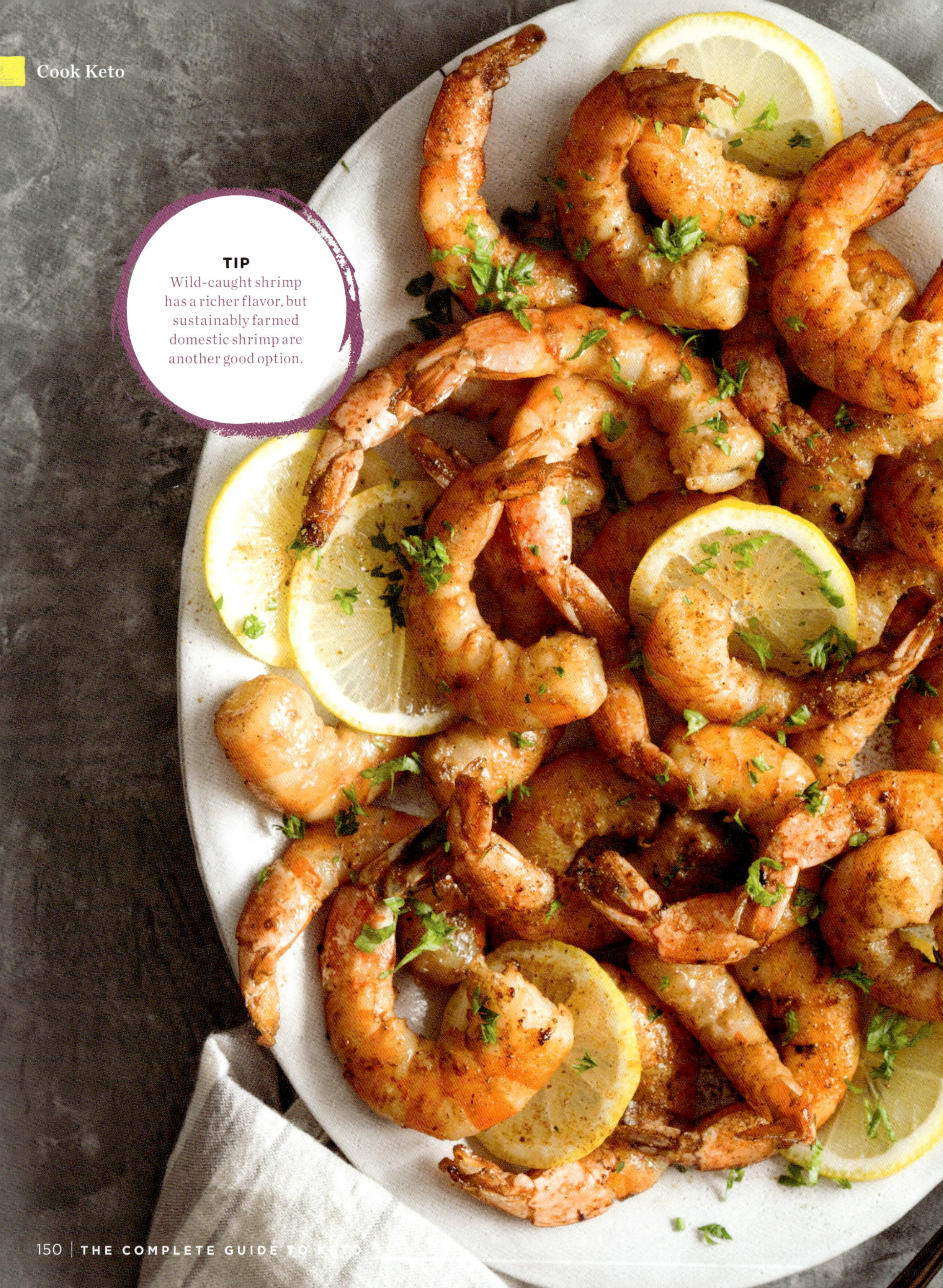

TIP
Wild-caught shrimp has a richer flavor, but sustainably farmed domestic shrimp are another good option.

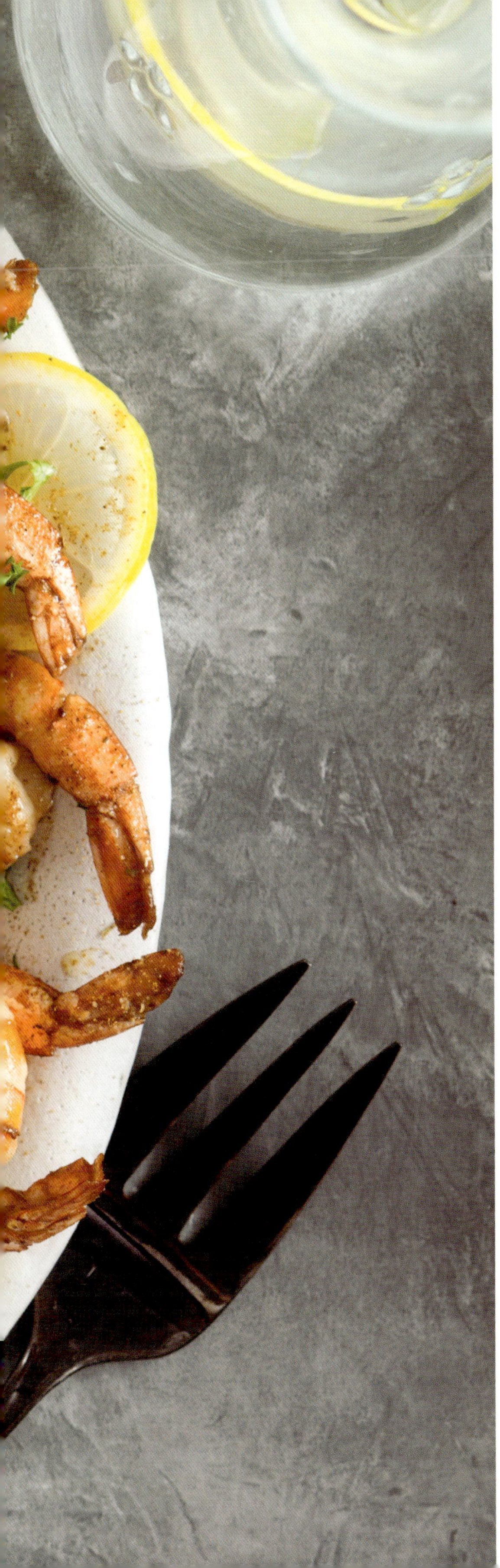

OVEN BBQ SHRIMP

START TO FINISH 45 minutes (15 minutes active)

SERVINGS 4

INGREDIENTS

- ½ cup butter
- ¼ cup Worcestershire sauce
- 1 tablespoon chopped garlic
- 1 teaspoon hot sauce
- 1 teaspoon Old Bay seasoning
- 2 pounds peeled jumbo shrimp, tails on

GARNISH lemon slices

DIRECTIONS

1 Melt butter in a medium saucepan over low heat. Add next 4 ingredients. Stir until well combined, remove from heat and let cool.

2 Place shrimp in a 13 x 9-inch baking dish. Pour cooled sauce over shrimp; cover with plastic wrap and refrigerate. Marinate for 30 minutes or longer.

3 Remove shrimp from refrigerator and spread onto sheet pan. Place pan in broiler; cook shrimp for 5 minutes then turn over and broil for 1 more minute. Serve with lemon slices.

NUTRITION INFORMATION

CALORIES 264; **PROTEIN** 46g; **FAT** 6.5g; **CARBS** 5g; **FIBER** 0g; **NET CARBS** 5g

LEMON BAKED SALMON FILLETS

START TO FINISH 30 minutes (5 minutes active)
SERVINGS 4

INGREDIENTS

- 4 (8-ounce) salmon fillets
- 1 teaspoon salt
- 1 teaspoon pepper
- ¼ cup melted butter
- ⅓ cup grated Parmesan
- 3 cloves garlic, minced
- 2 tablespoons chopped parsley

GARNISHES lemon slices, parsley leaves

DIRECTIONS

1 Preheat oven to 350°F.
2 Place parchment paper on a baking pan. Place salmon on top and sprinkle with salt and pepper.
3 In a small bowl, combine butter, Parmesan, garlic and parsley. Spread mixture evenly on salmon fillets.
4 Bake for 20-25 minutes or until salmon is cooked through.
5 Garnish with lemon slices and parsley leaves.

NUTRITION INFORMATION

CALORIES 218; **PROTEIN** 24g; **FAT** 12g; **CARBS** 2g; **FIBER** 0.25g; **NET CARBS** 1.75g

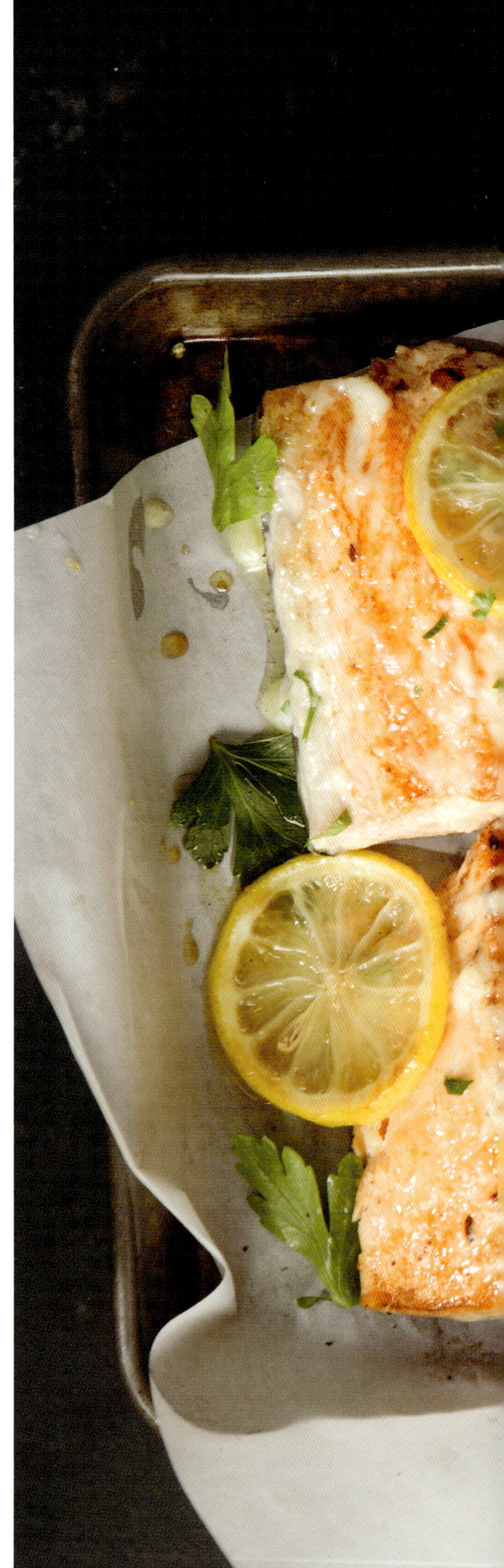

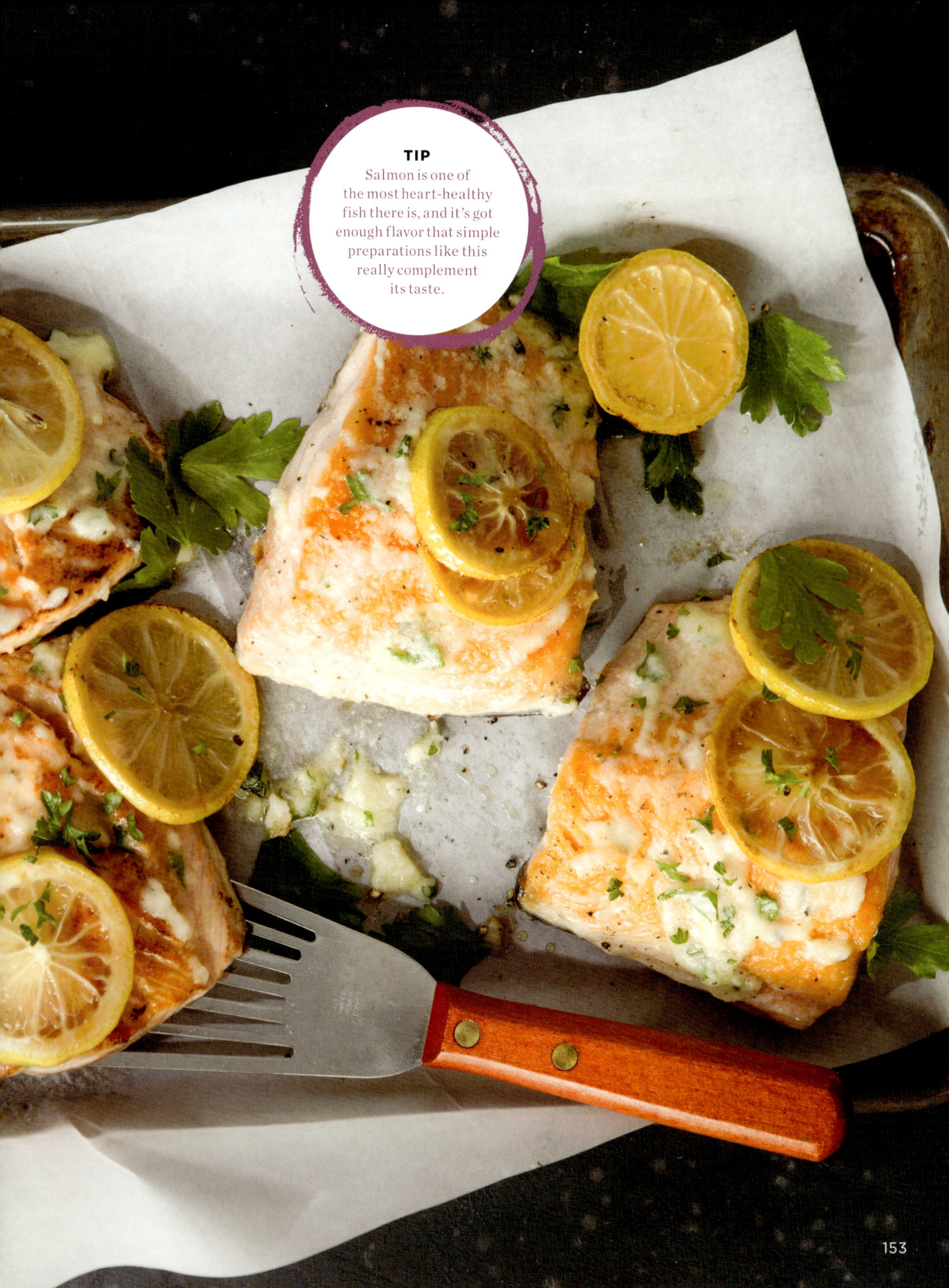

TIP
Salmon is one of the most heart-healthy fish there is, and it's got enough flavor that simple preparations like this really complement its taste.

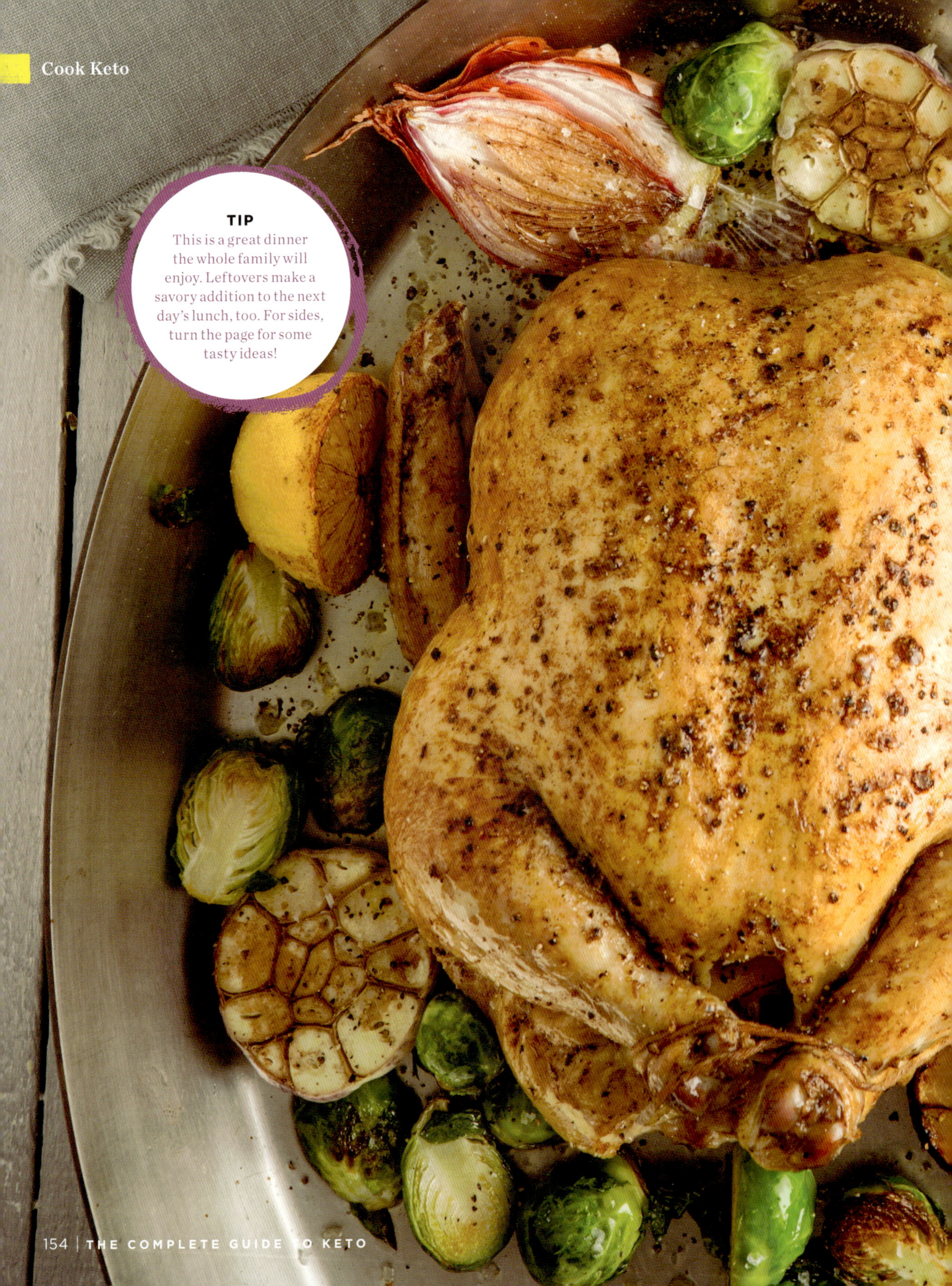

TIP

This is a great dinner the whole family will enjoy. Leftovers make a savory addition to the next day's lunch, too. For sides, turn the page for some tasty ideas!

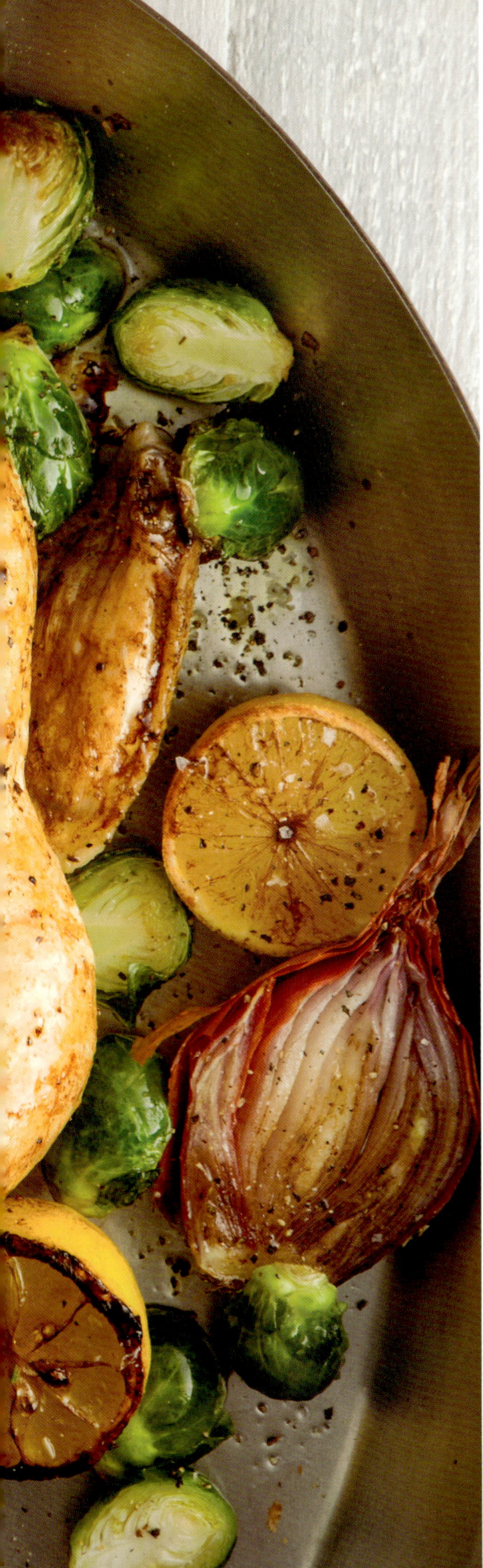

WHOLE ROASTED CHICKEN WITH BRUSSELS SPROUTS

START TO FINISH 1 hour 10 minutes (15 minutes active)

SERVINGS 4

INGREDIENTS

- ½ cup butter, softened
- 1 tablespoon chopped garlic
- 1 teaspoon salt
- 1 teaspoon pepper
- 1 4-pound whole chicken
- 1 cup chicken stock
- 2 shallots, quartered
- 2 garlic bulbs, halved
- 2 lemons, halved
- 1 cup Brussels sprouts, halved

DIRECTIONS

1 Preheat oven to 400°F.

2 In a small bowl, combine butter and next 4 ingredients until incorporated.

3 Place chicken in roasting pan breast side up. Add the chicken broth to the bottom of the pan. Add shallots, garlic, lemon and Brussels sprouts.

4 Rub butter mixture under the skin of chicken and all over the top of chicken.

5 Bake for 30 minutes and then baste. Roast an additional 30 to 45 minutes, basting every 15 minutes. Roast until thermometer reads 165°F.

NUTRITION INFORMATION

CALORIES 341; **PROTEIN** 27g; **FAT** 22g; **CARBS** 52g; **FIBER** 13g; **NET CARBS** 39g

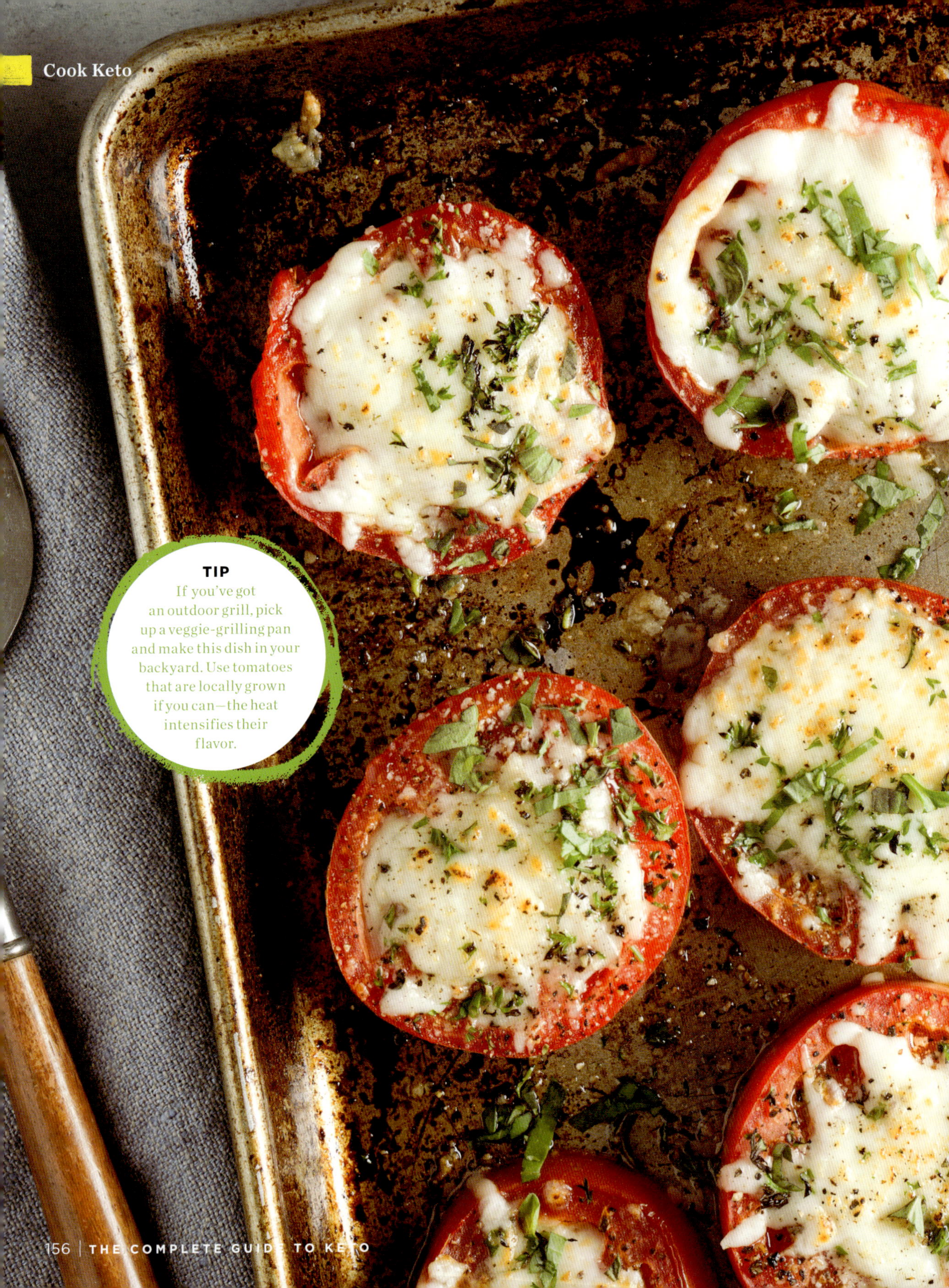

TIP
If you've got an outdoor grill, pick up a veggie-grilling pan and make this dish in your backyard. Use tomatoes that are locally grown if you can—the heat intensifies their flavor.

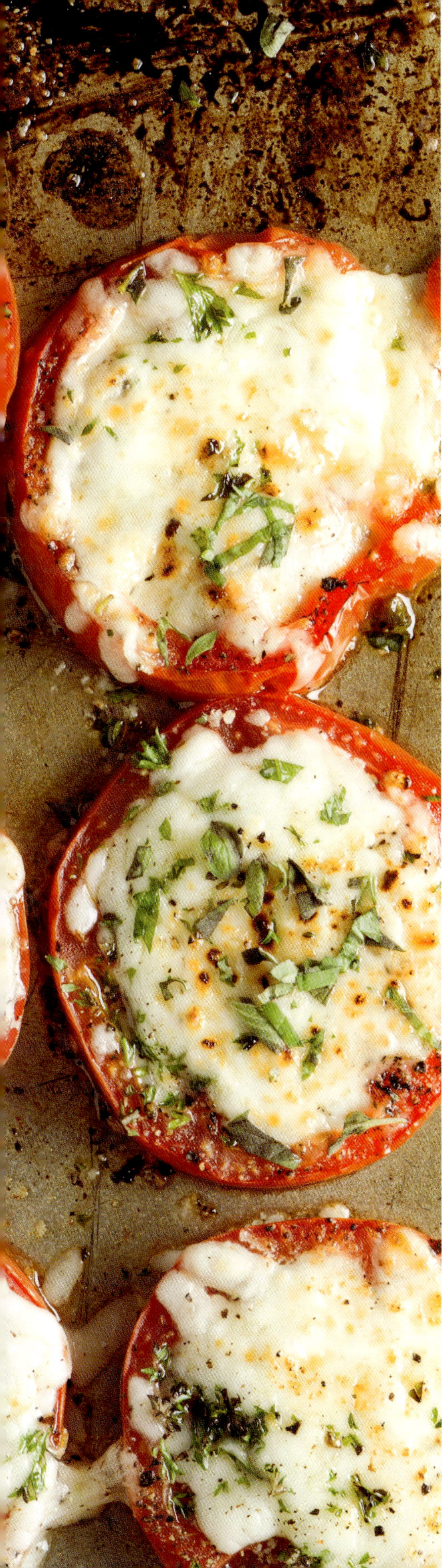

Sides

CHEESY BROILED TOMATOES WITH HERBS

START TO FINISH 15 minutes (10 minutes active)
SERVINGS 4

INGREDIENTS

- 4 medium tomatoes, sliced
- 1 ½ cups shredded mozzarella
- 1 cup grated Parmesan cheese
- 2 tablespoons chopped basil
- 1 tablespoon chopped parsley
- 1 tablespoon chopped oregano
- 2 tablespoons olive oil

DIRECTIONS

1 Preheat oven to 400°F.
2 On a greased baking sheet, arrange tomato slices. Top evenly with mozzarella and Parmesan. Sprinkle with fresh herbs and drizzle with olive oil.
3 Bake 8 minutes or until cheese melts. Broil for 2-3 minutes to brown.

NUTRITION INFORMATION

CALORIES 293; **PROTEIN** 21g; **FAT** 23.5g; **CARBS** 12g; **FIBER** 1.5g; **NET CARBS** 10.5g

STEAKHOUSE CREAMED SPINACH

START TO FINISH 15 minutes (5 minutes active)

SERVINGS 4

INGREDIENTS

- ¼ cup butter
- 2 tablespoons minced garlic
- 15 ounces baby spinach
- ½ cup heavy cream
- 8 ounces cream cheese, cubed
- ½ teaspoon salt
- ½ teaspoon pepper
- ½ cup grated Parmesan cheese

DIRECTIONS

1 Heat butter in a large nonstick sauté pan over medium heat. Add garlic and cook for 1-2 minutes.

2 Add spinach and sauté for 3-4 minutes or until wilted.

3 Add cream and next 3 ingredients. Stir until the cheese melts and mixture is thickened.

4 Sprinkle with Parmesan cheese and serve.

NUTRITION INFORMATION

CALORIES 154; **PROTEIN** 3g; **FAT** 13g; **CARBS** 5g; **FIBER** 3g; **NET CARBS** 2g

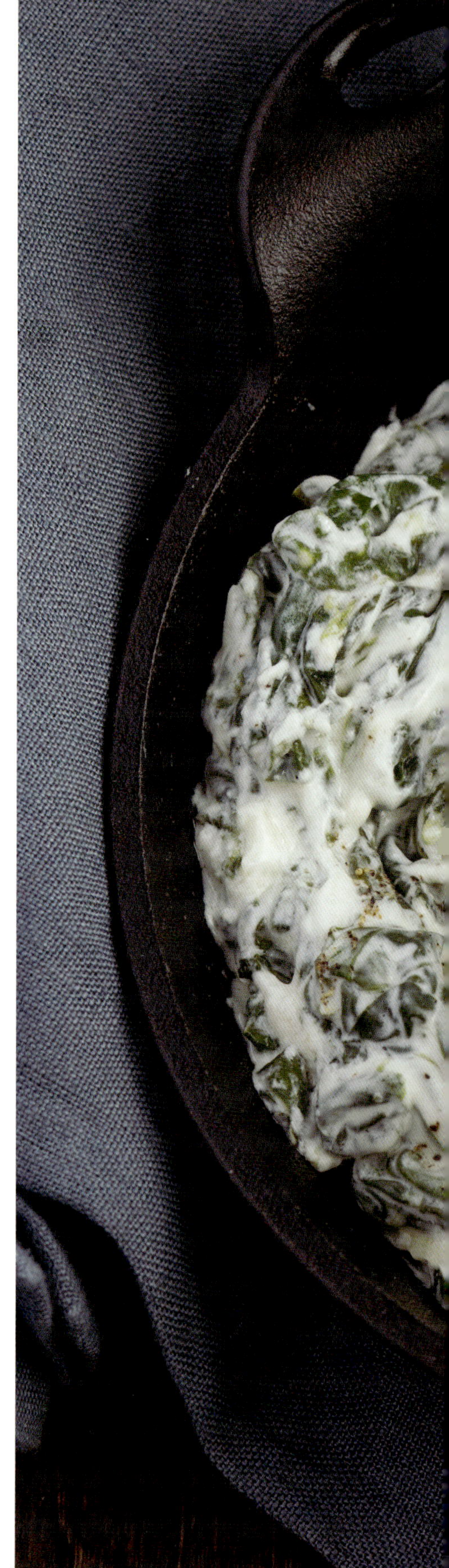

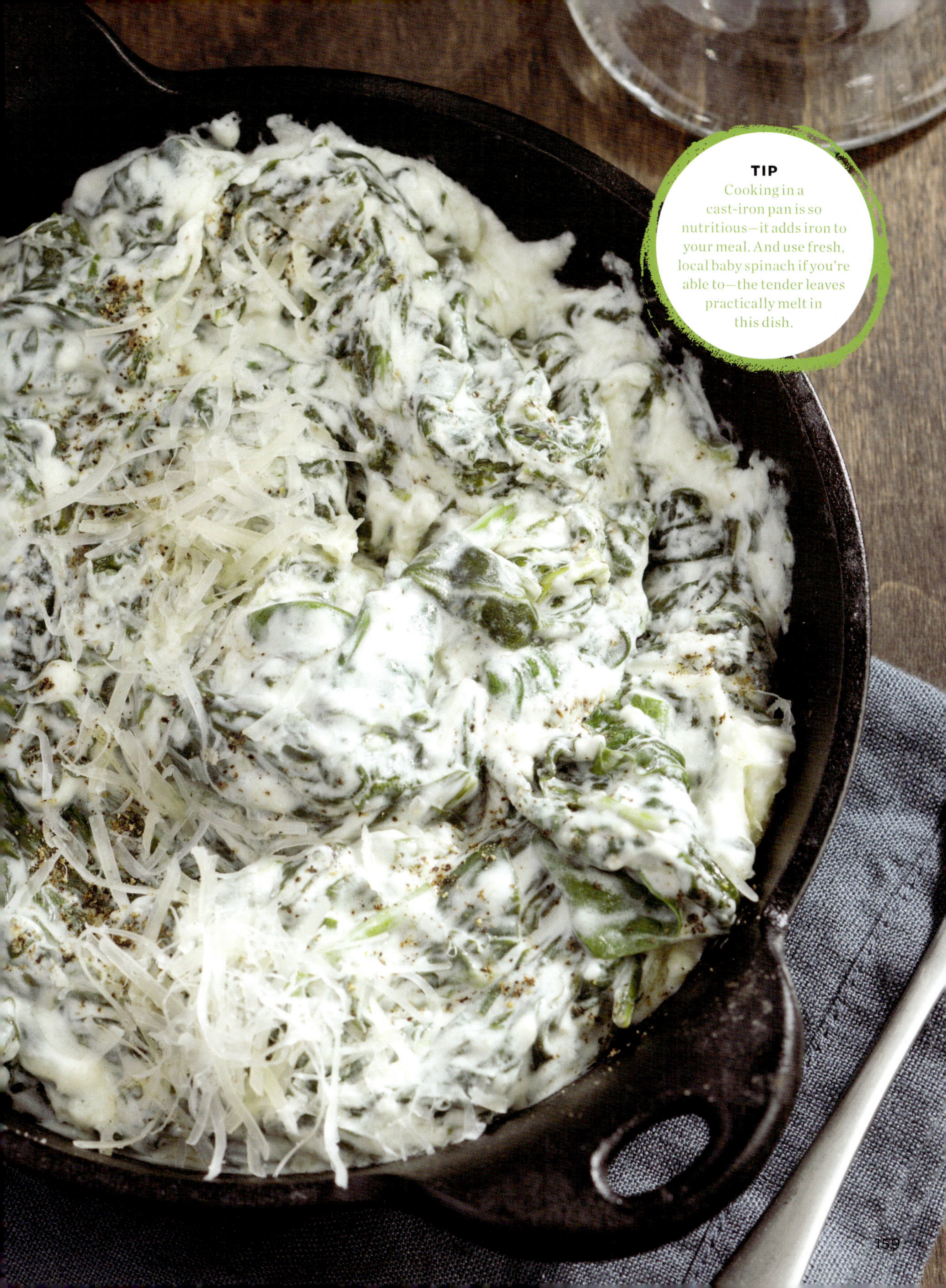

TIP
Cooking in a cast-iron pan is so nutritious—it adds iron to your meal. And use fresh, local baby spinach if you're able to—the tender leaves practically melt in this dish.

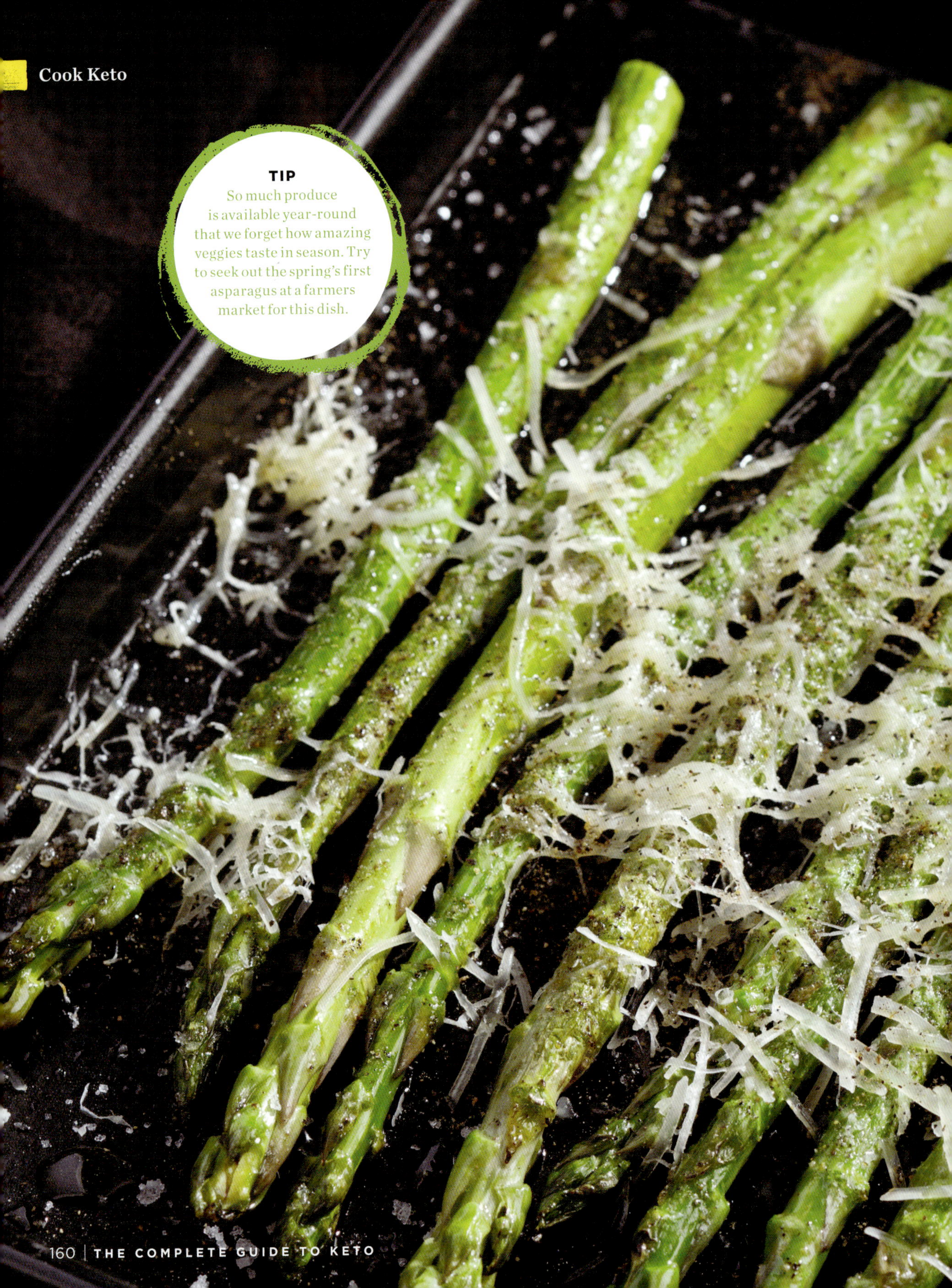

TIP

So much produce is available year-round that we forget how amazing veggies taste in season. Try to seek out the spring's first asparagus at a farmers market for this dish.

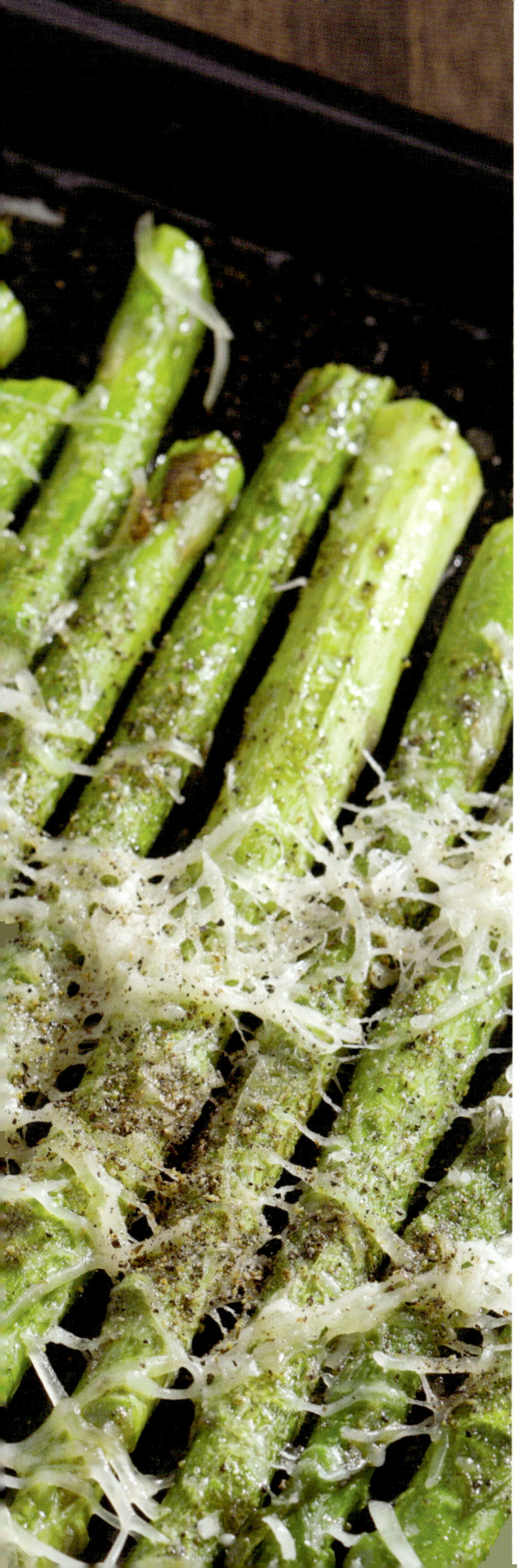

PARMESAN ROASTED ASPARAGUS

START TO FINISH 20 minutes (5 minutes active)
SERVINGS 4

INGREDIENTS

- 1 bunch asparagus, trimmed
- 2 tablespoons extra-virgin olive oil
- ½ cup shredded Parmesan cheese
- 2 tablespoons lemon juice
- 1 teaspoon sea salt
- 1 teaspoon pepper

DIRECTIONS

1 Preheat oven to 375°F.
2 On greased baking sheet, arrange asparagus.
3 Drizzle olive oil and lemon juice over asparagus. Toss to coat evenly.
4 Sprinkle shredded cheese over asparagus.
5 Season with salt and pepper.
6 Bake for 15 minutes.

NUTRITION INFORMATION

CALORIES 89; **PROTEIN** 2g; **FAT** 8g; **CARBS** 2g; **FIBER** 1g. **NET CARBS** 1g

CAULIFLOWER MASH WITH TOPPINGS

START TO FINISH 30 minutes (all active)
YIELD 8 servings

INGREDIENTS

2 (12 ounce) bags cauliflower florets
1 cup milk
1 cup cream
¼ cup butter
1 tablespoon minced garlic
1 teaspoon salt
1 teaspoon pepper

GARNISHES shredded cheddar, sour cream, green onions, chives, crumbled bacon

DIRECTIONS

1 Place cauliflower in a Dutch oven and cover with water. Bring to a boil and cook about 20 minutes or until tender. Drain and return to Dutch oven.
2 In a small saucepan combine milk and next 5 ingredients; bring to a simmer over medium heat.
3 Pour milk mixture over cauliflower mixture slowly, mashing with potato masher until desired consistency. Garnish with desired toppings.

NUTRITION INFORMATION

CALORIES 102; **PROTEIN** 2g; **FAT** 9g; **CARBS** 4g; **FIBER** 0.5g; **NET CARBS** 3.5g

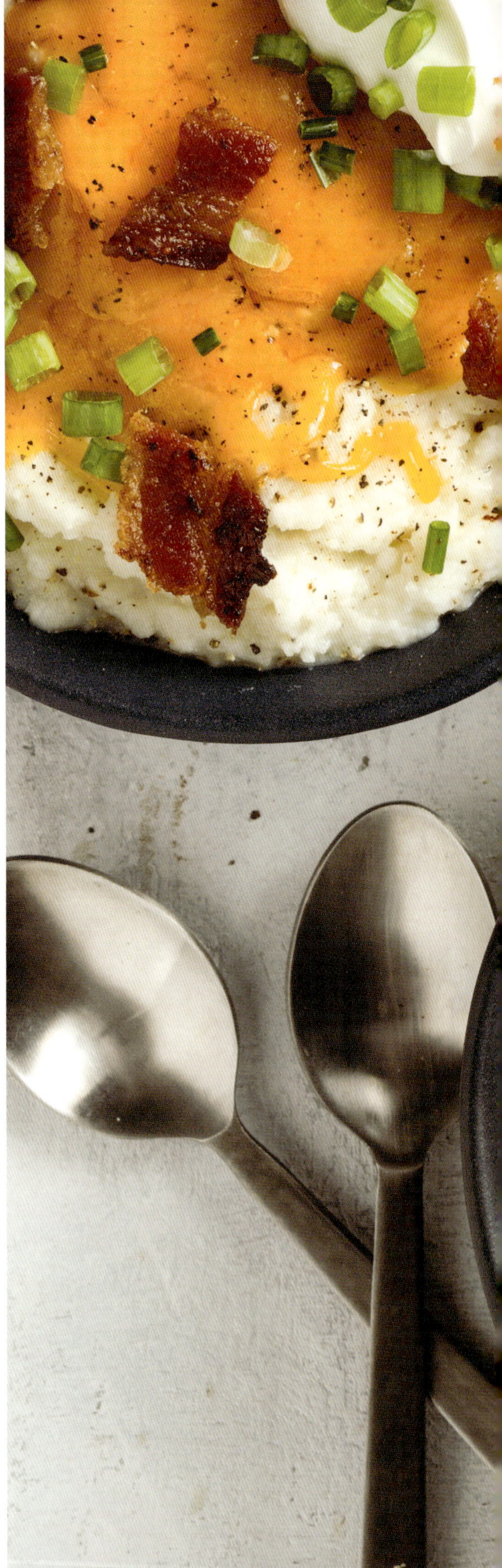

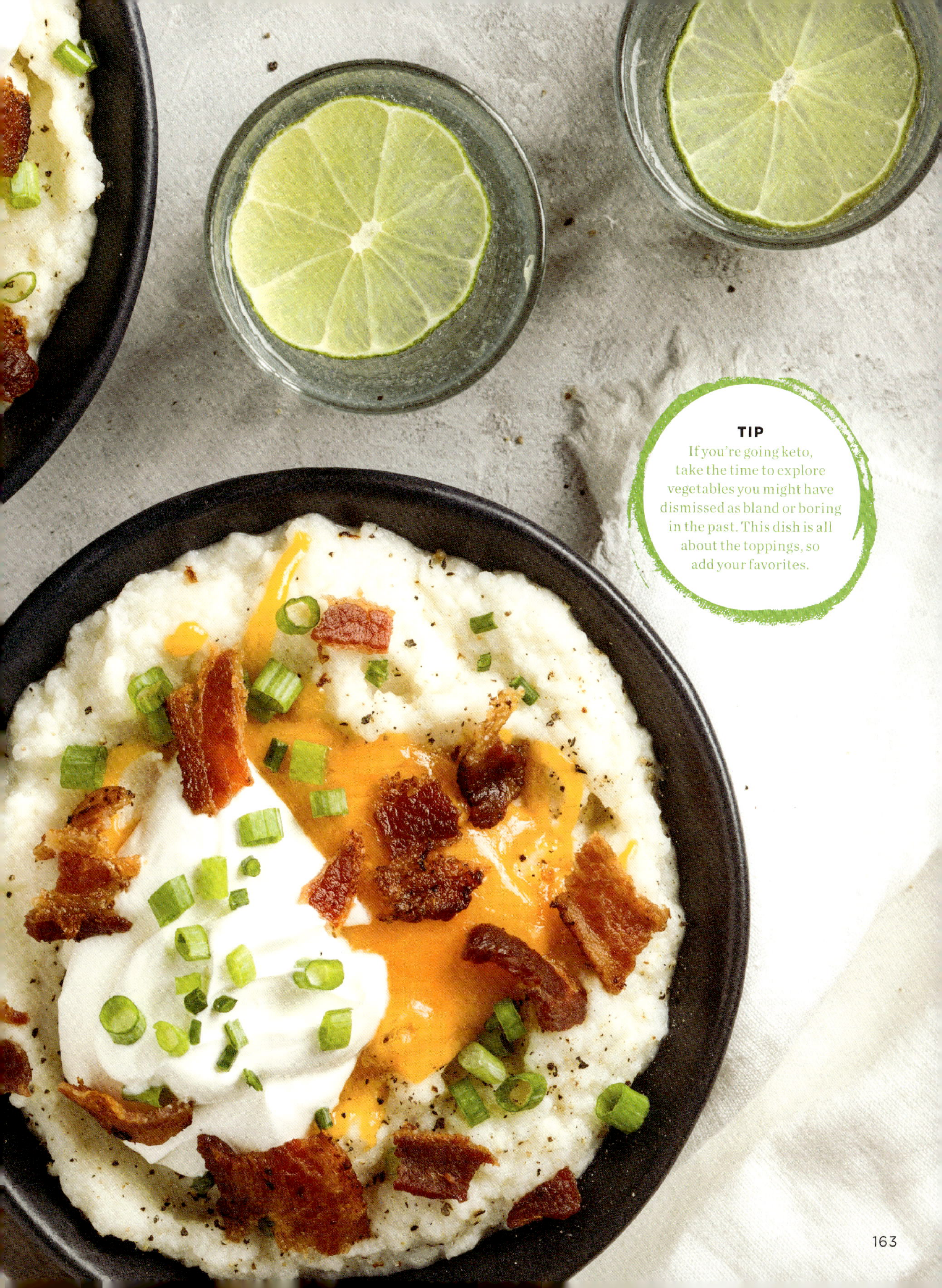

TIP

If you're going keto, take the time to explore vegetables you might have dismissed as bland or boring in the past. This dish is all about the toppings, so add your favorites.

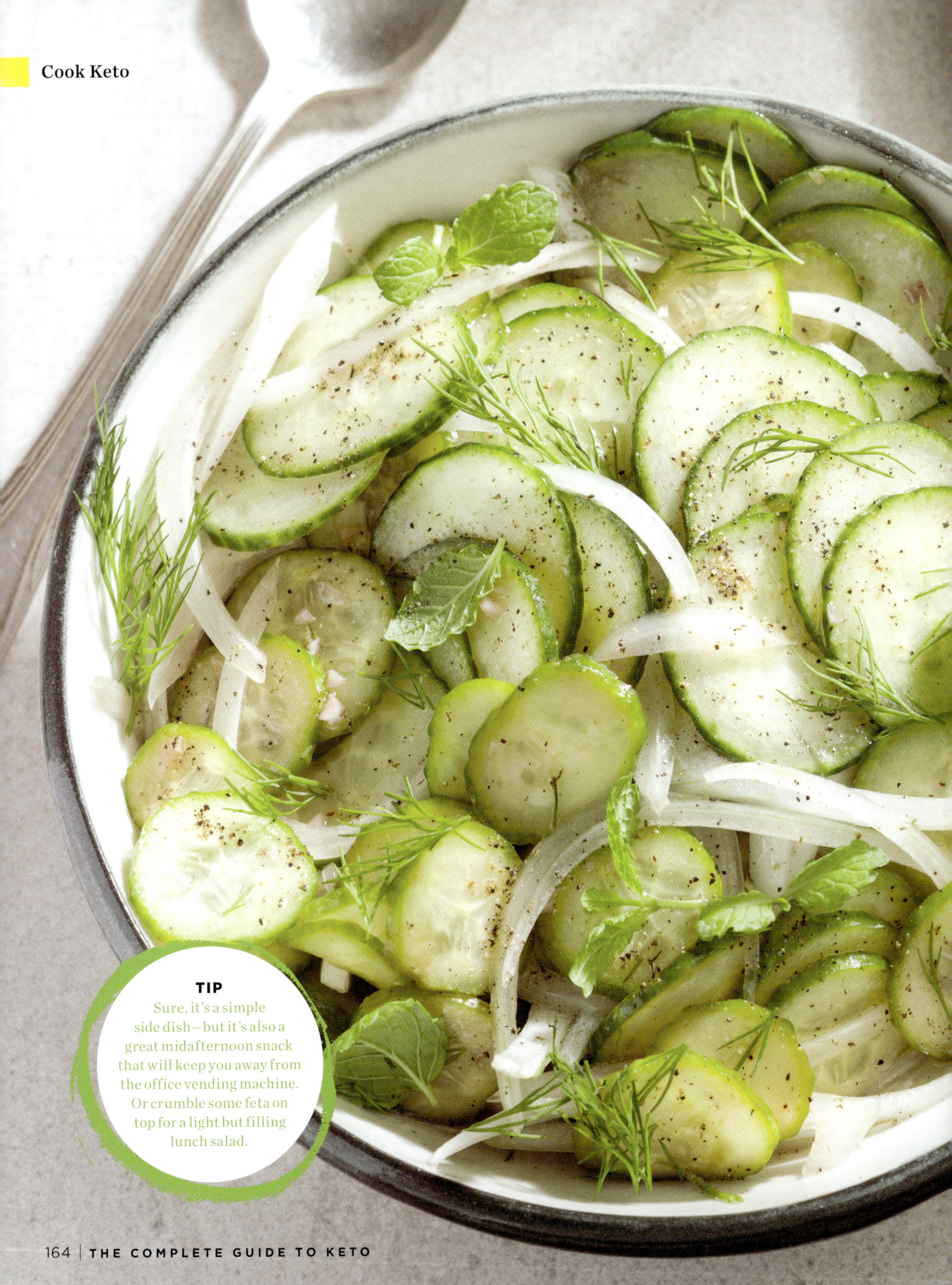

TIP

Sure, it's a simple side dish—but it's also a great midafternoon snack that will keep you away from the office vending machine. Or crumble some feta on top for a light but filling lunch salad.

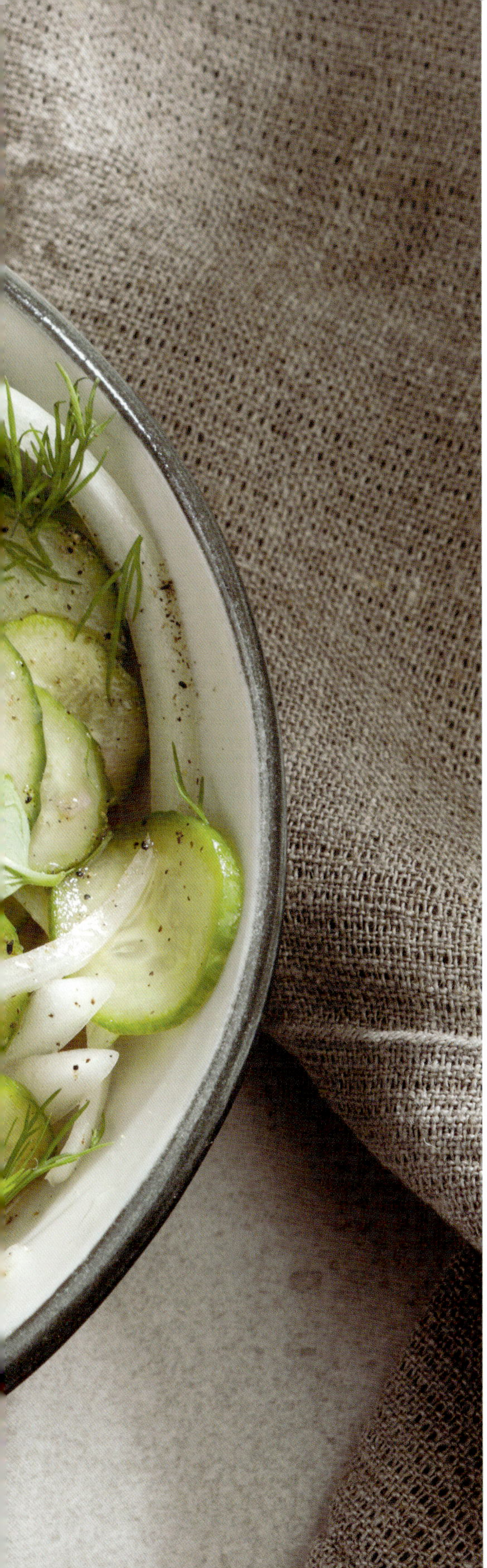

MARINATED CUCUMBERS

START TO FINISH 30 minutes (all active)
SERVES 6

INGREDIENTS

- 2 medium cucumbers, sliced
- 3 Persian cucumbers, sliced
- 1 cup sliced white onion
- 3 cloves garlic, minced
- ¾ cup red wine vinegar
- ½ cup olive oil
- 1 teaspoon salt
- 1 teaspoon pepper
- 1 teaspoon dill, chopped

GARNISHES dill sprigs, mint leaves

DIRECTIONS

1 In a large bowl, add cucumbers, onion and garlic. Set aside.
2 In a small bowl, combine vinegar, olive oil, salt and pepper. Stir in chopped dill.
3 Pour vinegar mixture over cumbers and chill until ready to serve. Garnish with dill and mint.

NUTRITION INFORMATION

CALORIES 36; **PROTEIN** 1.5g; **FAT** 1g; **CARBS** 6g; **FIBER** 1g; **NET CARBS** 5g

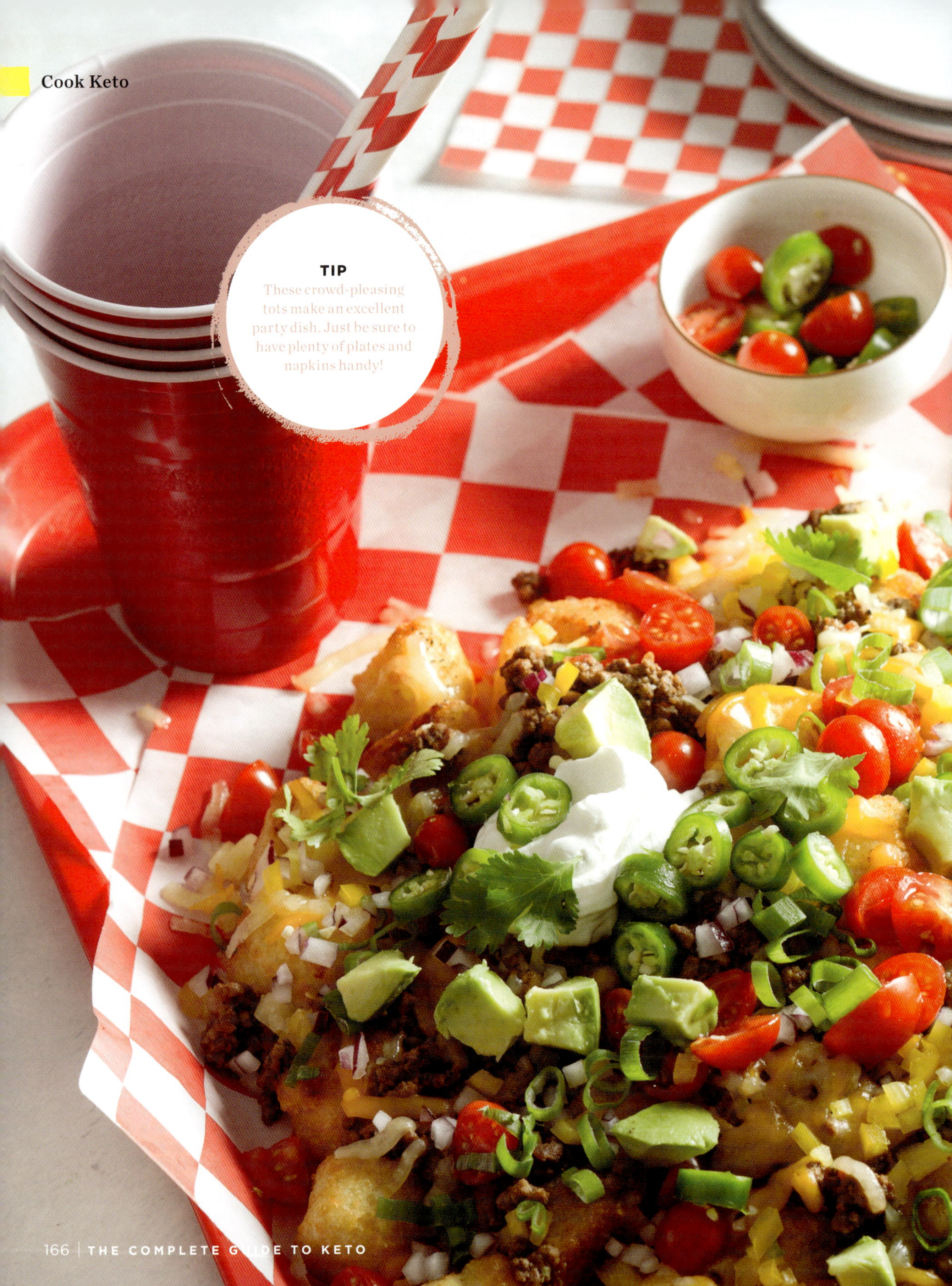

TIP

These crowd-pleasing tots make an excellent party dish. Just be sure to have plenty of plates and napkins handy!

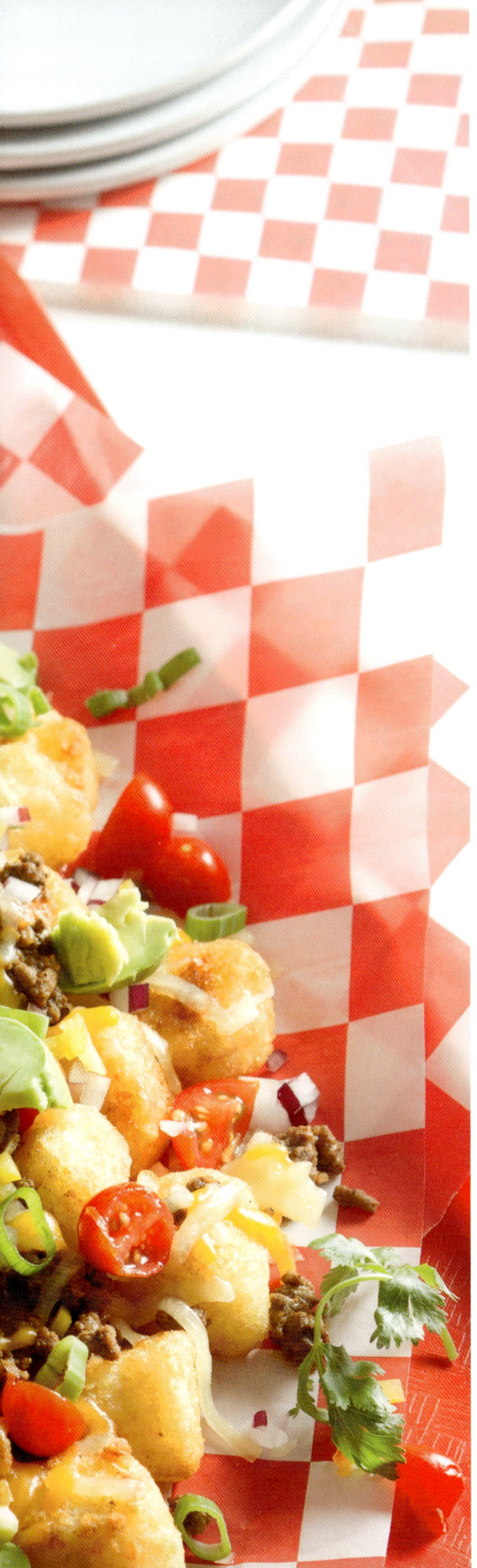

Snacks

CAULIFLOWER TOT-CHOS

START TO FINISH 20 minutes (10 minutes active)

SERVINGS 6

INGREDIENTS

- 1 (12-ounce) bag frozen cauliflower tots (Green Giant®)
- 1 pound ground sirloin
- 1 teaspoon salt
- 1 teaspoon cumin
- 1 teaspoon chili powder
- 1 cup salsa
- 2 cups shredded Mexican cheese blend
- 1 cup chopped tomato
- ½ cup diced red onion
- ½ cup diced avocado (or guacamole)
- ¼ cup diced yellow bell pepper
- ¼ cup sour cream

GARNISHES cilantro sprigs, green onions, jalapeño slices

DIRECTIONS

1 Prepare cauliflower tots according to package directions.
2 In a large skillet over medium-high heat, brown the sirloin until no longer pink; drain. Add salt, cumin, chili powder and salsa.
3 Spoon meat over hot, cooked tots. Top with cheese and remaining ingredients. Garnish with desired toppings.

NUTRITION INFORMATION

CALORIES: 73; **PROTEIN** 9g; **FAT** 12g; **CARBS** 7g; **FIBER** 2g; **NET CARBS** 5g

MINI BLT BITES

START TO FINISH 10 minutes (all active)
SERVINGS 1

INGREDIENTS

1 lettuce leaf (Little Gems)
2 Campari tomato slices
1 cooked bacon slice, broken in pieces
1 tablespoon Japanese mayonnaise
1 teaspoon pepper

DIRECTIONS

1 Top lettuce leaf with tomato slices, bacon pieces, mayonnaise and pepper to taste. For a party, make as many as you'd like, then fold and spear each one on a pick.

NUTRITION INFORMATION

CALORIES 111; **PROTEIN** 4g; **FAT** 7g; **CARBS** 8g; **FIBER** 2g; **NET CARBS** 6g

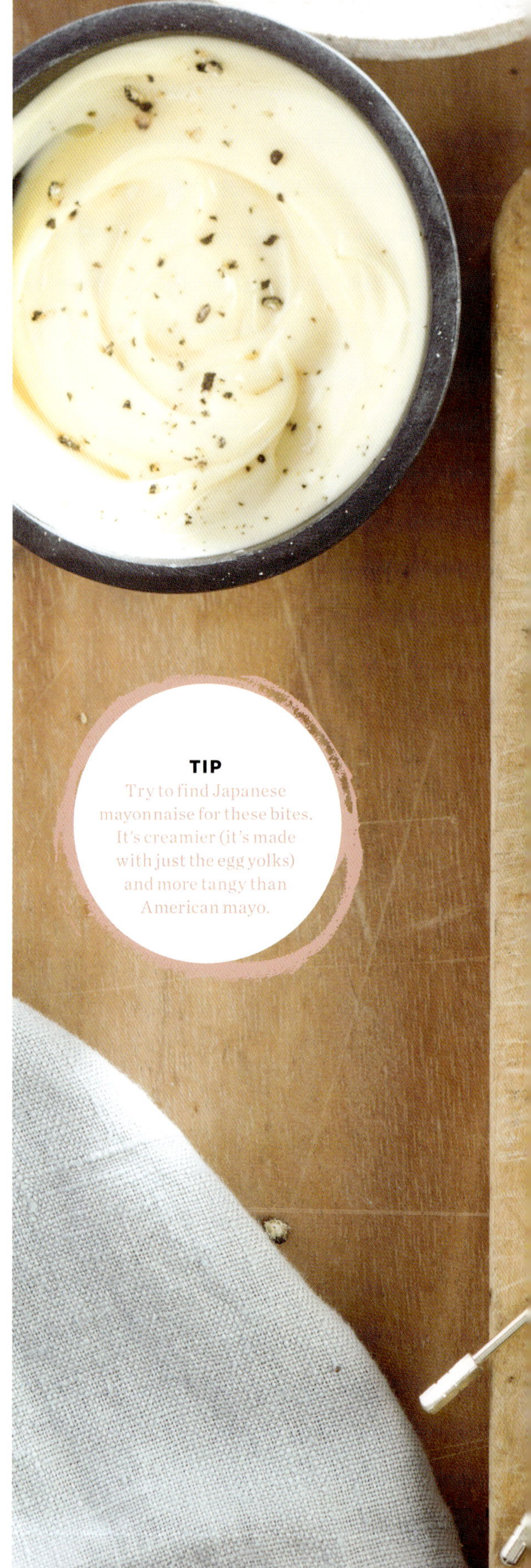

TIP
Try to find Japanese mayonnaise for these bites. It's creamier (it's made with just the egg yolks) and more tangy than American mayo.

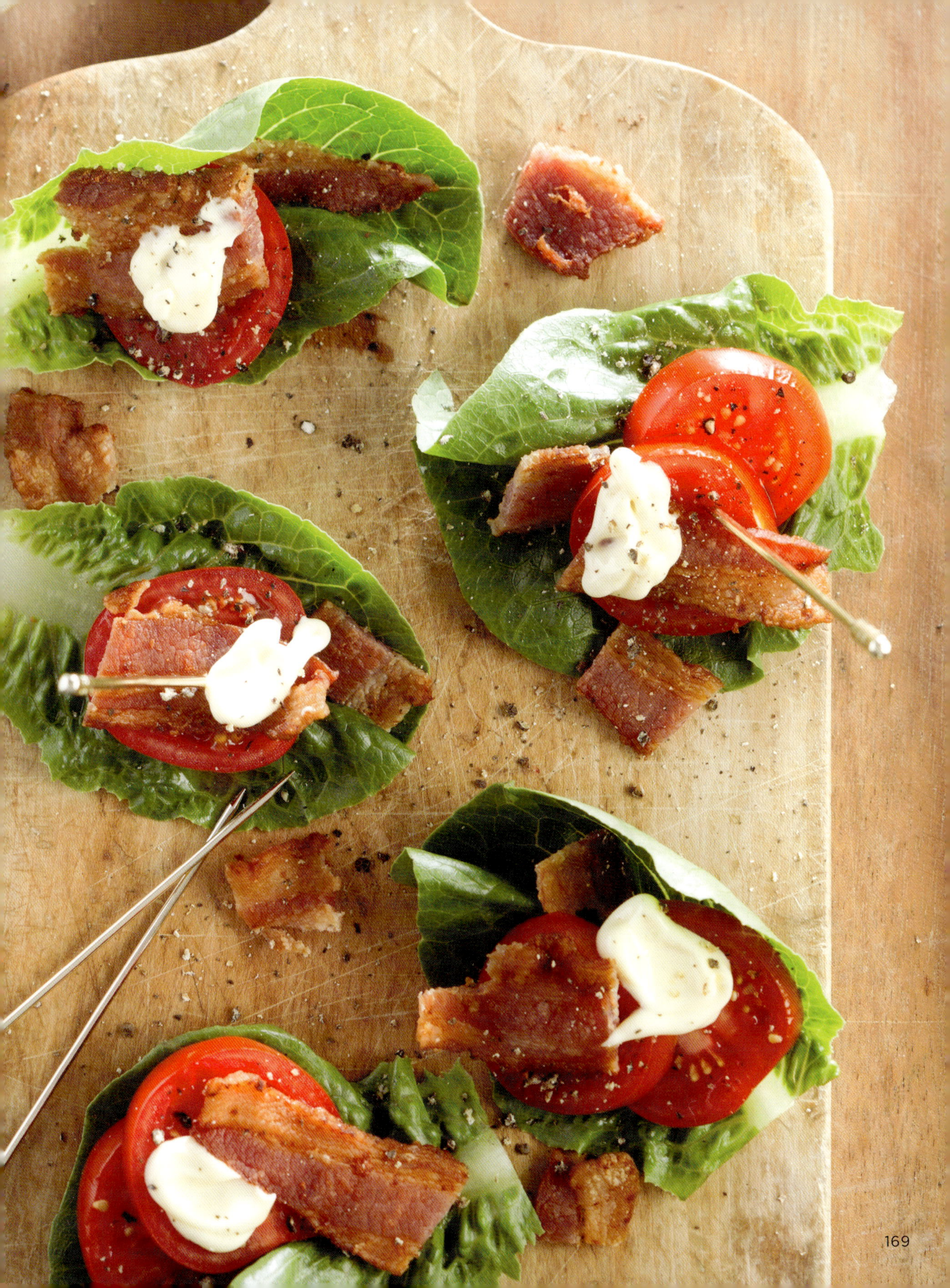

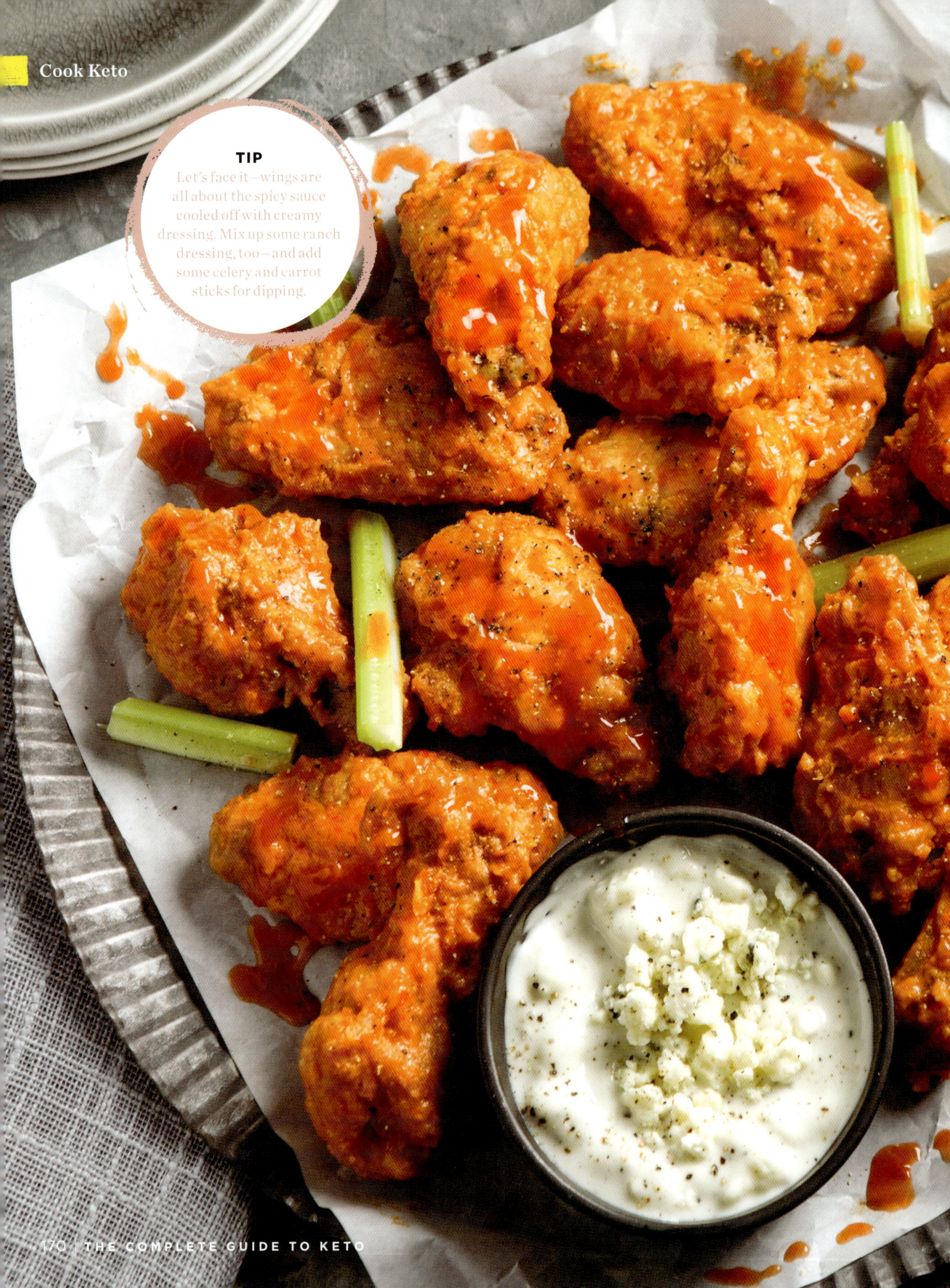

TIP

Let's face it—wings are all about the spicy sauce cooled off with creamy dressing. Mix up some ranch dressing, too—and add some celery and carrot sticks for dipping.

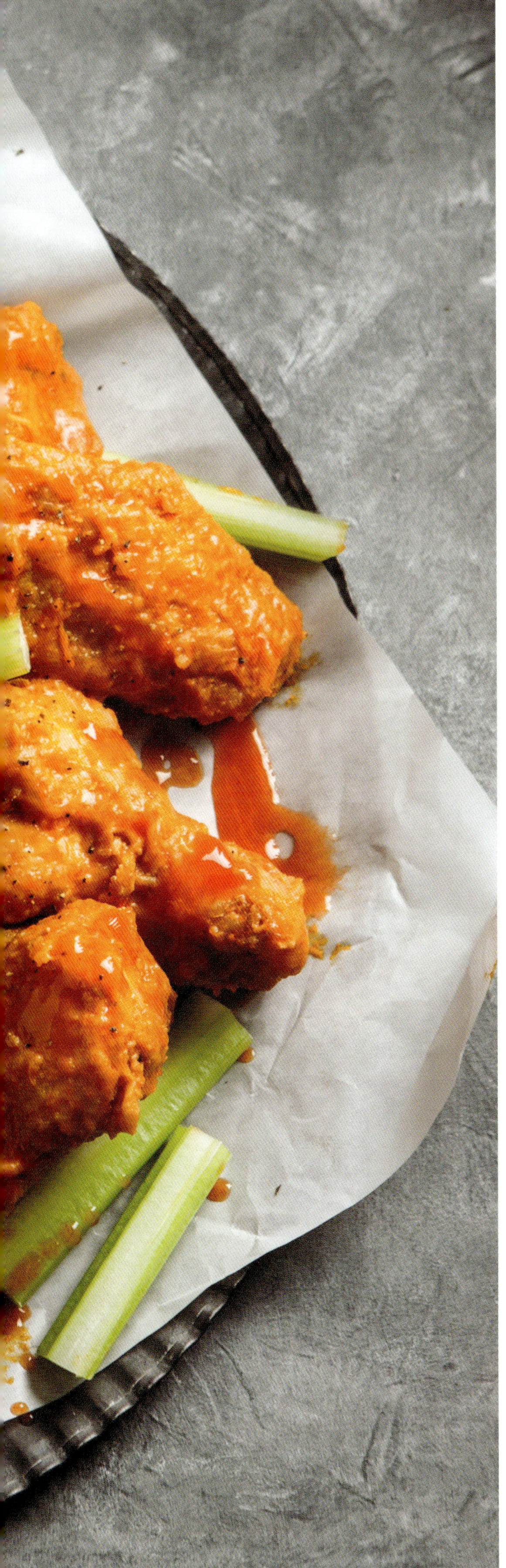

BAKED WINGS WITH BLUE CHEESE DRESSING

START TO FINISH 1 hour (10 minutes active)
SERVINGS 6 (about 6 wings per serving)

INGREDIENTS

- 4 pounds chicken wings
- 2 teaspoon baking powder
- 1 teaspoon salt
- 1 teaspoon pepper
- 1 teaspoon garlic powder
- 1 cup wing sauce (Frank's Red Hot)
- ¼ cup melted butter
- ½ cup cream
- ½ cup sour cream
- ½ cup mayonnaise
- 1 tablespoon vinegar
- 1 teaspoon salt
- ½ teaspoon pepper
- ½ cup crumbled blue cheese

DIRECTIONS

1 Preheat oven to 450°F.

2 Lightly grease two rimmed baking sheets with cooking spray.

3 In a large bowl combine baking powder and next 3 ingredients. Add wings and toss to coat.

4 Place wings on baking sheets. Bake for 30 minutes. Flip wings and bake an additional 20 minutes.

5 In another large bowl, mix hot sauce and melted butter. Toss cooked wings in sauce to coat.

6 In a medium bowl add remaining 6 ingredients until combined.

7 Serve wings with blue cheese sauce and celery sticks, if desired.

NUTRITION INFORMATION

CALORIES 216; **PROTEIN** 11g; **FAT** 16g; **CARBS** 7g; **FIBER** 0g; **NET CARBS** 7g

LOADED DEVILED EGGS

START TO FINISH 15 minutes (10 minutes active)
SERVINGS 6

INGREDIENTS

- 6 hard boiled eggs, halved
- ½ cup mayonnaise
- 1 tablespoon Dijon mustard
- 1 teaspoon Old Bay seasoning
- ½ teaspoon salt
- ½ teaspoon pepper

GARNISHES bacon pieces, green onions, sprinkle of Old Bay seasoning

DIRECTIONS

1 In a medium bowl, mix cooked egg yolks and mayonnaise. Combine until smooth. Stir in mustard, Old Bay, salt and pepper. Fill each egg-white half with yolk mixture. Refrigerate until ready to serve.
2 Garnish as desired before serving.

NUTRITION INFORMATION

CALORIES 162; **PROTEIN** 8g; **FAT** 12g; **CARBS** 5g; **FIBER** 0g; **NET CARBS** 5g

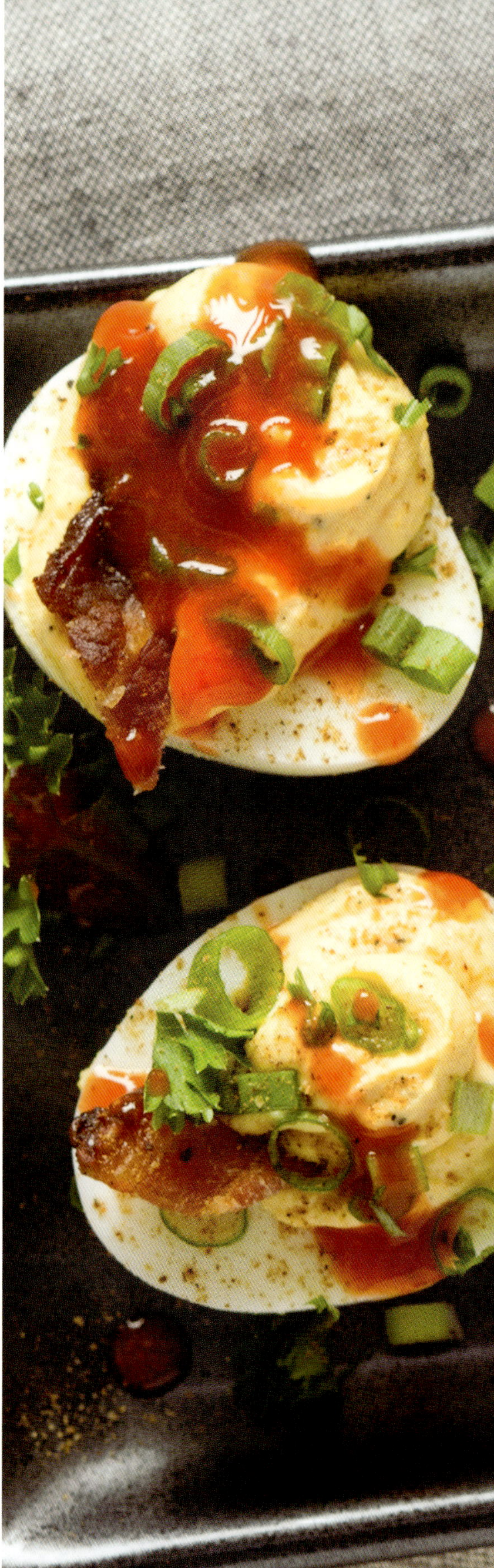

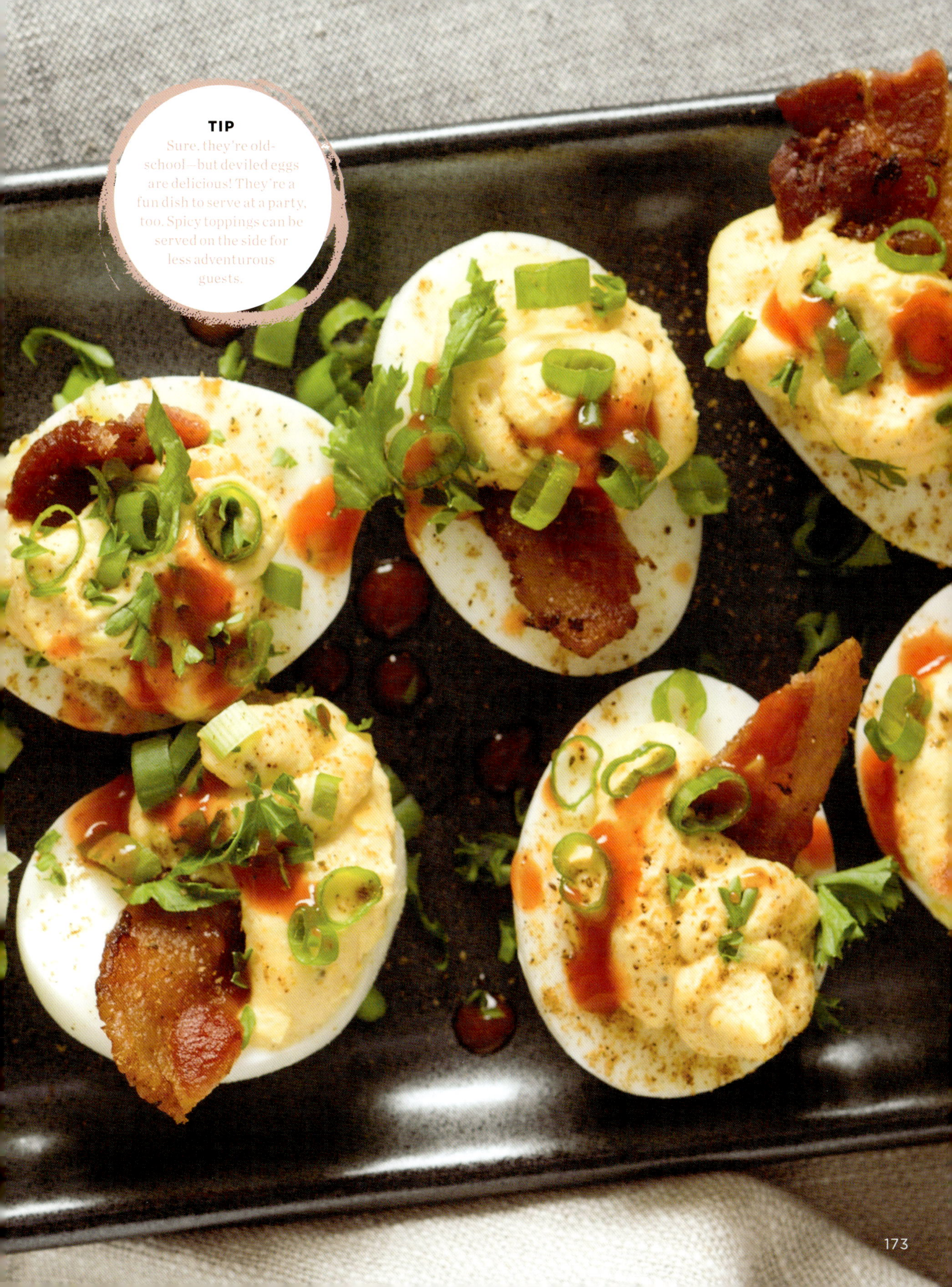

TIP

Sure, they're old-school—but deviled eggs are delicious! They're a fun dish to serve at a party, too. Spicy toppings can be served on the side for less adventurous guests.

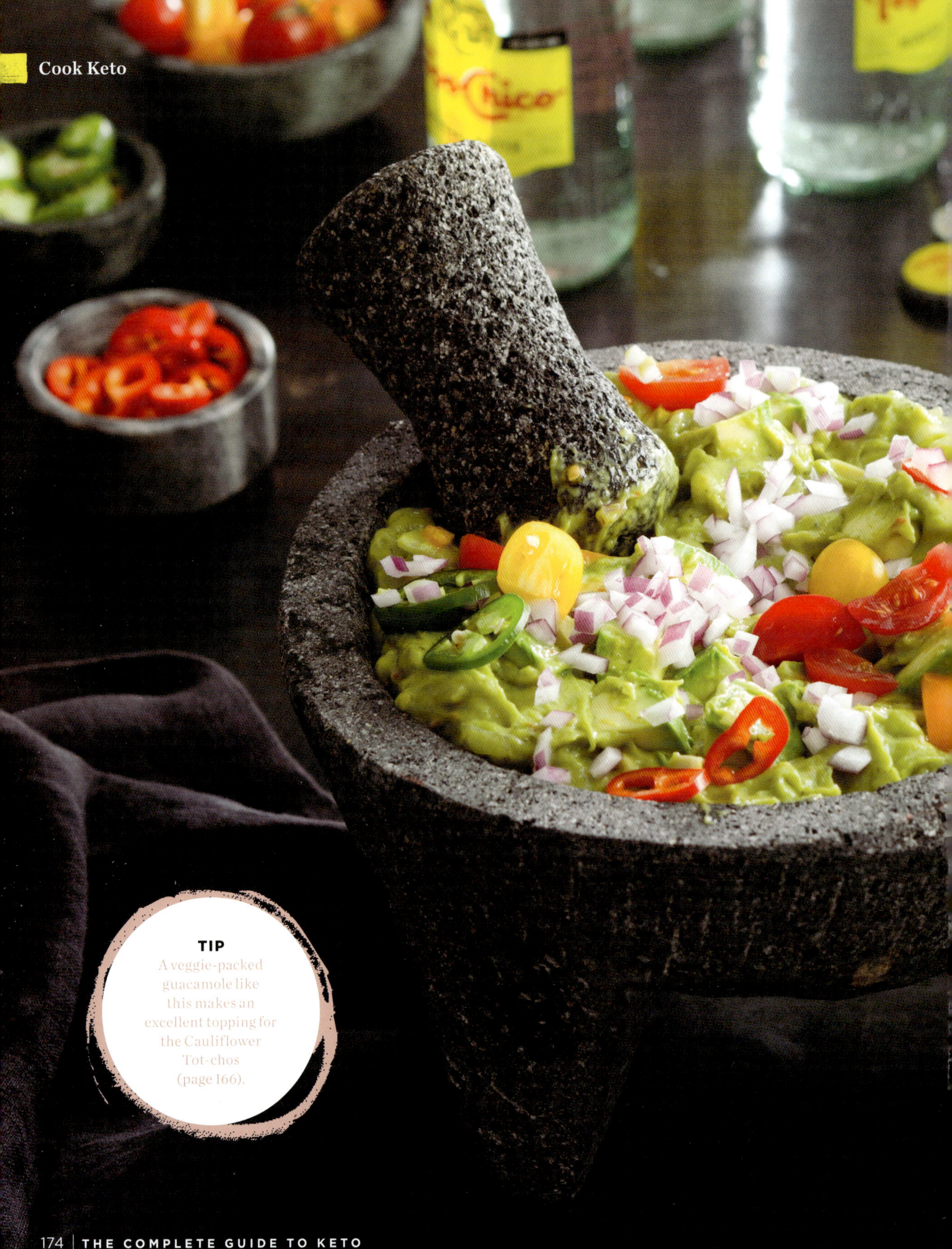

TIP
A veggie-packed guacamole like this makes an excellent topping for the Cauliflower Tot-chos (page 166).

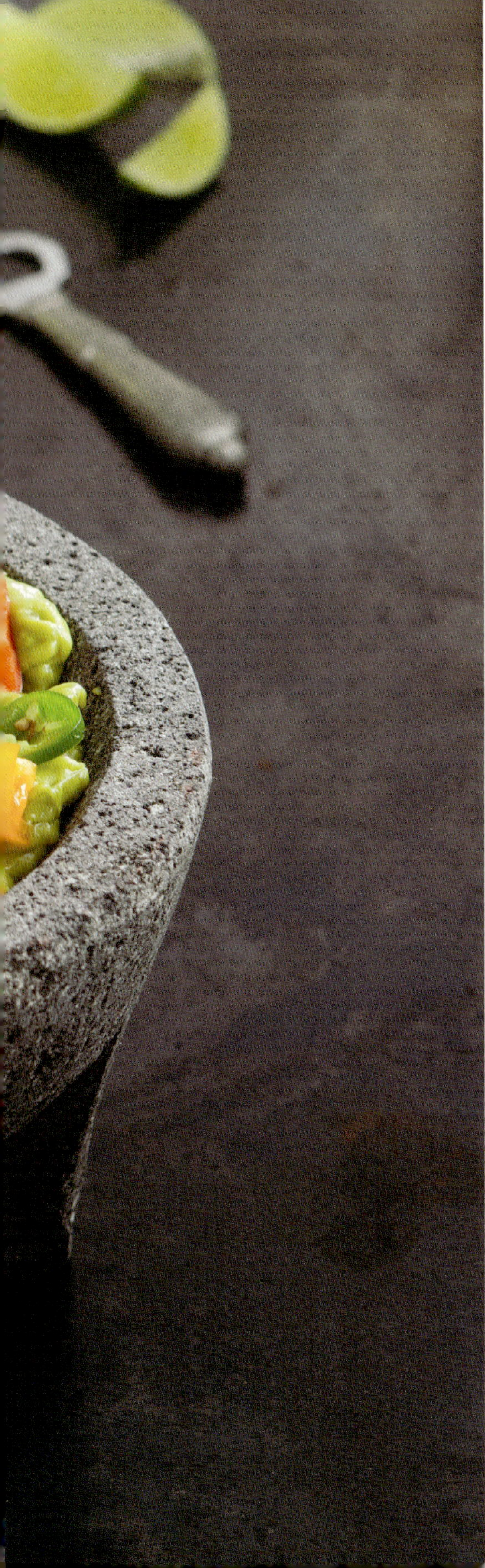

ULTIMATE GUACAMOLE

START TO FINISH 10 minutes (all active)
SERVINGS 2 servings

INGREDIENTS

- 2 ripe avocados
- 2 cloves garlic, minced
- 2 tablespoons fresh lime juice
- 1 cup chopped white onion
- 2 tablespoons chopped cilantro
- 1 jalapeño, chopped
- 1 Fresno pepper, chopped
- 2 scallions, chopped
- 1 teaspoon salt
- ½ teaspoon pepper
- Radish slices (for "chips")

GARNISHES diced red onion, jalapeño slices, Fresno pepper slices, quartered red and yellow cherry tomatoes

DIRECTIONS

1 In a medium bowl, mash avocado with a fork. Stir in remaining ingredients except radish chips.

2 Place guacamole in serving bowl and garnish as desired. Serve with radish chips on the side.

NUTRITION INFORMATION

CALORIES 371; **PROTEIN** 2g; **FAT** 30g; **CARBS** 27g; **FIBER** 15.5g; **NET CARBS** 11.5g

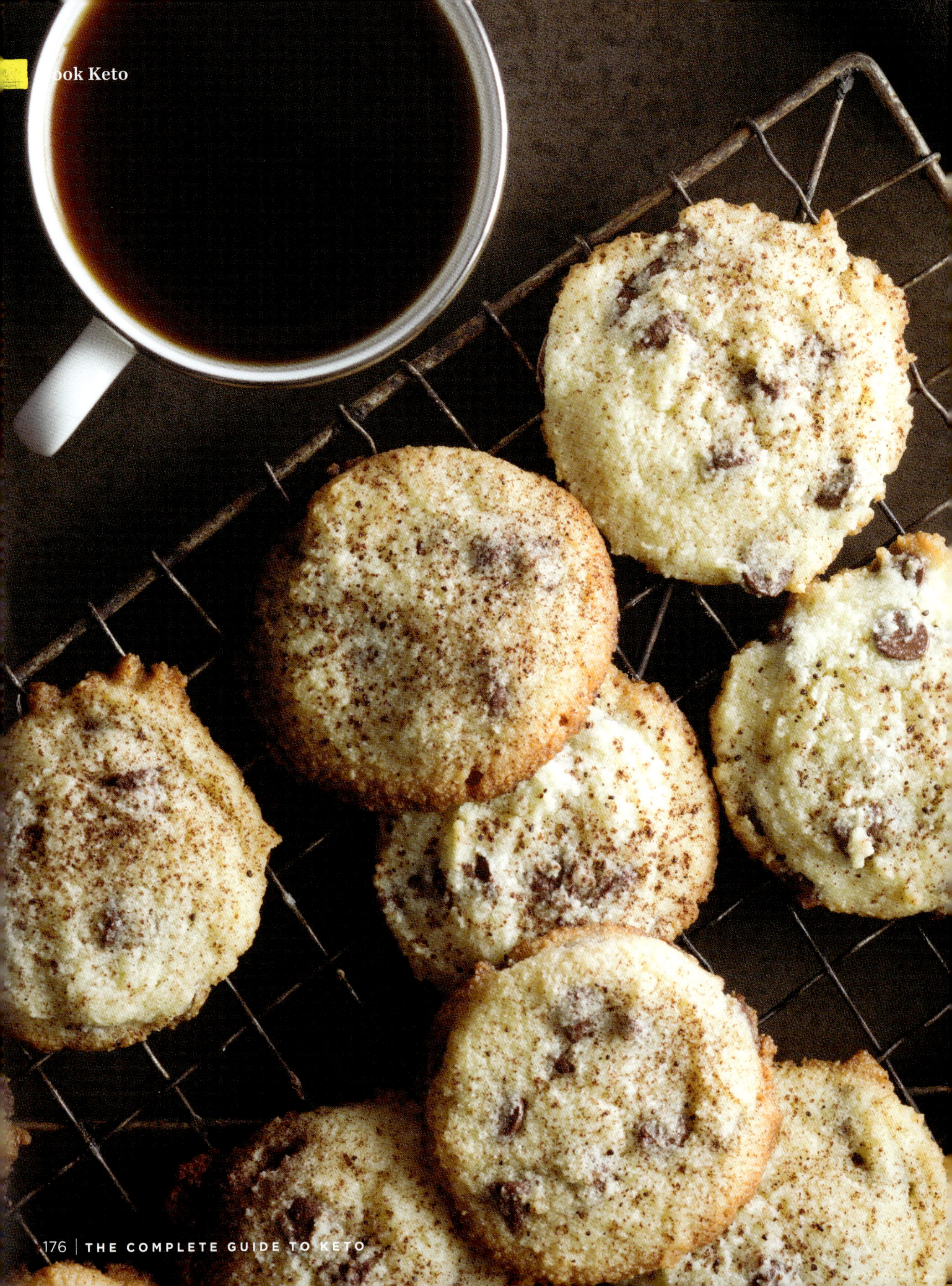

TIP
These cookies are delicious as is—but some chopped macadamias, almonds or walnuts will really bring them up a notch.

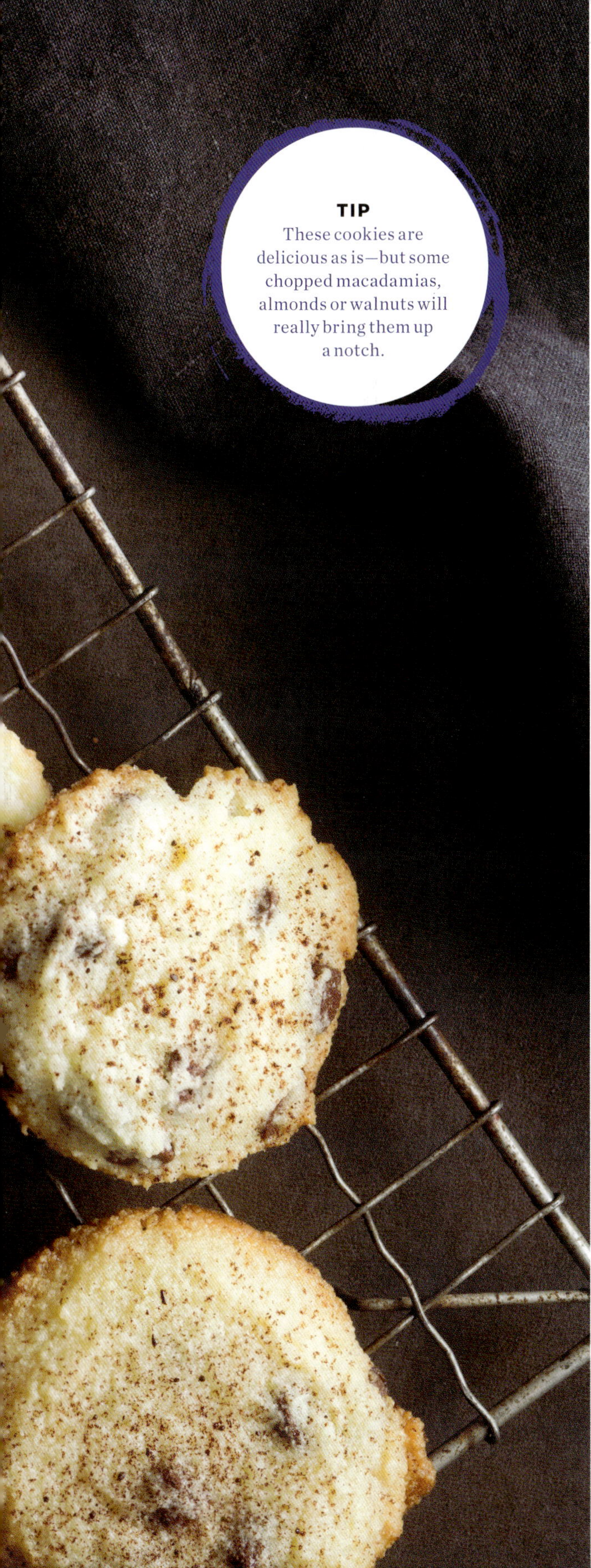

Desserts

CHOCOLATE CHIP COOKIES

START TO FINISH 50 minutes (10 minutes active)
SERVINGS 12 (1 cookie)

INGREDIENTS

- ½ cup butter
- ¾ cup granulated monk fruit sweetener
- 1 teaspoon vanilla extract
- 1 egg
- 1½ cups almond flour
- ½ teaspoon baking powder
- ½ teaspoon xanthan gum
- ¼ teaspoon salt
- 1 cup sugar-free chocolate chips (Lily's)

GARNISH cocoa powder

DIRECTIONS

1 Preheat oven to 350°F.
2 In a mixing bowl, cream butter and sweetener. Add vanilla and egg, beat on low until combined.
3 Add almond flour, baking powder, xanthan gum and salt. Beat until combined. Stir in chocolate chips.
4 Using a small ice cream scoop, make 12 balls and place on greased cookie sheets.
5 Bake for 10–11 minutes or until browned. Cool on wire rack. Dust with cocoa powder, if desired.

NUTRITION INFORMATION

CALORIES 50; **PROTEIN** 4g; **FAT** 1g
CARBS 8g; **FIBER** .15g; **NET CARBS** .65g

INDIVIDUAL STRAWBERRY SHORTCAKE TRIFLES

START TO FINISH 15 minutes (10 minutes active) **SERVINGS** 2

INGREDIENTS

- 2 tablespoons coconut flour
- 2 tablespoons sweetener (such as stevia)
- ¼ teaspoon baking powder
- ¾ cup heavy cream
- 1 egg
- 2 teaspoons vanilla
- ¼ cup sour cream
- 2 tablespoons sugar-free strawberry jam
- 1 cup strawberries, sliced

GARNISHES whipped cream, strawberry slices, mint sprigs

DIRECTIONS

1 In a medium bowl, combine coconut flour, 1 tablespoon sweetener, baking powder, ¼ cup of heavy cream, egg and 1 teaspoon vanilla. Let sit for 3 minutes.

2 Pour the dough into 2 greased coffee mugs and microwave on high for 1½ minutes. Let cool.

3 Turn cakes out onto a cutting board and tear into pieces. Set aside.

4 Pour remaining heavy cream into a mixing bowl; whip until stiff peaks form. Fold in sour cream, remaining vanilla and remaining sweetener.

5 Divide half of the cake pieces between 2 individual trifle dishes to line bottoms. Line the sides with strawberry slices. Add strawberry jam and top with cream mixture. Repeat layers. Top with cream, strawberry slices and mint sprigs, if desired.

NUTRITION INFORMATION

CALORIES 270; **PROTEIN** 5.5g; **FAT** 17.5g; **CARBS** 15.5g; **FIBER** 4g; **NET CARBS** 11.5g

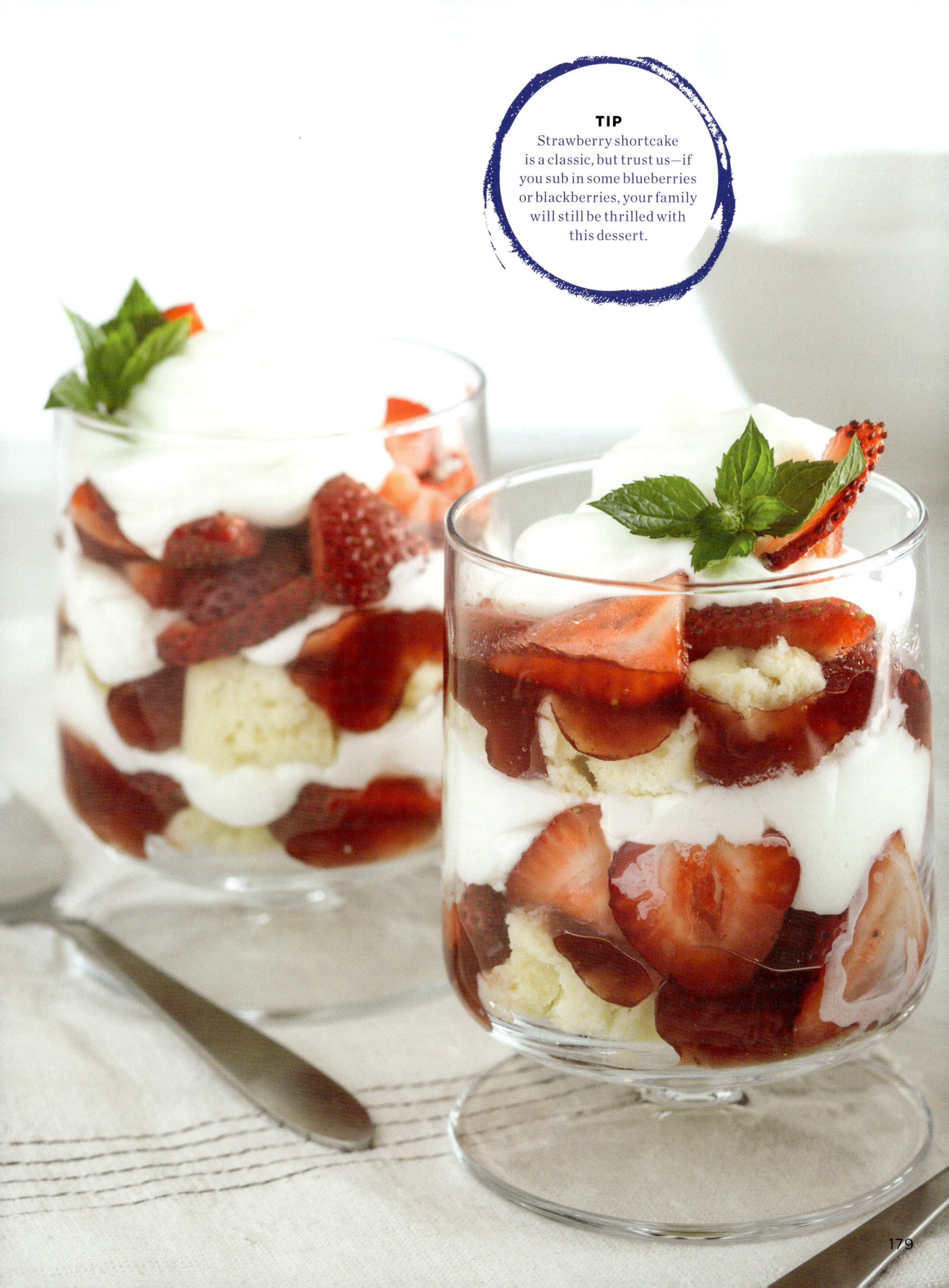
TIP
Strawberry shortcake
is a classic, but trust us—if
you sub in some blueberries
or blackberries, your family
will still be thrilled with
this dessert.

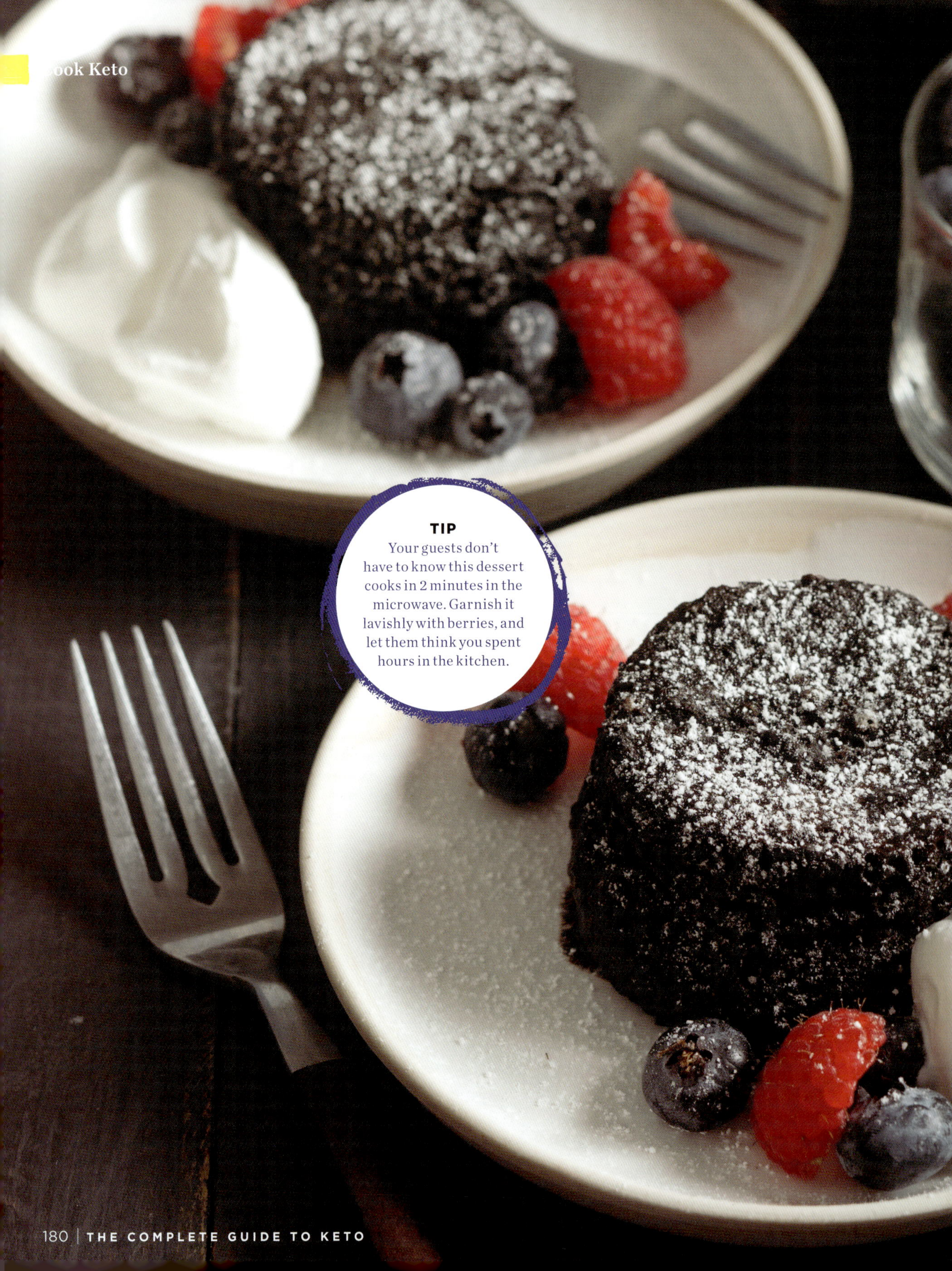

TIP
Your guests don't have to know this dessert cooks in 2 minutes in the microwave. Garnish it lavishly with berries, and let them think you spent hours in the kitchen.

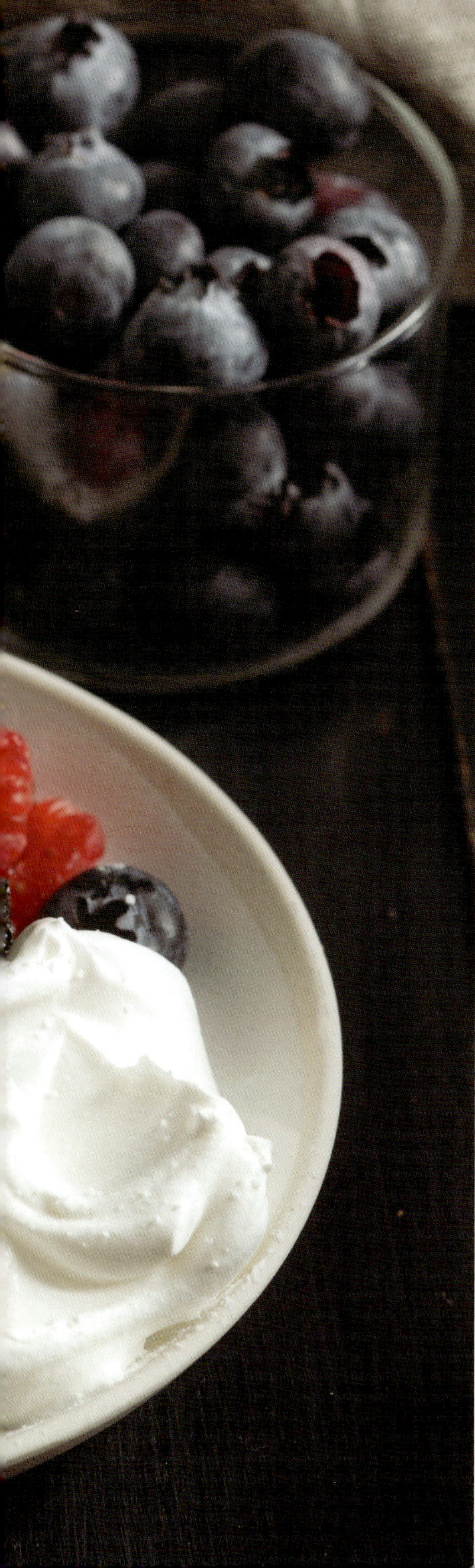

CHOCOLATE LAVA CAKE

START TO FINISH 5 minutes (2 minutes active)

SERVINGS 2

INGREDIENTS

- 2 tablespoons coconut or almond flour
- ½ teaspoon baking powder
- 2 tablespoons unsweetened cocoa powder
- 2 tablespoons granulated sweetener
- 1 egg
- ¼ cup heavy cream
- 2 teaspoons vanilla
- 2 tablespoons sugar-free chocolate chips (Lily's)
- 1 tablespoon butter, melted

GARNISHES whipped cream, berries

DIRECTIONS

1 In a bowl, add flour and next 3 ingredients. Stir in egg, cream and vanilla. Mix until smooth. Stir in chocolate chips.

2 Brush 2 standard coffee mugs with melted butter and pour batter in evenly.

3 Microwave for 1½ minutes on high. Let rest one minute and turn cakes out onto plate.

4 Garnish with cream and berries, if desired.

NUTRITION INFORMATION

CALORIES 574; **PROTEIN** 6.5g; **FAT** 23.5g; **CARBS** 22g; **FIBER** 4g; **NET CARBS** 18g

VANILLA PUDDING WITH CREAM AND MIXED BERRIES

START TO FINISH 15 minutes (5 minutes active)
SERVINGS 6

INGREDIENTS

- 1 cup heavy cream
- ½ cup unsweetened almond milk
- ⅓ cup granulated sweetener (Swerve or stevia)
- 1 tablespoon cornstarch
- 2 whole eggs
- 3 egg yolks
- 1 tablespoon water
- 1 teaspoon gelatin powder
- 1 teaspoon vanilla extract
- ¼ teaspoon liquid stevia
- 2 tablespoons butter

GARNISHES whipped cream, mixed berries

DIRECTIONS

1 In a small saucepan over medium-high heat, bring cream and almond milk to a simmer.
2 In a medium heat-proof bowl, combine the sweetener and cornstarch. Whisk in whole eggs and egg yolks.
3 In a small bowl add water and sprinkle gelatin over.
4 Pour the hot cream over the egg mixture, stirring constantly. Whisk in gelatin until smooth.
5 Cook over low heat until thickened. Stir in vanilla, liquid stevia and butter until smooth. Pour into serving cups or bowls.
6 Top with whipped cream and berries, if desired.

NUTRITION INFORMATION

CALORIES 204; **PROTEIN** 4g; **FAT** 18g; **CARBS** 5.5g; **FIBER** 0g; **NET CARBS** 5.5g

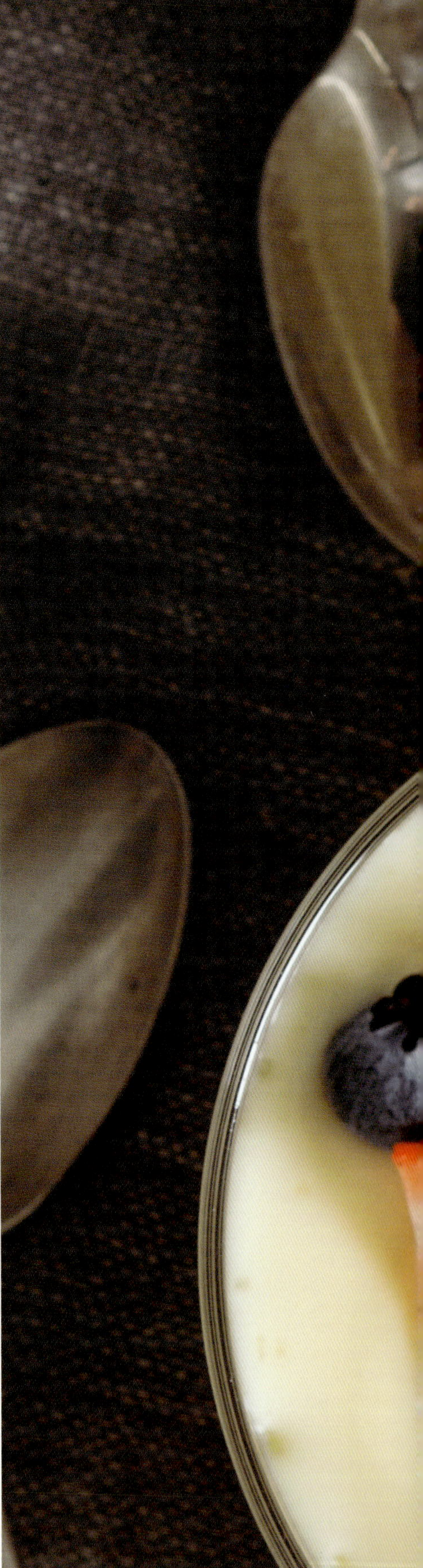

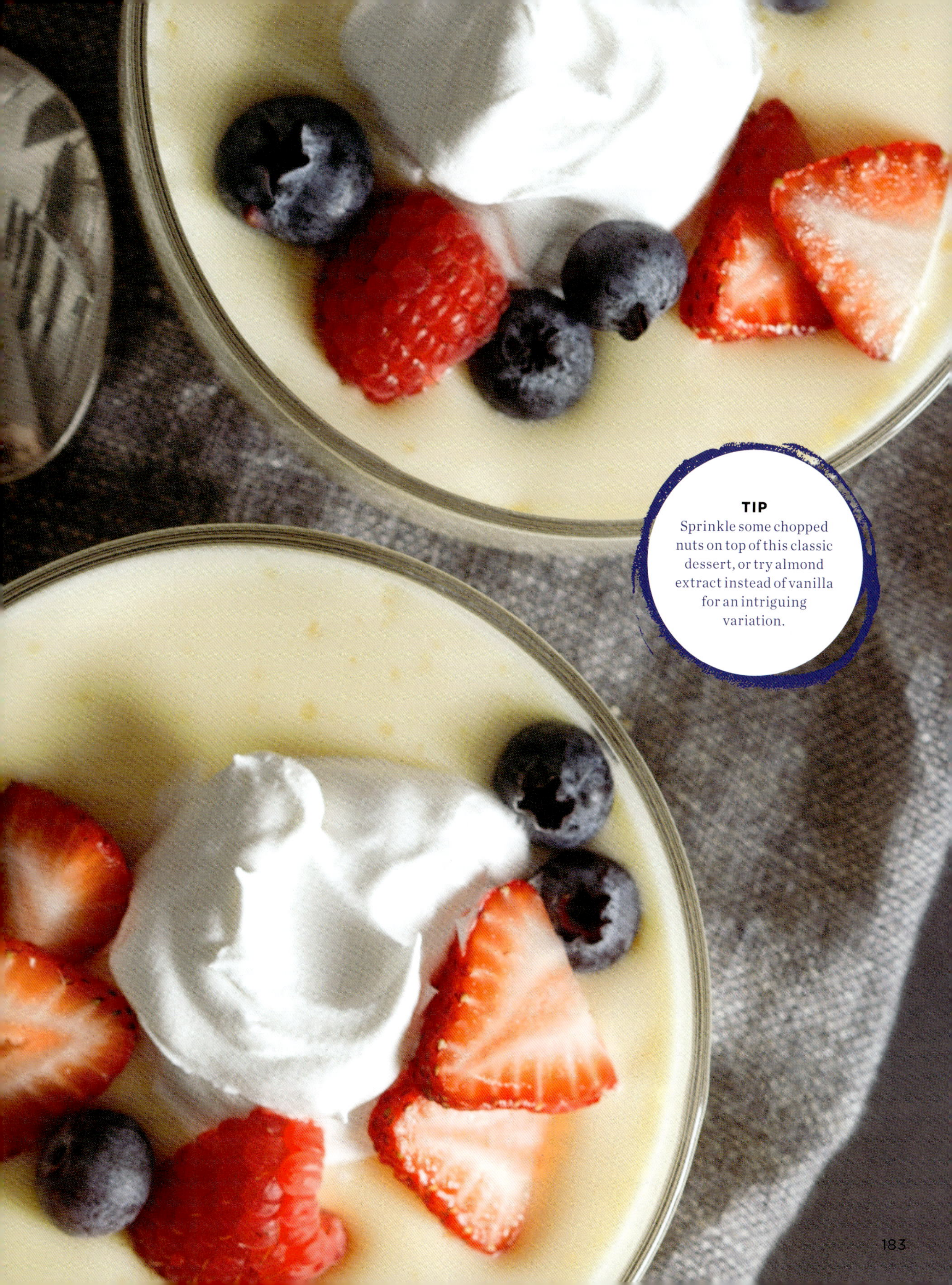

TIP

Sprinkle some chopped nuts on top of this classic dessert, or try almond extract instead of vanilla for an intriguing variation.

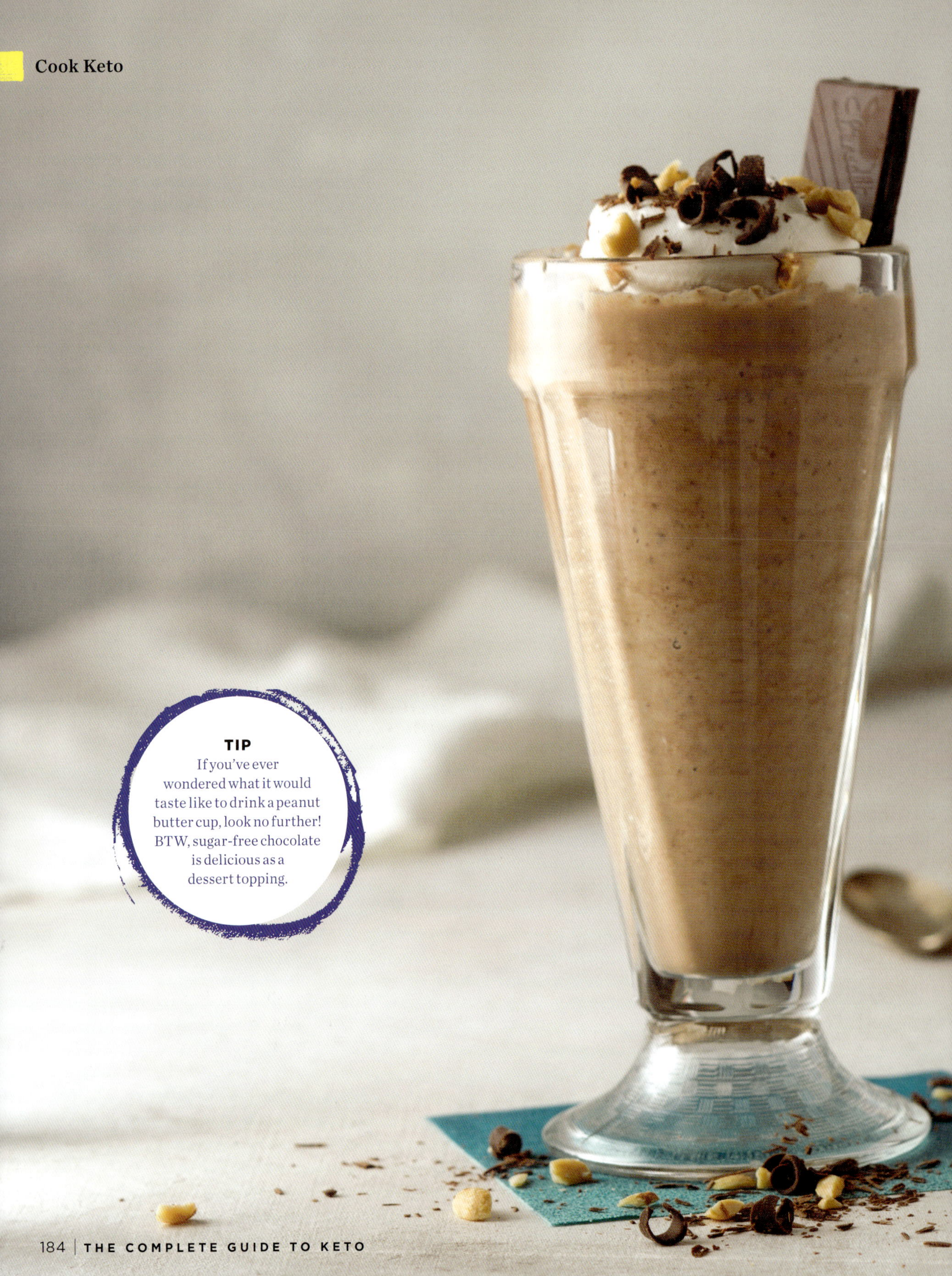

TIP
If you've ever wondered what it would taste like to drink a peanut butter cup, look no further! BTW, sugar-free chocolate is delicious as a dessert topping.

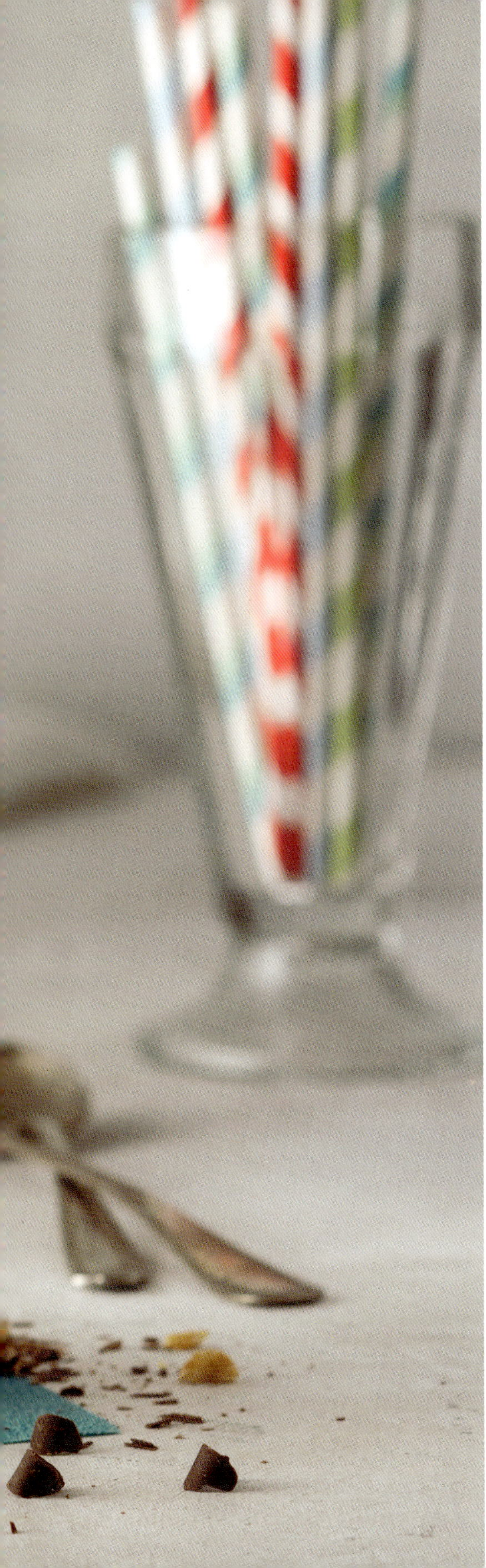

CHOCOLATE-PEANUT BUTTER MILKSHAKE

START TO FINISH 1 hour (5 minutes active)
SERVINGS 4

INGREDIENTS

- 2 cups heavy cream
- ¼ cup no-sugar-added peanut butter
- ¼ cup unsweetened cocoa powder
- 2 teaspoons granulated sweetener (stevia)
- 1 teaspoon vanilla

GARNISHES whipped cream, sugar-free chocolate shavings, chopped peanuts

DIRECTIONS

1 Add all ingredients together in blender. Mix until smooth.
2 Pour into freezer-safe containers and freeze for one hour.
3 Scoop into glasses; let soften slightly before serving. Garnish with whipped cream, chocolate shavings and chopped peanuts, if desired.

NUTRITION INFORMATION

CALORIES 520; **PROTEIN** 6.5g; **FAT** 53g; **CARBS** 8.5g; **FIBER** .5g; **NET CARBS** 8g

Index

Credits

Cover Shutterstock/GTS; Rob White/Getty Images; Shutterstock/Nattika; Shutterstock/Jiang Hongyan; Joff Lee/Getty Images; Dorling Kindersley/Getty Images; KLH49/Getty Images **2-3** Mike Kemp/Getty Images **4** Mike Kemp/Getty Images; Liam Franklin; Westend61/Getty Images; Science Photo Library/Getty Images; EyeEm/Getty Images **5** Liam Franklin; fcafotodigital/Getty Images; Foodcollection/Getty Images **6-7** Shutterstock/Sunvic **8** Shutterstock/SewCream **11** Shutterstock/picturepartners; Shutterstock/gresei; Shutterstock/maxpro **12-13** Moment/Getty Images **14-15** PeopleImages/Getty Images **17** Paper Boat Creative/Getty Images 18 Jim David/Getty Images; Westend61/Getty Images **19** Artem Varnitsin/EyeEm/Getty Images; Westend61/Getty Images; James And James/Getty Images; Steven Morris/Getty Images; PeopleImages/Getty Images; Frank Bean/Getty Images(2); Cathy Scola/Getty Images; James And James/Getty Images; Lew Robertson/Getty Images **20-21** SCIENCE PHOTO LIBRARY/Getty Images **22** Shutterstock/Billion Photos; Shutterstock/Lisovskaya Natalia **23** Shutterstock/Olgysha; Shutterstock/Africa Studio **24** TS Photography/Getty Images **25** EyeEm/Getty Images **26-27** Sally Anscombe/Getty Images **28** subjug/Getty Images **29** Siraphol Siricharattakul/Getty Images **30** DNY59/Getty Images **32-33** EyeEm/Getty Images **34** Nomad/Getty Images **35** Andrew Brookes/Getty Images **36-37** Shutterstock/unoL **38-39** Science Photo Library/Getty Images **40** Shutterstock/Alena Ozerova **42-43** Vladimir Godnik/Getty Images 45 Liam Norris/Getty Images **46** Foodcollection/Getty Images **47** evemilla/Getty Images **48-49** kyoshino/Getty Images; Foodcollection/Getty Images **50** Stockbyte/Getty Images **52-53** Caiaimage/Getty Images **54-55** E+/Getty Images **57** RoBeDeRo/Getty Images **58-59** Peter Dazeley/Getty Images **60** Getty Images/Westend61 **61** Shutterstock/Olga Miltsova **62-63** Steve Debenport/Getty Images **65** duckycards/Getty Images; Shutterstock/Elovich; Shutterstock/Jiri Hera **66-67** jamesharrison/Getty Images **68-69** Steve Debenport/Getty Images **70-71** Shutterstock/ltummy **72** Shutterstock/Drozhzhina Elena; Shutterstock/Vladislav Noseek; Shutterstock/Hong Vo **73** Shutterstock/Africa Studio; Shutterstock/bogdan ionescu; Shutterstock/Igor Dutina **74** StockFood/Peters,Ina **77** Diana Miller/Getty Images **78-79** PeopleImages/Getty Images **80** Claudia Totir/Getty Images **81** ma-k/Getty Images **82** MirageC/Getty Images **84-85** Getty Images/Foodcollection **86-87** skaman306/Getty Images **88** Tim Roberts/Getty Images **90** kemalbas/Getty Images **92** Lartal/Getty Images **94-95** EyeEm/Getty Images **97** Education Images/Getty Images **98-99** fcafotodigital/Getty Images **100-101** Foodcollection/Getty Images **103** RICOWde/Getty Images **104-105** Shutterstock/Jacob Lund **107** Johner/Getty Images **109** E+/Getty Images **110** Westend61/Getty Images **112-113** Shutterstock/Volodymyr Krasyuk **114-115** Shana Novak/Getty Images **116-117** Shutterstock/Boontoom Sae-Kor 119 Shutterstock/Suto Norbert Zsolt **120** Westend61/Getty Images **121** Matt Lincoln/Getty Images; Rosemary Calvert/Getty Images **122-123** Shutterstock/Vicuschka **124** Vicuschka/Getty Images; MelindaSiklosi/Getty Images; StockFood/News Life Media; Anna Kurzaeva/Getty Images; Igor Golovniov/EyeEm/Getty Images; StockFood/Comet, Renée; Westend61/Getty Images; StockFood/Castilho, Rua/Getty Images; The Picture Pantry/Getty Images; Westend61/Getty Images; Claudia Totir/Getty Images; Annabelle Breakey/Getty Images; Mike Kemp/Getty Images; Pinkybird/Getty Images; EyeEm/Getty Images (2); Westend61/Getty Images; Claudia Totir/Getty Images; dlerick/Getty Images; Studio/Getty Images; rudisill/Getty Images **126-185** Liam Franklin/Recipe styling and development: Margaret Monroe Dickey (30) **Back cover and Spine** alle12/Getty Images; Tiina &Geir/Getty Images; Shutterstock/Cosma; ugurhan/Getty Images; Brian Hagiwara/Getty Images (2); Tony Robbins/Getty Images; NickS/Getty Images

---

SPECIAL THANKS TO CONTRIBUTING WRITERS:
Erin Alexander, Margaret Monroe Dickey, Diana Kelly Levey, Stacy Baker Massand, SJ McShane, Gina Roberts-Grey, Jenn Sinrich, Brittany Smith

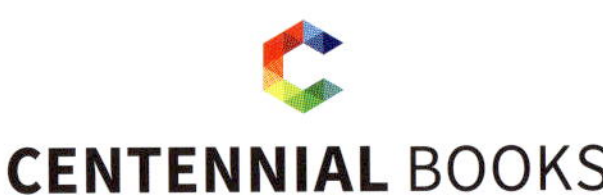

An Imprint of
Centennial Media, LLC
40 Worth St., 10th Floor
New York, NY 10013, U.S.A.

CENTENNIAL BOOKS is a trademark of Centennial Media, LLC

ISBN 978-1-951274-10-8

Distributed by
Simon & Schuster, Inc.
1230 Avenue of the Americas
New York, NY 10020, U.S.A.

For information about custom editions, special sales and premium and corporate purchases, please contact Centennial Media at contact@centennialmedia.com.

Manufactured in China

Publishers & Co-Founders Ben Harris, Sebastian Raatz
Editorial Director Annabel Vered
Creative Director Jessica Power
Executive Editor Janet Giovanelli
Deputy Editor Alyssa Shaffer
Design Director Ben Margherita
Senior Art Director Laurene Chavez
Art Directors Natali Suasnavas, Joseph Ulatowski
Production Manager Paul Rodina
Production Assistant Alyssa Swiderski
Editorial Assistant Tiana Schippa
Sales & Marketing Jeremy Nurnberg